Cosmeceuticals

Procedures in Cosmetic Dermatology
Series Editor: Jeffrey S. Dover MD FRCPC
Associate Editor: Murad Alam MD

Botulinum Toxin
*Alastair Carruthers MABM BCh FRCPC FRCP(Lon) and
Jean Carruthers MD FRCS(C) FRC(OPHTH)
ISBN 1 4160 2470 0*

Soft Tissue Augmentation
*Jean Carruthers MD FRCS(C) FRC(OPHTH) and
Alastair Carruthers MABM BCh FRCPC FRCP(Lon)
ISBN 1 4160 2469 7*

Cosmeceuticals
*Zoe Diana Draelos MD
ISBN 1 4160 0244 8*

Laser and Lights: Volume 1
Vascular • Pigmentation • Scars • Medical Applications
*David J. Goldberg MD JD
ISBN 1 4160 2386 0*

Laser and Lights: Volume 2
Rejuvenation • Resurfacing • Hair Removal • Treatment of Ethnic Skin
*David J. Goldberg MD JD
ISBN 1 4160 2387 9*

Photodynamic Therapy
*Mitchel P. Goldman MD
ISBN 1 4160 2360 7*

Liposuction
*C. William Hanke MD MPH FACP and Gerhard Sattler MD
ISBN 1 4160 2208 2*

Treatment of Scars
Kenneth A. Arndt MD

Chemical Peels
Mark Rubin MD

Hair Restoration
Dowling B. Stough MD and Robert S. Haber MD

Leg Veins
Tri H. Nguyen MD

Blepharoplasty
Ronald L. Moy MD

Face Lifting
Ronald L. Moy MD

PROCEDURES IN COSMETIC DERMATOLOGY

Series Editor: Jeffrey S. Dover MD FRCPC

Associate Editor: Murad Alam MD

Cosmeceuticals

Edited by

Zoe Diana Draelos MD

Clinical Associate Professor, Department of Dermatology, Wake Forest University School of Medicine, Winston-Salem, NC; Dermatology Consulting Services, High Point, NC, USA

Series Editor

Jeffrey S. Dover MD FRCPC

Associate Professor of Clinical Dermatology, Yale University School of Medicine, Adjunct Professor of Medicine (Dermatology), Dartmouth Medical School, Director, SkinCare Physicians of Chestnut Hill, Chestnut Hill, MA, USA

Associate Editor

Murad Alam MD

Chief, Section of Cutaneous and Aesthetic Surgery, Department of Dermatology, Northwestern University, Chicago, IL, USA

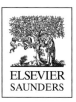

ELSEVIER
SAUNDERS

ELSEVIER
SAUNDERS

An imprint of Elsevier Inc.
© 2005, Elsevier Inc. All rights reserved.
First published 2005

ISBN: 1 4160 0244 8

British Library Cataloguing in Publication Data
A catalogue record for this book is available from the British Library

Library of Congress Cataloging in Publication Data
A catalog record for this book is available from the Library of Congress

---

Notice

Medical knowledge is constantly changing. Standard safety precautions must be followed, but as new research and clinical experience broaden our knowledge, changes in treatment and drug therapy may become necessary or appropriate. Readers are advised to check the most current product information provided by the manufacturer of each drug to be administered to verify the recommended dose, the method and duration of administration, and contraindications. It is the responsibility of the practitioner, relying on experience and knowledge of the patient, to determine dosages and the best treatment for each individual patient. Neither the Publisher nor the editor assumes any liability for any injury and/or damage to persons or property arising from this publication.

The Publisher

Printed in China
Last digit is the print number : 9 8 7 6 5 4 3 2 1

Commissioning Editors: **Sue Hodgson, Shuet-Kei Cheung**
Project Development Managers: **Martin Mellor Publishing Services Ltd, Louise Cook**
Project Managers: **Naughton Project Management, Cheryl Brant**
Illustration Manager: **Mick Ruddy**
Design Manager: **Andy Chapman**
Illustrators: **Richard Prime, Tim Loughhead**

Contents

Part 3: The Application of Cosmeceuticals to Dermatologic Practice

This section was compiled by Zoe Diana Draelos, MD, on behalf of the individual chapter authors

Part 4: Cosmeceutical Myths

Part 5: New Research in Cosmeceuticals

Series Foreword
Procedures in Cosmetic Dermatology

While dermatologists have been procedurally inclined since the beginning of the specialty, particularly rapid change has occurred in the past quarter century. The advent of frozen section technique and the golden age of Mohs skin cancer surgery has led to the formal incorporation of surgery within the dermatology curriculum. More recently technological breakthroughs in minimally invasive procedural dermatology have offered an aging population new options for improving the appearance of damaged skin.

Procedures for rejuvenating the skin and adjacent regions are actively sought by our patients. Significantly, dermatologists have pioneered devices, technologies and medications, which have continued to evolve at a startling pace. Numerous major advances, including virtually all cutaneous lasers and light-source based procedures, botulinum exotoxin, soft-tissue augmentation, dilute anesthesia liposuction, leg vein treatments, chemical peels, and hair transplants, have been invented, or developed and enhanced by dermatologists. Dermatologists understand procedures, and we have special insight into the structure, function, and working of skin. Cosmetic dermatologists have made rejuvenation accessible to risk-averse patients by emphasizing safety and reducing operative trauma. No specialty is better positioned than dermatology to lead the field of cutaneous surgery while meeting patient needs.

As dermatology grows as a specialty, an ever-increasing proportion of dermatologists will become proficient in the delivery of different procedures. Not all dermatologists will perform all procedures, and some will perform very few, but even the less procedurally directed amongst us must be well-versed in the details to be able to guide and educate our patients. Whether you are a skilled dermatologic surgeon interested in further expanding your surgical repertoire, a complete surgical novice wishing to learn a few simple procedures, or somewhere in between, this book and this series is for you.

The volume you are holding is one of a series entitled "Procedures in Cosmetic Dermatology." The purpose of each book is to serve as a practical primer on a major topic area in procedural dermatology.

If you want make sure you find the right book for your needs, you may wish to know what this book is and what it is not. It is not a comprehensive text grounded in theoretical underpinnings. It is not exhaustively referenced. It is not designed to be a completely unbiased review of the world's literature on the subject. At the same time, it is not an overview of cosmetic procedures that describes these in generalities without providing enough specific information to actually permit someone to perform the procedures. And importantly, it is not so heavy that it can serve as a doorstop or a shelf filler.

What this book and this series offer is a step-by-step, practical guide to performing cutaneous surgical procedures. Each volume in the series has been edited by a known authority in that subfield. Each editor has recruited other equally practical-minded, technically skilled, hands-on clinicians to write the constituent chapters. Most chapters have two authors to ensure that different approaches and a broad range of opinions are incorporated. On the other hand, the two authors and the editors also collectively provide a consistency of tone. A uniform template has been used within each chapter so that the reader will be easily able to navigate all the books in the series. Within every chapter, the authors succinctly tell it like they do it. The emphasis is on therapeutic technique; treatment methods are discussed with an eye to appropriate indications, adverse events, and unusual cases. Finally, this book is short and can be read in its entirety on a long plane ride. We believe that brevity paradoxically results in greater information transfer because cover-to-cover mastery is practicable.

We hope you enjoy this book and the rest of the books in the series and that you benefit from the many hours of clinical wisdom that have been distilled to produce it. Please keep it nearby, where you can reach for it when you need it.

Jeffrey S. Dover MD FRCPC and Murad Alam MD

To the women in my life

My grandmothers, Bertha and Lillian
My mother, Nina
My daughters, Sophie and Isabel
And especially to my wife, Tania

For their never-ending encouragement, patience, support, love, and friendship

To my father, Mark
A great teacher and role model

To my mentor, Kenneth A. Arndt for his generosity, kindness, sense of humor, joie de vivre, and above all else curiosity and enthusiasm

At Elsevier, Sue Hodgson who conceptualized the series and brought it to reality

and

Martin Mellor for polite, persistent, and dogged determination.

Jeffrey S. Dover

The professionalism of the dedicated editorial staff at Elsevier has made this ambitious project possible. Guided by the creative vision of Sue Hodgson, Martin Mellor and Shuet-Kei Cheung have attended to the myriad tasks required to produce a state-of-the-art resource. In this, they have been ably supported by the graphics team, which has maintained production quality while ensuring portability. We are also deeply grateful to the volume editors, who have generously found time in their schedules, cheerfully accepted our guidelines, and recruited the most knowledgeable chapter authors. Finally, we thank the chapter contributors, without whose work there would be no books at all. Whatever successes are herein are due to the efforts of the above, and of my teachers, Kenneth Arndt, Jeffrey Dover, Michael Kaminer, Leonard Goldberg, and David Bickers, and of my parents, Rahat and Rehana Alam.

Murad Alam

Preface

Cosmeceuticals are becoming an increasingly important area of dermatology. Underlying this trend is growth in our fund of knowledge regarding skin physiology and a plethora of novel raw materials that can alter the structure and function of the skin. Even though cosmeceuticals as a category are not officially recognized from a regulatory standpoint, their dominance in the skin care marketplace is unmistakable. This body of information cannot be ignored by the dermatologist. Some cosmeceuticals complement traditional textbook treatments of skin disease while others are popular among patients, but lacking in scientific data. In this text, we explore both types.

We open with a discussion by Albert Kligman, MD, PhD – the father of cosmeceuticals. Dr. Kligman became interested in this area when he realized that even water – not to mention other common topical substances such as petrolatum, mineral oil, lanolin, vitamins, minerals – can profoundly alter the structure of the skin. Dr. Kligman was the first to realize that the skin can be impacted by substances other than those requiring prescriptions. Next, this book briefly considers key elements of cosmeceutical design, including barrier function, formulation, efficacy, and marketing, before entering into a detailed scientific analysis of the most relevant cosmeceuticals. The data is presented by category to cover all the major cosmeceuticals in the current marketplace, from vitamins to botanicals, lipids, metals, exfoliants, antioxidants, growth factors, and sunscreens.

We then present treatment regimens organized by skin condition and type of cosmeceutical to help the dermatologist appreciate how cosmeceuticals might be incorporated into daily medical practice. Some of the more common myths regarding cosmeceuticals are dispelled. We conclude with a look into the future of the cosmeceutical category, now clearly still in its infancy.

The intent of this book is to familiarize dermatologists with the theory and practical use of cosmeceuticals. This information will not only help practitioners scientific analysis of products found on the store shelf and at the cosmetic counter, but it will also supply them with knowledge in a concise format to answer patient questions regarding topical cosmeceuticals. Conveying accurate, timely information to patients is crucial, since lay people turn to dermatologists as the physicians trained to understand the effects of all topically applied substances, both those in the prescription and nonprescription realms.

This text brings together experts from the industry, manufacturing, research, and dermatologic communities to provide the reader with a state-of-the-art, comprehensive review of cosmeceuticals. It was a pleasure to meet the challenge of working with the many authors who contributed their time and expertise to produce this unique book, simultaneously dense and concise, packed with practical tips and rich in relevant background knowledge. I hope that you will enjoy learning from this book as much as I enjoyed organizing and editing this effort!

Zoe Diana Draelos MD

List of Contributors

Cynthia A. Berge BS
Clinical Research Associate, Skin Care, Procter & Gamble, Miami Valley Laboratories, Cincinnati, OH, USA

Donald L. Bissett PhD
Research Fellow, Skin Care, Procter and Gamble, Miami Valley Laboratories, Cincinnati, OH, USA

M. Elizabeth Briden MD
Medical Director, Advanced Dermatology and Cosmetic Institute, Edina, MN, USA

Karen E. Burke MD PhD
Assistant Attending Physician, Department of Dermatology, The Mount Sinai Medical Center, New York, NY; Attending Physician, Department of Medicine, Cabrini Medical Center, New York, NY, USA

Jonn Damia
Technical Support Specialist, cyberDERM Inc., Media, PA, USA

James Q. Del Rosso DO FAOCD
Clinical Associate Professor, Department of Dermatology, University of Nevada School of Medicine, Las Vegas, NV, USA

Cherie M. Ditre MD
Director, Cosmetic Dermatology and Skin Enhancement Center, Penn Medicine at Radnor, PA, USA; Assistant Professor of Dermatology, University of Pennsylvania School of Medicine, PA, USA

Zoe Diana Draelos MD
Clinical Associate Professor, Department of Dermatology, Wake Forest University School of Medicine, Winston-Salem, NC; Dermatology Consulting Services, High Point, NC, USA

Swarna Ekanayake-Mudiyanselage MD
Postdoctoral Fellow, Department of Dermatology, Northwestern University, Feinberg School of Medicine, Chicago, IL, USA

Peter M. Elias MD
Professor of Dermatology, University of California; Staff Physician, Veteran Affairs Medical Center, San Francisco, CA, USA

Patricia Farris MD
Clinical Assistant Professor, Department of Dermatology, Tulane University School of Medicine, New Orleans, LA, USA

Richard E. Fitzpatrick MD
Associate Clinical Professor of Dermatology, University of California, San Diego, CA, USA

Bryan B. Fuller PhD
Associate Professor, Department of Biochemistry and Molecular Biology, University of Oklahoma Health Sciences Center, Oklahoma City, OK, USA

Jorge I. Gaviria MD
Hair Transplant Surgeon; Clinical Research Fellow, Dermatology & Aesthetic Center, Boca Raton, FL, USA

Ellen C. Gendler MD
Clinical Associate Professor, Dermatology Division, New York University School of Medicine, New York, NY, USA

Dee Anna Glaser MD
Associate Professor and Vice Chairman, Department of Dermatology, Saint Louis University School of Medicine, Saint Louis, MO, USA

Barbara A. Green RpH MS
Executive Director, Technical & Consumer Affairs, Neostrata Company Inc., Princeton, NJ, USA

Gary L. Grove PhD
Vice President of Research and Development, cyberDERM Inc., Media, PA, USA

Sherry N. Hsieh PhD
Postdoctoral Fellow, Department of Dermatology, Northwestern University, Chicago, IL, USA

Anthony W. Johnson BSc PhD DipRCPath
Director of Clinical Evaluation, Skin Global Innovation Center, Unilever HPC-NA, Trumbull, CT, USA

Kenneth Klein BS MS
President, Cosmetech Laboratories Inc., Fairfield, NJ, USA

Albert M. Kligman MD PhD
Professor Emeritus of Dermatology,
University of Pennsylvania,
Department of Dermatology,
Philadelphia, PA, USA

Mary P. Lupo MD FAAD
Clinical Professor of Dermatology,
Tulane Medical School, New Orleans,
LA, USA

Christen M. Mowad MD
Assistant Professor, Department of
Dermatology, Geisinger Medical Center,
Danville, PA, USA

Carla G. Nugent MBA
Consultant, the BIG idea group, Concept
and Product Development, New York,
NY, USA

John E. Oblong PhD
Principal Scientist, Personal Beauty Care
Technology Division, Procter and Gamble,
Miami Valley Laboratories, Cincinnati,
OH, USA

Brian K. Pilcher PhD
Director of Research, Cutanix
Corporation, Oklahoma, OK, USA

Marta I. Rendon MD FAAD FACP
Associate Clinical Professor of
Dermatology, University of Miami;
Medical Director, Dermatology and
Aesthetic Center, Boca Raton, FL, USA

Neil S. Sadick MD FACP FAACS
Clinical Professor of Dermatology,
Weill Medical College of Cornell
University, New York, NY, USA

James R. Schwartz PhD
Research Fellow, Procter and Gamble,
Sharon Woods Technical Center,
Cincinnati, OH, USA

Dustin R. Smith
BS Graduate Student, Department
of Biochemistry & Molecular Biology,
University of Oklahoma Health
Sciences Center, Oklahoma City,
OK, USA

Doug Stuckey BA MBA
Senior Manager, Professional Marketing,
Procter and Gamble, Cincinnati, OH, USA

Jens J. Thiele MD
Research Associate, Department of
Dermatology, Northwestern University,
Feinberg School of Medicine, Chicago,
IL, USA

Carl R. Thornfeldt MD
Associate Professor, Department of
Dermatology, University of Oregon Health
Sciences Center, Portland, Oregon and
CT Derm Fruitland, Fruitland, ID, USA

Heidi A. Waldorf MD
Associate Clinical Professor, Mount Sinai
School of Medicine; Director of Laser and
Cosmetic Dermatology, Department of
Dermatology, Mount Sinai Medical Center,
New York, NY, USA

Charles Zerweck PhD
Senior Research Scientist, KGL Inc.,
Skin Study Center, Broomall, PA, USA

Introduction

What are Cosmeceuticals?

Albert M. Kligman

I coined the term cosmeceuticals 25 years ago at a presentation I gave at the annual meeting of the Society of Cosmetic Chemists. To my astonishment the response was not only negative but downright hostile and derisive. Unwittingly, I started a controversy, which continues to this very day. European writers have been especially derogatory, some arguing that 'having a separate classification is neither helpful, scientifically suitable, nor juridically necessary. Further, the cosmeceutical concept is superfluous and should be abandoned.' One prominent European dermatologist decries cosmeceuticals as 'cosmeceutical chaos'.

Nonetheless, wherever one comes down in this argument, the term has permanently entered the vocabulary, evidently having enough pragmatic value to require major trade blocks (USA, Japan, and Europe) and legislative bodies to weigh in on the subject. The current economic tensions regarding globalization of international commerce has forced each block to come to grips with how it defines and regulates topical products. The Japanese category of 'quasi-drugs' comes closest to my original concept.

Like it or not, cosmeceuticals are here to stay. It does not matter what semantic contrivances are created to duck the pesky problem of 'what is a cosmeceutical'? There now exists a choice among synonymous niceties, instead of the term cosmeceutical. These alternatives include 'dermaceuticals', 'active cosmetics', 'functional cosmetics', having in common acknowledgement that the product contains 'active' ingredients that go beyond mere camouflage such as rouge and lipstick.

Cosmeceuticals are in any case a reality, as evidenced by multiple international symposia and seminars, a growing library of textbooks titled cosmeceuticals, and common usage of the term by marketers who perceive that consumers want products that are functional as well as ornamental. The most balanced, practical and scholarly account of the cosmeceutical imbroglio is to be found in the enlightening article by two outstanding dermatologists, Vermeer and Gilchrest.

The historical circumstances that led me to invent the term cosmeceutical may be briefly summarized as follows. In 1938, Congress passed the Food, Drug and Cosmetic Act, which by statutory law defined how a topical product should be classified. Only two categories were recognized: drugs and cosmetics. These stood at opposite poles regarding their intended use. If the purpose of the product was to mitigate, prevent or treat a disease, it automatically fell into the drug category, requiring the manufacturer to demonstrate safety and efficacy before approval by the Food and Drug Administration. By contrast, a product that was simply intended to beautify or improve appearance would be assigned to the category of a cosmetic and could be sold without the necessity to establish safety and efficacy before marketing. However, there was one further caveat attached to the definition of a cosmetic; namely, that it should have no demonstrable effect on the structure and function of skin. In 1938 this stricture seemed reasonable. Looked at 50 years later, it was an oxymoron that flies in the face of biologic reality. During that time, methods for studying the impact of exogenous substances on the physiology and anatomy of human skin had become extremely sophisticated and sensitive. Experimental studies showed that everything applied to skin would inevitably alter it in some measurable way. Water, the most benign and innocent of all known substances, provided the most dramatic example. Water applied occlusively to normal skin for a few hours greatly swells the horny layer, promotes shedding of corneocytes, releases stores of proinflammatory cytokines, induces cytotoxic damage to Langerhans' cells and keratinocytes, enhances permeability, increases blood flow, among other changes. Water is a basic ingredient of water–oil emulsions that comprise the general class of moisturizers whose beneficial effects have been celebrated for centuries. It would be a bureaucratic idiocy to call water a drug.

Another supposedly inert substance, petrolatum, actually permeates the intercellular spaces between corneocytes, becoming part of the stratum corneum, thereby altering its structure with attendant beneficial moisturizing effects. A strict interpretation of the 1938 act would require the reclassification of practically all topical substances as drugs, an unwelcome, unnecessary change, harmful to the development of novel products. To reconcile modern science with the obsolescent 1938 law, I thought it necessary for the sake of rationality to establish a third category, which would span the region lying between drugs and cosmetics. I viewed cosmeceuticals as hybrids, intermediate between both poles. Some lie closer to what are universally regarded as cosmetics in the sense of adornments, while others lie closer to the category of drugs. In the latter category are products that contain 'active' ingredients that help to maintain skin and might even protect skin from various insults.

These distinctions are not academic musings but have profound implications regarding international trade. For example, sunscreens and antiperspirants are regulated as drugs in the USA but not in Europe where they are classified as cosmetics. This has the unfortunate consequence of keeping out of the US market certain broad spectrum European sunscreens that are superior to American products.

Some American patients with extremely photosensitive skin disorders, such as subacute lupus erythematosus, resort to the internet in order to buy more effective European sunscreens from Canada and Mexico.

Then, too, legalistic interpretation creates further controversies. For instance, when the FDA thinks that the advertising claims for a cosmetic have crossed the line and are really drugs in disguise, it will then send out warning letters to the manufacturer to modify the claims it makes in its marketing strategies. It turns out that it is not simply the ingredients of a product that determine its status but its intended use. The same component can be a drug in one instance and a cosmetic in another. For example, if the advertisements claim that the product improves appearance, it is a cosmetic. On the other hand, if the same product is marketed as having antiaging effects, it becomes a drug. This implies that 'you are what you say you are'.

Contradictions and confused policies are so prevalent that it is timely for international regulatory authorities and scientists to come together to lay out standards and guidelines that can resolve these thorny problems. Cosmeceuticals are here to stay because they make biological sense and have practical advantages for rational interactions between manufacturers, regulators, and skin care specialists.

Further Reading

Kligman AM 1998 Cosmeceuticals as a third category. Cosmetics and Toiletries 113:33

Vermeer BJ, Gilchrest BA 1996 Cosmeceuticals. A proposal for rational definition, evaluation and regulation. Archives of Dermatology 132:337

Part 1

Defining the Cosmeceutical Realm

Part I of this text presents the elements necessary to understand the cosmeceutical realm as defined by Dr Kligman. The functioning of these biologically active ingredients on the skin barrier and the health of the skin characterize the cosmeceutical realm. The ability of these ingredients to enhance skin functioning depends on how they are formulated into creams, lotions etc. that can maintain the integrity of the active, deliver it in a biologically active form to the skin, reach the target site in sufficient quantity to exert an effect, and properly release from the carrier vehicle. Cosmeceuticals are sold as cosmetics, making marketing an important consideration. These marketing claims must be substantiated by clinical testing, however clinical testing is also important to establish cosmeceutical efficacy. The recognition that there are limitations on efficacy claims means that cosmeceuticals can only be assessed in terms of their ability to improve skin appearance, but not function. Herein lies the challenge of defining the cosmeceutical realm.

1

Cosmeceuticals and the Practice of Dermatology

Ellen C. Gendler

The Cosmeceutical Phenomenon

America's 78 million baby boomers have taken a very proactive approach to combating the signs of aging. As the 45+ age bracket is set to grow at three times the rate of the general population, 'anti-aging' products and services proliferate dramatically, a trend that is expected to continue over the next two decades. While the demand for aesthetic medical treatments such as botulinum toxin A, soft tissue augmentation, and laser or chemical resurfacing is considerable, many people prefer a more economical or less invasive approach. Cosmeceuticals, or cosmetic products promoted as having 'biologically active' ingredients, are increasingly being used in place of or in addition to medical procedures. The cosmeceutical phenomenon has had a profound impact on the cosmetic industry and the practice of dermatology. As our profession's involvement in this arena increases, so does the need for a knowledge base allowing a rational, scientific approach.

Medical marketing

A tremendous amount of hype surrounds cosmeceuticals as consumers are exposed to products from a variety of sources. Interactions with retail sales clerks and editorials or advertisements in the popular press are the primary means of communication. On television, cosmeceuticals are featured on commercials, talk show beauty segments, news programs, home shopping networks, and infomercials, an advertisement vehicle with a prolonged and highly detailed sales message. Increasing use is being made of print advertorials, or sponsored editorials, which are essentially advertisements designed to resemble editorial content. The Internet is an extremely powerful and important source of information. Chat rooms and message boards devoted to health and aesthetic concerns frequently feature discussions on the latest skincare products.

In all these venues, savvy marketers capitalize on every possible scientific angle to promote cosmeceutical products. While the concept of scientific skincare and medicinal cosmetics is nothing new, therapeutic positioning has accelerated dramatically in recent years, and its appeal has firmly taken hold in the minds of marketers and consumers. Claims are made for efficacy based on 'scientific studies' and consumers are led to believe that products are backed by solid medical evidence. Such claims are rarely distributed through scientific channels, seemingly because manufacturers are concerned about protecting proprietary formulations but mostly due to fear of negative results. Clinical props such as sales clerks in white lab coats, pharmaceutical-like bottles and packaging, and even black doctors' bags, are employed to enhance the impression of scientifically formulated products.

Complicating the situation for consumers as well as physicians is the fact that many of these claims do have some foundation in scientific plausibility. However, most consumers do not have the knowledge to judge an advertisement's veracity and may not understand that cosmetics, unlike drugs, have no pre-market requirement for proof of safety or efficacy.

The Cosmetics Marketplace

Growing demand

Points of sale for cosmeceutical products include department stores, specialty stores, apothecaries, chain drugstores, mass volume retailers, home shopping networks, Internet sites, spas, beauty salons, and, increasingly, doctors' clinics. It is estimated

US spending on beauty products, 2003

Category	$ billions
Color cosmetics	15.2
Skin care	15
Body and bath products	6.4
Women's fragrances	6.2
Men's products	2.6

Table 1.1 US spending on beauty products, 2003. Source: CosmeticIndustry.com

that around 40% of dermatologists are currently dispensing products from their clinics, and doctors of every other specialty are getting involved as well.

In 2003, the total US cosmetics market was valued at $45.5 billion with skincare products accounting for $15 billion alone. Within this category, anti-aging and sun protection products are at the top of the demand and drive the overall industry. Table 1.1 depicts a further breakdown of spending by cate-

gory. According to the NPD Group, department store sales for cosmeceuticals, or clinical brands as they are sometimes referred to, grew at a phenomenal 77% in 2003, relative to 6% for the entire skincare category. A study by the Freedonia Group estimates that US demand for cosmeceutical products will exceed $5 billion by 2007.

Regulatory issues and product development

From a regulatory perspective, cosmeceuticals do not really exist. It is a functional but not legal term used primarily for marketing purposes by cosmetic manufacturers, who cannot claim drug-like ingredients or benefits for their products. Yet, cosmeceutical products contain an endless list of supposedly active substances. (A partial listing of agents by category is provided in Table 1.2.) Most of these ingredients do not meet Kligman's definition of efficacy—namely proof of penetration, identifiable mechanism of action, and evidence of clinical value.

Common cosmeceutical agents by category

Category	Agent	
Vitamins	Beta-carotene Coenzyme Q10 (ubiquinone) Niacinamide (nicotinamide) panthenol Pro-vitamin B_5 (panthenol) Retinaldehyde Retinol Retinyl acetate Retinyl esters	Retinyl palmitate Retinyl propionate Vitamin A (retinoic acid) Vitamin B Vitamin B_3 (niacinamide) Vitamin C (L-ascorbic acid) Vitamin E (alpha-tocopherol)
Synthetic vitamins	Adapalene Tazarotene Tretinoin	
Minerals	Copper Selenium Zinc	
Antioxidants	Alpha-lipoic acid (ALA) Catalase Dimethylaminoethanol (DMAE)	Glutathione Idebenone Ubiquinone
Hydroxy acids	Alpha-hydroxy acids (glycolic, lactic, malic acids) Beta-hydroxy acids (salicylic acid) Dihydroxyacetone 4-Hydroxy-retinoic acid	Lanolin 4-Oxo-retinoic acid Polyhydroxy acids (gluconolactone, lactobionic acid) Salicyclic acid
Growth factors	Epidermal growth factor (EGF) Granulocyte colony stimulating factor Hepatocyte growth factor Interleukin	Keratinocyte growth factor Platelet-derived growth factor Transforming growth factor (TGF) Vascular endothelial growth factor

Table 1.2 Common cosmeceutical agents by category

Continued

Common cosmeceutical agents by category—cont'd		
Category	**Agent**	
Lipids	Glucosylceramide	
Proteins	Copper peptides Oligopeptides (Pal-KTTKS) Pentapeptides	
Glycosaminoglycans	Hyaluronic acid	
Botanicals	Allantoin Aloe vera Aloesin Arnica Bearberry Beeswax Bisbolol Black tea Capsaicin Ceramides Chamomile Cinnimate Curcumin Echinacea Garlic Genestein Ginseng *Ginkgo biloba*	Grape Green tea Lavender Licorice extract May apple Oolong tea Papaya Paper mulberry extract Pomegranate Pycnogenol Silymarin Soy St John's Wort Tea tree oil White tea White willow Witch hazel
Moisturizers	Acylceramide Cholesterol Linoleic acid	Petrolatum Sodium PCA Squalene
Pigment lightening agents	Azelaic acid Hydroquinone Kojic acid	
Sunscreens	Anthranilate Padimate A	Padimate O p-Aminobenzoic acid

Table 1.2 Common cosmeceutical agents by category

In addition to scientifically demonstrable efficacy, characteristics of the ideal cosmeceutical product would include immediate and long-lasting results, a low side effect profile, preventive benefits, and application to a variety of skin concerns including texture, pigmentation, and laxity.

The regulatory situation is a dilemma for cosmetic manufacturers and prevents them from developing products containing truly active ingredients. Efficacy claims must be carefully worded so as not to attract the attention of regulators. Expensive and lengthy clinical trials are unfeasible for a highly competitive industry that must respond quickly to changing fashion. Pharmaceutical companies have not yet been major players in the cosmeceutical arena as dermatologic drugs per se are a comparatively small therapeutic area for the industry. However, if drug companies believed that truly effective cosmetic agents could be developed to blockbuster potential, the manufacturing landscape could change very quickly.

Best Practices for Dermatologists

Challenges and opportunities

Cosmeceuticals are a good news, bad news story for dermatologists. Many of us feel a growing sense of frustration with some of the outrageous claims made by purveyors of skincare products, including our own colleagues in the medical profession. We spend precious time explaining to confused patients why the $600 jar of 'anti-aging' skin cream may not be the major discovery that it claims to be, or why it's usually not necessary to layer on five different types of products. On the other hand, when patients use products with proven benefits (e.g. tretinoin), compliance with other maintenance and preventive regimens may be enhanced.

While some new agents in development sound very exciting, our immediate concern is to help patients choose the best products available today. To this end, education and communication are more important than ever, which has led to the development of this reference text on cosmeceuticals.

Patient education and compliance

When using cosmeceuticals as part of a dermatologic practice, it is important to maintain the professionalism of a physician. Critical issues to consider include:

1. **Managing patient expectations is important.** Fully explain the type of improvement that can realistically be achieved as well as any potential side effects. Instruct patients on proper application, cautioning against the common tendency for overuse. Always remind patients that a product that may be safe and effective in the right dose can provoke clogged pores, redness, or irritation if used inappropriately. Always take the opportunity to emphasize the importance of prevention, and encourage regular follow-up to monitor progress.
2. **Beware of recommending anything that will undermine objectivity.** When uncomfortable about overly enthusiastic commercial claims, counter such messages with clear, straightforward rebuttals. If you feel that you do not have adequate time to fully discuss these issues with patients, try to provide handouts or suggested reading so that patients can learn more on their own.
3. **Guide patients on how to incorporate cosmeceuticals into their daily skin care regimen.** As much as possible, consider your patients' ability to stick with the program from a practical as well as an economic point of view. Most patients will quickly lose patience with complex and expensive regimens that don't deliver promised results—and physicians lose credibility for recommending such products.

4. **Diligently keep abreast of reported reactions from new agents, including those with natural and botanical ingredients.** In addition to the medical literature, the Cosmetic, Toiletry and Fragrance Association's Cosmetic Ingredient Review expert panel listing of unsafe ingredients is a good source of information (http://www.cir-safety.org/). The greatest risk to patients may be in wasting their money—not a life-threatening situation, but something to try to avoid nonetheless. Discouraged patients can be lost to follow-up, making it all the more difficult to judge overall outcomes.

Dispensing products

There is a lot of debate about the appropriateness of selling products in the office. Dermatologists have always compounded medicinal products, and this is considered to be a valuable and accepted aspect of medical practice. Dispensing cosmetic products, despite potential conflicts of interest, can provide patients with a value-added service. If products are sold in a medical office, it is important to be aware of ethical boundaries. The American Academy of Dermatology has developed dispensing guidelines for prescription and non-prescription products (summarized in Box 1.1), which set the standard for the in-office sale of cosmeceuticals.

American Academy of Dermatology Office Dispensing Guidelines for Prescription and Non-Prescription Products

- DO NOT place your own financial interests above the well-being of patients
- DO NOT price products at an excessive mark-up
- DO NOT create an atmosphere of coercive selling
- DO NOT sell products whose claims of benefit lack validity
- DO NOT represent products as 'special formulations' not available elsewhere if this is not the case
- DO clearly list all ingredients, including generic names of drugs
- DO advise patients of alternative purchase options if products are available elsewhere
- DO provide prescription refills that can be filled outside the office if patients so choose

Box 1.1 American Academy of Dermatology Office Dispensing Guidelines for Prescription and Non-Prescription Products. Source: American Academy of Dermatology, 2003. Available http://www.aadassociation.org/Policy/dispensing.html

Summary

A youthful healthy appearance is important in modern society. Consequently, many people feel a sense of anxiety about the visible signs of aging and seek dermatologic advice. As dermatologists, we understand that the preservation of healthy and attractive skin is of great value to the happiness and well-being of our patients. Therefore, we have a unique and important role in the growing use of cosmeceuticals and must address this phenomenon collectively as a profession and in our daily interactions with patients. This text provides the necessary material to gain a state-of-the-art understanding of cosmeceuticals and their role in dermatology.

Further Reading

American Academy of Dermatology 1999 Position Statement on Dispensing. September 26, 1999. American Academy of Dermatology, Schaumberg, Illinois.

Farris PK 2000 Office dispensing: a responsible approach. Seminars in Cutaneous Medicine and Surgery 19:195–100

Kligma A 2000 A dermatologist looks to the future: promises and problems. Dermatologic Clinics 18:699–709

Kligman D 2000 Cosmeceuticals. Dermatologic Clinics 18: 609–615

Lamberg L 2001 'Treatment' cosmetics: hype or help? Journal of the American Medical Association 279:1595–1596

Millikan LE 2001 Cosmetology, cosmetics, cosmeceuticals: definitions and regulations. Clinics in Dermatology 19:371–374

Moore A 2002 The biochemistry of beauty. The science and pseudo-science of beautiful skin. EMBO Reports 3:714–717

Ogbogu P, Fleischer AB, Brodell RT, et al 2001 Physicians' and patients' perspectives on office-based dispensing: the central role of the physician–patient relationship. Archives of Dermatology 137:151–154

Pearson H 2003 Drug discovery; in the eye of the beholder. Nature August 28 424:990–991

Sadick N 2003 Cosmeceuticals: their role in dermatology practice. Journal of Drugs in Dermatology 2:529–537

2

Cosmeceuticals: Function and the Skin Barrier

Anthony W. Johnson

Introduction

Much of the research to identify the activities and mechanisms of actives proposed as cosmeceuticals for the skin is carried out in vitro. What happens when these actives are applied to skin in vivo, bearing in mind that skin has evolved to exclude the entry of exogenous materials into the body whether chemicals or microorganisms? In cosmetology as in medicine delivery of actives across the skin barrier is a major challenge and usually seriously limits the physiologic usefulness of topically applied substances. Consider how few transdermal drugs exist after 30 years of intensive delivery research by the pharmaceutical industry. It is the structure and daily renewal of the stratum corneum that enables the skin to be a remarkably effective barrier for a lifetime.

The Stratum Corneum Structure and Function

The stratum corneum has a simple structure of pancake-like cells stacked in layers with a thin coating of fat between the layers (Fig. 2.1). The underlying biology, mostly worked out in the last 20 years, reveals a series of interrelated processes that start with a dividing cell in the basal layer of the living epidermis and complete with a spent squame shed from the skin surface 4–6 weeks later. The process of change and maturation during this journey appears complex but reduces to four key processes (Fig. 2.2). The main features of these four processes are summarized in Table 2.1. When all four processes are functioning optimally the stratum corneum is not only an excellent moisture barrier (without which all mammals would quickly dehydrate and perish) but also an effective barrier to microorganisms and chemicals.

The Stratum Corneum Barrier and the Environment

Although an excellent and resilient barrier the stratum corneum is usually in a state of minor dysfunction because of daily insults from the

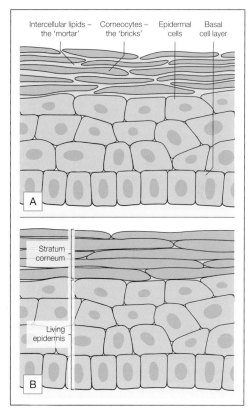

Fig. 2.1 The stratum corneum sitting above the living epidermal layers: (**A**) a typical bricks and mortar representation that does not reflect the relative proportions of skin cells and (**B**) a truer to life representation of the stratum corneum structure with closely opposed and heavily cross-linked corneocytes and intercellular lipids. Corneocyte length is 50–100 times greater than thickness

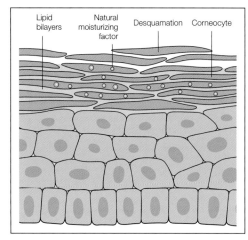

Fig. 2.2 The four key processes for the formation and functioning of the stratum corneum

environment. Low humidity, wind, the sun, and cleansing agents are all capable of lowering the water concentration in the superficial layers of the stratum corneum to less than the level required to allow desquamating enzymes to function. The result is dry skin. In fact, what we experience as dry skin is not simply skin that lacks water but is dysfunctional skin where there is an accumulation of attached corneocytes at the skin surface (Fig. 2.3). The skin feels rough; looks dull because light is scattered by the uneven surface; looks pale because the pinky glow from the microcirculation is obscured; may show visible scaling and is susceptible to irritation. Such are the consequences of a little dehydration at the skin surface!

Water is also important for maintaining the elasticity of the stratum corneum. Without this the skin feels tight and may crack in regions subject to stretching forces (e.g. knuckles). UV radiation, which we mostly associate with sunburn in the short term and photoaging over time, may also damage the stratum corneum and in particular disrupt the skin's natural moisturizing process. As little as one MED (minimal erythemal dose) of UV is sufficient to disrupt enzymic breakdown of filaggrin to NMF (natural moisturizing factor) amino acids.

The variations of skin and the stratum corneum barrier

Cosmetic scientists, like dermatologists, are aware that normal skin structure and function as described in textbooks is seldom found in the real world. One measure of the great variation in human skin types and conditions is the surprising number of classifications that have been developed to describe normal skin. Consumer skin is traditionally categorized as normal, dry, oily, or combination. The great variation in sensitivity of skin to sunlight is captured in the six phototypes of the Fitzpatrick photosensitivity classification. In recent years sensitive skin has emerged as another axis of variation that seemingly cuts across other categories and reflects the ease or otherwise with which skin reacts negatively to products and environmental challenges. The Glogau four-point scale of skin photoaging is yet another classification of skin condition as it is encountered in practice. Added to or superimposed on these variations are those due to age, sex, hormonal status, lifestyle, and environment. It is clear that normal skin varies greatly in type, condition, and functioning.

Alongside the clinical variations of skin, consumer research reveals an associated great variety of consumer habits and attitudes towards their skin and its care. There are many opportunities for cosmetics and cosmeceutical products to impact and improve the condition of normal consumer skin. While most of the variations of normal skin described above are

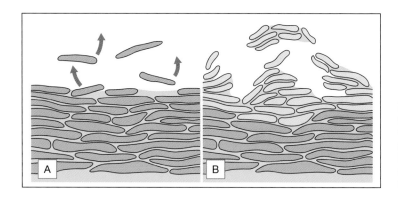

Fig. 2.3 (A) Stratum corneum fully hydrated at the skin surface with normal desquamation and release of effete corneocytes. **(B)** Stratum corneum with reduced hydration in the superficial layers leading to incomplete desquamation and a build up of attached cells at the skin surface (skin dryness)

Four key processes for the formation and functioning of the stratum corneum

Key process	Essential features	Significant function	Schematic
Corneocyte process Corneocytes are cells of the stratum corneum—protein structures bounded by a cornified envelope and containing natural moisturizing factor (NMF)	Keratinocytes (KC) formed by cell division in the basal layer of epidermis migrate upwards. As they enter the stratum corneum (SC) they transform to flat enucleated proteinaceous cells (corneocytes). The corneocytes (CTs) continue upward migration and mature with extensive cross-linking of the cell membrane to produce a highly resistant and insoluble outer envelope. CTs are joined together by multiple protein links called corneodesmosomes. A covalently bound layer of lipid on the outer surface of the CT provides the correct template for organization of the lamellar lipid structure of the intercellular lipids	Corneocytes provide the framework of the stratum corneum barrier—the 'bricks' in the 'bricks and mortar' structural analogy. It resists physical insult. They provide a physical barrier to water loss and entry of chemicals and microorganisms. Hydrated corneocytes provide elasticity to the SC	 Corneodesmosomes Corneocyte Corneocyte Keratinocytes Basal layer
Stratum corneum lipid process Forming the lipid matrix of the stratum corneum	Specialized lipids occupy the intercellular space of the stratum corneum. They are produced within KCs and discharged at the base of the stratum corneum as the KCs transform to corneocytes. There are three major lipid classes; ceramides, fatty acids, cholesterol, that spontaneously arrange in multiple bilayers (lamellar structure). Also called stratum corneum barrier lipids	The stratum corneum lipid bilayers are the moisture barrier of the SC. The lipid barrier prevents penetration of many classes of chemical. However, most materials that penetrate the stratum corneum do so via the hydrophobic or hydrophilic regions of the lipid bilayers	 Bipolar lipids stored in lamellar bodies of keratinocytes Barrier lipid bilayers

Continued

Table 2.1 Four key processes for the formation and functioning of the stratum corneum

Four key processes for the formation and functioning of the stratum corneum—cont'd

Key process	Essential features	Significant function	Schematic
NMF process Natural moisturizing factor occurs within the corneocyte—in the protein matrix	A mix of low MW hygroscopic molecules that reside in the corneocyte structure and enable CTs to remain hydrated. NMF is approximately 50 : 50 amino acids: salts including lactic acid and urea. The amino acids are primarily derived from the protein filaggrin formed as a precursor protein in the KCs and subsequently processed into amino acids within the CTs	NMF is the skin's natural mechanism to keep the stratum corneum hydrated. The conversion of filaggrin to constituent amino acids is controlled by the water activity of the SC. If external humidity is low NMF is produced lower in the SC than if humidity is high	Corneocytes contain filaggrin (protein) Profilaggrin stored in keratohyalin granule of keratinocytes Filaggrin degraded to NMF amino acids
Desquamation process Detachment and shedding of spent corneocytes from the skin surface	Desquamation is the process of enzymic degradation of protein links (corneodesmosomes) that attach CTs one to another. Hydrolytic enzymes that degrade corneodesmosomes require a high water activity and do not function if the SC surface is dry—leading to accumulation of CTs at the skin surface and the well known symptoms of dry skin	Orderly release of spent CTs at the skin surface is required for skin to be soft smooth and looking attractive. If desquamation is inhibited (e.g. by skin dryness) CTs accumulate at the skin surface and provide the signs of dry skin	Shedding corneocytes Degrading desmosomes Intact desmosomes

Table 2.1 Four key processes for the formation and functioning of the stratum corneum

widely recognized, it is less well known that there are differences in skin barrier effectiveness associated with most of these different categories. This means that particular cosmeceuticals ostensibly aimed at the same end benefit will be better suited and be more effective for some consumers than for others.

The Stratum Corneum As a Target for Cosmeceuticals

Although moisturization is not the most dramatic or exciting effect of skin care products it is a benefit delivered with greatest certainty and maximum extent. An effective moisturizer contains a good humectant, such as glycerol, to hold water in the stratum corneum, and lipid emollients that seal in moisture and prevent the wash out of humectant when the skin is next in contact with water. Moisturizers reverse the negative effects of dryness leaving skin soft and smooth with a natural looking healthy glow. Moisture restores the elasticity of the stratum corneum, making skin feel firmer and more vibrant. Skin looks better, looks healthier, and looks rejuvenated. All this from using a good moisturizer!

Effects beyond the stratum corneum

Cosmetic moisturizers have a profound effect on skin quality by providing the moisture-retaining ability required to maintain optimum activity of stratum corneum function. To do this moisturizers need only penetrate the superficial layers of the stratum corneum.

To exert effects on the deeper living layers of skin requires that cosmeceuticals penetrate the stratum corneum barrier and reach the target tissue in sufficient concentration to be effective. Penetrating the barrier is not easy. Penetrating at a rate sufficient to deliver an effective concentration at a target site below the stratum corneum is even more difficult.

Before moving on to consider how cosmeceuticals may impact the skin at deeper levels it is important to realize that skin has remarkable rejuvenating ability in its own right. In many placebo controlled studies the placebo formulation produces a significant benefit relative to baseline and often not much less of a benefit than seen with the active formulation. It seems that placebo formulations that do not have actives to penetrate the stratum corneum can have effects and benefits below the stratum corneum. Why is this?

Natural Rejuvenation of Skin

As indicated above and confirmed by many studies in the literature, the skin has remarkable ability to repair and compensate for environment insults. The healing of wounds after an injury is not usually considered rejuvenation. However, most of the skin rejuvenation techniques used in cosmetic dermatology, such as chemical peels, ablative laser therapies, and dermabrasion, involve controlled injury of 'bad skin' with the expectation that wound healing processes will replace the damaged skin with new skin that looks and functions better. The biologic mechanisms involved are simple in concept although complex in detail. Injury to skin kills some cells and damages others. Many chemical messengers (cytokines) are released which activate and recruit wound healing cells (immune, inflammatory, hematopoietic) to the damaged area. Scavenger cells remove the debris and the tissue remodeling cells rebuild the structure.

The same processes of damage and repair, degradation and synthesis operate at the molecular level in the skin. The pioneering work of John Vorhees' group in Michigan reveals that photoaging induced by solar UV reflects a balance between tissue degradation and tissue rebuilding at the level of molecular genetics. UV light promotes the induction of genes for the biochemical reactions that degrade collagen and inhibits the molecular interactions leading to repair and replacement. By simply reducing UV exposure there is not only less damage but also an increase in collagen synthesis. So it is possible to induce positive changes in the dermis without having to use a product let alone a product with an active. Moisturization also has benefits below the barrier. If skin is spared the perturbation of stratum corneum drying and dysfunction there are fewer distress signals to the living layers of skin, leaving it free to concentrate on repair and remodeling of the dermis.

The Barrier is a Challenge for Cosmeceuticals

Normal skin is seldom entirely normal because of a daily battery of environment insults ranging from unavoidable exposure to surfactants during daily cleansing to exposure to solar UV, which is largely avoidable. Minor defects accumulate over time and produce a noticeable deterioration of skin function and appearance. Cosmeceutical products to address these issues must somehow penetrate the stratum corneum barrier.

Examination of Figure 2.1b suggests that a route through the linked corneocytes is the most direct way across the stratum corneum barrier. However, the corneocyte outer membrane, the cornified envelope, is so extensively cross-linked and insoluble that very few substances are able to penetrate. It is now accepted that most substances that cross the stratum corneum barrier do so by taking a tortuous path through the lipid matrix between the corneocytes. There are three types of lipid in the stratum corneum, fatty acids, ceramides, and cholesterol (Fig. 2.4). These are bipolar lipids that spontaneously arrange in multiple bilayers between and around the corneocytes (Fig. 2.5). They create a formidable barrier to water and many chemical types. There has been extensive research to find methods to enhance delivery of actives through the stratum corneum. Many penetration enhancers have been developed that function by temporarily disrupting the lipid bilayer structures of the stratum corneum to allow easier passage of active molecules. However, the most effective chemical penetration enhancers are generally unsuitable for use in cosmeceuticals because they tend to be irritating at the concentrations required to enhance penetration.

The challenge to deliver actives beyond the stratum corneum barrier has stimulated several new lines of research. This includes high throughput screening to identify Synergists Combinations of Penetration Enhancers (SCOPE), development of new techniques like micro-needles and microchip controlled micro-electrode arrays, and a re-examination of older techniques such as iontophoresis and sonophoresis.

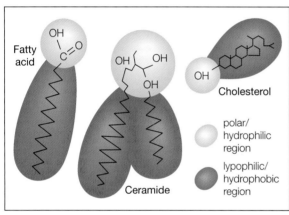

Fig. 2.4 Three classes of polar lipids, ceramides, fatty acids, and cholesterol, are the main constituents of the lipid matrix of the stratum corneum

Further Reading

Barry BW 2004 Breaching the skin's barrier to drugs. Nature Biotechnology 22 165–167

Bos JD, Meinardi MM 2000 The 500 Dalton rule for the skin penetration of chemical compounds and drugs. Experimental Dermatology 9:165–169

Coderch L, De Pera M, Fonollosa J, De La Maza A, Parra J 2002 Efficacy of stratum corneum lipid supplementation on human skin. Contact Dermatitis 47:139–146

Current Stratum Corneum Research 2004 Optimizing barrier function through fundamental skin care. Dermatological Therapy 17:1–68 [a full issue of the journal (9 papers) dedicated to the biology of the stratum corneum barrier and the impact of cleansing and moisturizing products]

Forster T (ed) 2002 Cosmetic lipids and the skin barrier. Marcel Dekker, New York

Kanikkannan N, Kandimalla K, Lamba SS, Singh M 2000 Structure–activity relationship of chemical penetration enhancers in transdermal drug delivery. Current Medicinal Chemistry 7:593–608

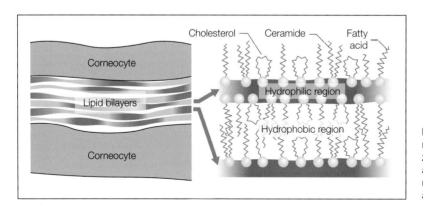

Fig. 2.5 The stratum corneum lipid matrix has a multiple bilayer organization formed by the spontaneous alignment of polar and non-polar regions of the ceramide, cholesterol, and fatty acid molecules

Karande P, Jain A, Mitragotri S 2004 Discovery of transdermal penetration enhancers by high-throughput screening. Nature Biotechnology 22:192–197

Leyden JJ, Rawlings AV (eds) 2002 Skin moisturiization. Marcel Dekker, New York

Loden M, Maibach HI (eds) 2000 Dry skin and moisturizers: chemistry and function. CRC Press, Boca Raton

McAllister DV, Allen MG, Prausnitz MR 2000 Microfabricated microneedles for gene and drug delivery. Annual Review of Biomedical Engineering 2:289–313

Mitragotri S 2001 Effect of bilayer disruption on transdermal transport of low molecular weight hydrophobic solutes. Pharmacological Research 18:1018–1025

Morgan CJ, Renwick AG, Friedmann PS 2003 The role of stratum corneum and dermal microvascular perfusion in penetration and tissue levels of water-soluble drugs investigated by microdialysis. British Journal of Dermatology 148:434–443

Smith EW, Maibach HI (eds) 1995 Percutaneous penetration enhancers. CRC Press, Boca Raton

Tamarkin D 2004 Using iontophoresis to enhance cosmetics delivery. Cosmetics and Toiletries 119:63–74

3

Cosmeceutical Formulation Considerations

Kenneth Klein

Introduction

The formulation of cosmeceutical products presents cosmetic chemists with a myriad of opportunities normally not encountered. By definition, a cosmetic is intended to have a short term topical effect. It is not intended to treat any 'disease' or have any systemic effect. With this in mind, cosmetic chemists go to great lengths to insure that the products they design are formulated to minimize skin penetration of any ingredients that are present in their formula. They now need to rethink that strategy in light of the development of cosmeceutical actives.

Vehicles

The most important part of any cosmeceutical is the vehicle that carries the active to the skin. The vehicle can enhance the efficacy of the active, make the active completely inactive, enhance the skin barrier, or induce allergic contact dermatitis. This section of the chapter reviews the important types of vehicles currently in the cosmeceutical marketplace.

Emulsions

Oil-in-water emulsions

While there are many vehicles from which to choose, emulsions are by far the most popular delivery form (Fig. 3.1). Most emulsions consist of droplets, which form the internal or dispersed phase, that are uniformly distributed into a continuous phase. Generally, the dispersed phase is composed of oil or oil soluble ingredients and the continuous phase is composed of water or water soluble ingredients. This is considered an oil-in-water emulsion. Since water soluble and oil soluble ingredients do not mix, an emulsifier is incorporated to reduce the interfacial tension between the oil and water phase by adsorbing to the oil/water boundary and thus acting as a barrier to coalescence. Table 3.1 presents typical components of an oil-in-water emulsion. Even though the cosmeceutical active is dissolved in the emulsion, the emulsion is a very important part of the formulation. The active can either reside amongst the water soluble or oil soluble ingredients.

Water-in-oil emulsions

Water-in-oil emulsions consist of the water phase, which is the internal/dispersed phase, mixed with oil, which is the continuous phase This emulsion type is often more difficult to prepare and stabilize since it is most often based on totally non-ionic emulsifiers. However, recent advances in silicone chemistry and polymer chemistry have allowed preparation of excellent water-in-oil (w/o) emulsions. A real benefit of these vehicle emulsions is that they are readily spread onto the lipophilic skin and provide a film which is very resistant to water wash off. This

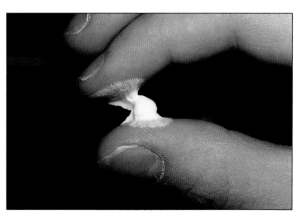

Fig. 3.1 The physical appearance of an oil-in-water emulsion

Components of an oil-in-water emulsion			
Material	**Examples**	**%**	**Function**
Water		60–95	Diluent
Humectant	Propylene glycol, glycerin, butylene glycol, sorbitol, hexylene glycol	2–5	Improves stability, affects skin feel, solubilizer for preservatives, and 'actives'
Emollient (water soluble)	PEG/PPG dimethicone, PEG-7 glyceryl cocoate	1–2	Improves skin feel, reduces tackiness
Thickener	Carbomer, xanthan gum, modified cellulose, guar gum	0.2–1.0	Improves stability, modifies skin feel, suspending agent
Preservative	Methylparaben (and its analogues), quaternium-15, phenoxyethanol, benzyl alcohol, DMDM hydantoin	0.1–1.0	Preservative
Emulsifier (primary and secondary)	TEA-stearate, laureth-23, steareth-21, glyceryl stearate (and) PEG-100 stearate	2.0–5.0	Stabilizes emulsion
Emollient (oil soluble)	Mineral oil, ethylhexyl palmitate, isopropyl myristate, isocetyl alcohol	5–15	Improves skin feel, may solubilize 'actives'
Silicone	Cyclopentasiloxane, dimethicone	2–5	Reduces skin whitening (soaping), improves skin feel, solubilizes 'actives'
Wax	Microcrystalline wax, cetyl alcohol, paraffin, candelilla, polyethylene	1–3	Affects skin feel
Color	Blue 1, yellow 5, etc.	As needed	Consumer appeal
Fragrance	Fragrance	0.15–0.5	Consumer appeal
Alcohol	Alcohol	0.0–20.0	Reduces tackiness, provides cooling effects, may solubilize 'actives'

Table 3.1 Components of an oil-in-water emulsion

is how water resistant moisturizing cosmeceuticals are created. Additionally, if the cosmeceutical 'active' is oil soluble, the w/o emulsion will insure it is uniformly deposited onto the skin surface ensuring the highest degree of efficacy. Since the emulsifiers used for these emulsions are lipophilic, meaning oil loving, they do not upset the lipid bilayer and thus will not damage the skin barrier.

Liquid crystal stabilized emulsions

Liquid crystal stabilized emulsions have become popular in recent years due to their intrinsic mildness. Additionally, they can be used to effectively transport 'actives' which can become trapped between the emulsifier bilayers. These emulsions are used to minimize skin irritation.

Multiple emulsions

Multiple emulsions have never gained much popularity. This is due to the difficulty in preparing them and considerable stability issues, most evident at elevated temperatures (45°C and higher). Multiple emulsions are formed by creating a water-in-oil emulsion and then using the oil phase to form a second oil-in-water emulsion. The resulting emulsion is categorized as a water in oil-in-water emulsion. If one puts an 'active' in the water phase of the water in oil pre-emulsion and then makes a water in oil-in-water emulsion, a controlled released cosmeceutical can be created. It is the kinetics and rate from migration of the active from one phase to another that allows the controlled release emulsion to be created. This is how some actives can be targeted to reach specific parts of the skin in specific concentrations.

Considerations in cosmeceutical emulsion technology

Many aspects must be considered when designing an emulsion which contains a cosmeceutical material to insure that it is not inactivated and loses functionality.

pH

The pH of most emulsions is slightly above 7.0, but they may be prepared at pH values as low as 3.5. pH levels that are too high or too low, meaning too acidic or too basic, are not compatible with the neutral acid mantle pH of the skin at 5.2–5.4.

Temperature

Generally emulsions are prepared at 75°C and designed to function optimally at room temperature.

Particle size

Cosmeceuticals must be mixed properly to insure the proper size of the droplets in the emulsion. While most emulsions are manufactured using low shear mixing, it is quite common to subject them to a final high shear mixing to insure that the particle size is small, somewhere between 2 and 5 microns.

Electrolyte considerations

As a general rule electrolytes are not incorporated into emulsions, since they usually have a negative effect on emulsion stability. This means that all the materials used to manufacture the comeceutical must be pure and free of electrolyte contaminants. This includes the water from which the cosmeceutical is manufactured. However, there are several instances where electrolytes can have a beneficial emulsion stabilizing effect. This is present in water-in-oil emulsions where the emulsifier has a positive cationic charge. If the cosmeceutical active is affected by the presence of electrolytes, they must be eliminated to prevent the emulsion from becoming unstable. Occasionally, the cosmeceutical may be the source of electrolytes which can destabilize the emulsion.

Electrical charge ingredient considerations

Emulsions often use emulsifiers that are uncharged or non-ionic. In this situation, the formulator should have no concern regarding inactivation of the cosme-ceutical active. However, anionic negatively charged emulsifiers are also widely employed. Most typical are the 'soap' emulsifiers, such as triethanolamine which is added to stearic acid to form TEA-stearate. Other anionic emulsifiers include sulfates, other carboxylates, and phosphates. Occasionally, formulators use emulsifiers which have a net cationic positive charge. These emulsions are substantive to the skin, can be very mild, and are almost self-preserving. However, if the cosmeceutical active is anionic then a reaction may occur which destabilizes the emulsion and does not allow release of the active to the skin. While charge considerations can be somewhat complex, this brief discussion serves to point out the intricacies of formulating with ingredients of the proper charge.

Preservation considerations

Great care must be taken to insure that the emulsion is adequately preserved. As a general rule the preservative should be soluble in the water phase. During product manufacture great care should be taken to insure that the preservative is not overheated which might degrade its performance. Many preservatives release formaldehyde, so it is important to be sure that the cosmeceutical active does not react with formaldehyde. Additionally, if the cosmeceutical active contains a primary or secondary amine, it will react with formaldehyde to form a Schiff base which will degrade the performance of the preservative, degrade the performance of the cosmeceutical active, and discolor the finished product. Products manufactured with gums, thickeners, or natural extracts require the use of more robust preservative systems. Product preservation is a careful science. Many products do not pass stability testing due to preservative failure.

Vehicle delivery systems

Emulsions are the most popular delivery systems, but other vehicles can also be employed. These include mousses, ointments, sticks, and gels.

Mousses

Mousses are a convenient, expensive delivery mode. They can be dispensed by aerosol propellant or a pump. When exposure to air or recontamination presents a problem for the cosmeceutical active, an aerosolized mousse presents a good delivery system.

Stability testing	
Storage condition	**Time period**
20°C	2 years
37°C	120 days
45°C	90 days
4°C	2 years
−10°C–20°C	5 cycles (24 hours at each temperature)
Exposure to sunlight	3 months

Table 3.2 Stability testing

Considerations for stability evaluation
■ Odor/color (compared to a refrigerated sample)
■ pH
■ Viscosity
■ Particle size change (for emulsions)
■ Weight loss (in the commercial package) not to exceed 1% per month when stored at 45°C
■ Preservative %
■ Cosmeceutical actives %

Box 3.1 Considerations for stability evaluation

Mousses also are advantageous because they require a low level of surfactant to create the foam effect. This low surfactant level may minimize skin irritation.

Ointments/sticks

Ointments and sticks are generally anhydrous vehicles, meaning they contain no water, with high concentrations of waxes or other oily thickeners. They can deliver a thick film to the skin but often are quite oily and greasy. They are good for delivery of the cosmeceutical active to a small targeted area such as the eyes or lips.

Gels

Typically gels are aqueous based utilizing a quality thickener. Carbomers or other polyacrylate chemistry is generally preferred because of its excellent clarity and low cost. Care must be taken to insure good preservation when employing cosmeceuticals in gel formulations. Gels are quite susceptible to the presence of electrolytes, as discussed previously, which may degrade the gel. Thus, cosmeceutical actives that contain electrolytes cannot be formulated as stable gels.

Stability Considerations

When formulating drug products in the United States an expiration date is required unless the product has a proven shelf-life of at least 3 years. Since cosmeceuticals are cosmetics and not drugs, no expiration dating is required. However, stability testing should be undertaken to insure that the product as sold to consumers is suitable for use. While it is difficult to predict long term stability, given the myriad of

possible storage conditions, many companies have developed testing that has been shown to be quite effective in judging shelf stability. It has been suggested that if a product is stored at 45°C for a period of 90 days, and no product degradation is seen, it is likely that the product will exhibit a shelf life of at least 2 years. The typical stability testing performed on cosmeceuticals is given in Table 3.2.

All stability testing must be conducted both in glass and the commercial packaging. In addition to looking for signs of physical instability, consideration should be given to the factors listed in Box 3.1.

Summary

The cosmetic chemist is endeavoring to deliver a cosmeceutical that is designed to provide some positive consumer benefit. A quality cosmeceutical active must be incorporated into a well formulated vehicle designed to closely mesh with the concept of the cosmeceutical. It would be foolhardy to spend time, money and effort launching a product where the benefit was not realized because the 'active' never actually did anything because it could not be released by the vehicle. While it may be advantageous to maximize penetration of the cosmeceutical active, care must be taken that the penetration enhancers do not also enhance irritation or sensitization. Often choice of the vehicle is one of the most important steps in the formulation process. 'Go down the wrong road' and failure of the cosmeceutical is assured.

Further Reading

Balsam MS, Sagarin E (eds) 1972 Cosmetics: science and technology, vol 1. Wiley-Interscience, New York
Klein K 1984 Improving emulsion stability. Journal of Cosmetics and Toiletries 99:121–126

4

The Cosmeceutical Marketplace

Doug Stuckey

Introduction

The value of marketing is sometimes not obvious to physicians. But, without marketing, physicians would have a much more difficult time learning about the treatments they use. Marketing allows manufacturers to educate consumers and/or physicians about the products they make and their benefits. A poor product will not succeed just due to marketing, but many good products have failed as result of lack of marketing, or from poor marketing.

So, what constitutes good marketing? Concisely, effective marketing helps the physician provide a better outcome for the patient by persuading her to use the promoted product. But, when digging just a little deeper into that statement, one will see the challenges of marketing. Which physicians are targeted for promotion? What outcome is sought? Which patient is the right one for this product, likely to have the targeted condition, and seen by the targeted physician? What product should the manufacturer promote? What makes a product worthy of promotion and likely to succeed, and conversely which ones should not be promoted to physicians? Done well, and for a good product, marketing can be a win for manufacturers, physicians, and, ultimately, for the patient.

The physician's challenge is to sort out from a number of products' marketing efforts, those products deserving of his/her support. How can the physician make that determination? First, with an admitted bias, it seems a larger company has more resources to commit to testing to prove their products worthy of support, and more to risk if they were to market a product that does not meet high standards.

There are three categories of concern for any health product, whether intended for skin health or for any other health condition. These categories are safety, efficacy and compliance. This framework works well for the physician trying to decide which products to support. The manufacturer must make a product that performs well in each regard and persuade the professional and the patient of that fact.

Safety

Safety testing done by a research-driven company begins with a four step process of selecting the right ingredients. First, screening is done on potential new ingredients for a variety of acute and/or chronic toxic endpoints. Examples of screening include tests for acute toxicity, neurotoxicity, developmental and reproductive toxicity, mutagenecity, carcinogenicity, eye and skin irritation, and skin allergic response.

Once a critical toxic event is identified (generally the toxic effect seen at the lower doses of the ingredient), dose–response studies are used to determine the highest dose at which no toxicity is seen. Next, use of a product is studied to calculate the actual exposure to the ingredient a consumer will encounter. Finally, a mathematical analysis will determine a margin of safety, which would compare the level of an ingredient where no adverse event was detected with the expected level of human exposure usage in the real world. If the margin of safety is high, the ingredient can be used.

This ingredient testing is just an example of the thoroughness with which leading companies test products. In addition to ingredient testing, before formulating a product, testing is done for ecological safety. Specifically, testing is done for ecotoxicity and biodegradability. It is not enough to determine a product has a high margin of safety in use, but also the environment needs to be considered and protected.

Finally, a finished product will be tested for irritancy and sensitization potential. Irritancy is tested for both diluted and undiluted products in repeated exposure. Sensitization is tested using models such as a Repeat Insult Patch Test. Because light can exacerbate allergic responses in some instances, testing combining ingredient exposure with light exposure is done. The product will be tested for stability (does it work as labeled even after exposure to extreme temperature) and to be sure the product and packaging prevent bacterial growth from occurring in real world circumstances.

Efficacy

Efficacy is evaluated in numerous ways. There are two primary categories of measurement for 'anti-aging' moisturizers: 'health' benefits (how good a moisturizer it is) and 'beauty' benefits (its effect on appearance of fine lines and wrinkles, skin tone and texture, etc.). For 'health' benefits, TEWL (trans-epidermal water loss) can be measured objectively, as can capacitance, an indirect measure with a correlation to moisturizer efficacy. Expert grading is carried out to evaluate visual dryness and redness.

In the beauty category, leading edge measurement uses digital photography with carefully controlled lighting and facial positioning which allows either naïve graders or expert graders to view side by side pre- and post-treatment images to evaluate improvement. Computer imaging can also be used to evaluate skin topography and tonality changes. To understand how advanced corporate progress is in this regard, the Canfield Visia® computerized imaging system was developed from Procter & Gamble technology. Other measures include the traditional skin turnover evaluation using dye and tracking number of days until the dye is not visible. This can be evaluated either by a trained grader or using imaging technology to identify the presence of dye.

The leaders in the field, who have written chapters elsewhere in this volume, should be relied upon to understand how these measurements work. But, from a marketing perspective, how can a provider digest what proof is offered if they are not expert in all the measurement methodologies? The following questions may aid in evaluating the quality of the data:

- Is the product from a reputable company? As a general rule, large companies have much more stringent self-regulation on claims than smaller companies.
- Is proof offered via some professional interchange? If the manufacturer will not invest in a

clinical study, rule out the product. It is possible, but unlikely, that a manufacturer with a great product just chooses not to prove it.

- What is the quality of the proof? The manufacturer's dilemma is that opportunities to profit from sales of new technology occur in the here and now, and publishing in some journals happens 'in the future', if at all. If the manufacturer has made reasonable attempts to do quality studies and has exposed them to peer review in some manner, they should be viewed favorably (posters at medical meetings, or engaging reputable dermatologists in the design and implementation of a clinical study would qualify). The term 'data on file' means a study was done, usually by the manufacturer, but not published, and so there is no citation to offer. If the reputation of the manufacturer is good, then this represents quality research.

Compliance

The compliance benefit in this category is achieved by making a final product that is cosmetically elegant (Fig. 4.1). It must absorb readily into the skin and have a nice feel, and improve the appearance of the skin immediately in a cosmetic or superficial way. It also must have some chronic or longer term benefit. However, patients will never learn about the ultimate benefit of a non-medical product if it does not improve appearance immediately, feel good while being applied, or absorb readily.

Compliance is an overlooked product aspect by both prescription and over-the-counter product manufacturers. Acute benefits are critical to consumer

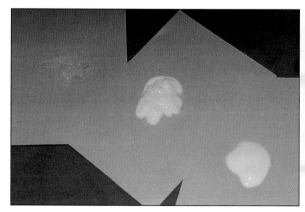

Fig. 4.1 The esthetics of a cosmeceutical influences compliance

satisfaction. The product may contain light diffusers, like titanium dioxide, which reduce the appearance of lines and wrinkles immediately by diffusing the light, and reducing the shininess. The product should have a nice skin feel, since to the consumer this is a quality of a good product. If a product has these qualities, the consumer will be encouraged to use the product long enough to achieve the chronic benefits.

The industry will never turn back from anti-aging, as the average price of an anti-aging product is substantially higher than that of basic moisturizers.

And, since product news is a key way to sell products, the market will always change rapidly. Physicians may view that as bad news, because it makes it difficult to stay up to speed with the market. However, it also represents an opportunity. Patients can readily assess whether a moisturizer has caused their dry skin to stop itching or look better in the short term. However, they are ill equipped to know whether a particular anti-aging product delivers on the advertising claims. For this information, they will always rely on the opinion of a well informed expert. For most, that expert is the dermatologist.

5

Evaluating Cosmeceutical Efficiency

Gary L. Grove, Jonn Damia, Charles Zerweck

Introduction

This chapter is intended to provide a brief, introductory survey of instrumental methods for evaluating cosmeceutical efficacy on human skin. Although the emphasis will be on instrumental methods, it is strongly recommended that a three pronged approach that includes expert graders' evaluations and panelists' self-appraisals, in addition to the instrumental measurements, are utilized to evaluate the effects of various cosmeceuticals on skin condition whenever possible.

Box 5.1 provides an alphabetical listing of the instruments that have been used over the years to noninvasively measure cosmeceutical effects on human skin. This is a very active area of research and there are a number of methods currently being developed.

Rather than discuss the various instruments in alphabetical order as they are presented in Box 5.1, a better approach is to start with those methods that measure aspects of the skin that are directly related to how the dermatologist and/or patients evaluate skin condition. That is, primarily to look with their eyes and feel with their fingers. Other instrumental techniques measure properties that cannot readily be appreciated by either visual or tactile means. These include assessments based on physiologic processes such as blood flow or transepidermal water loss rates.

Instrumental Methods that are Related to Visual Assessments

Image analysis

One of the more popular claims currently being made for most cosmeceuticals is that they are 'anti-aging and help restore a more youthful skin', or words to that effect. One highly desirable outcome of such a treatment would be to reduce the appearance of facial wrinkles, such as those in the crow's feet region. Although such changes can be documented by standardized clinical photographs, it is more desirable to cast a replica of the skin surface by using a silicone rubber impression material, such as Silflo. Figure 5.1 shows representative specimens

Instruments that have been used to noninvasively evaluate the skin of human volunteers		
Ballistometer	Image analysis	Resonance frequency analyzer
Calipers	Impedance meter	Rheometer
Chromameter	IR spectrometer	Scratch resistance device
Coefficient of friction	Laser Doppler velocimeter	Sebumeter/Sebu-Tape
Cohesograph	Load cells	Skin sensor
Ellipsiometer	NMR	Sonic wave propagation device
Evaporimeter	pH meter	Squametry and exfoliative cytology
Extensiometer	Photo-acoustic spectroscope	Suction cup device
Galvanic skin response	Photo-plethysmograph	Thermometers/thermography
Gas-bearing electrodynamometer	Photo-mechanical analyzer	Twistometer/dermal torque meter
Identometer/levelometer	Profilometer/surfometer	UltraSound—A, B, C, and M modes

Box 5.1 Instruments that have been used to noninvasively evaluate the skin of human volunteers

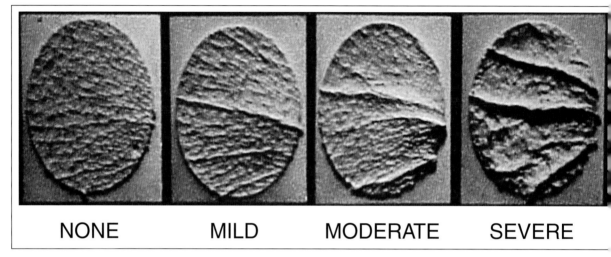

Fig. 5.1 Representative skin specimens obtained from individuals with varying degrees of photodamage

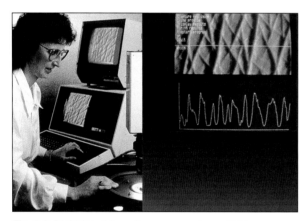

Fig. 5.2 Digitizing skin replicas can create a reliable noninvasive method for wrinkle assessment

---

Nonintrusive methods based on image analysis

- Silicon rubber impression of skin surface
- Clinical photographs:
  Psoriasis lesions
  Acne lesions
  Weal and flare response
  Wounds and ulcers
- Sticky tape specimens/D-Squame Discs
- Exfoliative cytology
- SebuTape specimens
- Sweat gland patterns

Box 5.2 Nonintrusive methods based on image analysis

---

obtained from individuals with varying degrees of photodamage, the differences in wrinkle depth are readily appreciated. However, by using Optical Profilometry one can objectively measure changes in skin surface topography due to effective cosmeceutical treatments. This technique involves computer imaging techniques in which a digitized image is taken of the replica that is illuminated from a fixed low angle. This causes various surface features to be highlighted or shadowed in such a way that a graphic representation of the surface topography can be generated and subsequently analyzed for wrinkling, roughness, and other textural features (Fig. 5.2).

This is but one example of how computerized image analysis can be used to objectively extract quantitative information from images. Box 5.2 pro-

vides a listing of some of the more common applications of image analysis that have been used to study skin structure and function. The basic rule seems to be that anything that can be seen by the unaided eye can easily be measured. Moreover, by using specialized lighting techniques such as Wood's lamp illumination, things that cannot be directly visualized can be detected and measured in the specially created images.

Skin coloration

Another important visual clue to the condition of the skin after cosmeceutical application is its color, which depends upon a number of factors, including pigmentation, blood perfusion, and desquamation patterns. Experienced dermatologists frequently use color information in several ways. First, they can

Instrumental methods for assessing skin surface color
■ CIE colorimeters: Minolta Chromameter Dr Lange Microcolor Hunter Labscan Photovolt ■ Two wave length method of Diffey et al: Dia-Stron Erythema Meter Cortex Technology Dermaspectrophotometer

Box 5.3 Instrumental methods for assessing skin surface color

Instrumental methods for evaluating skin biomechanics
■ Dia-Stron Ballistometer (impacts) ■ DermaLab Suction Cup (lifts) ■ C-K Cutometer (lifts) ■ Extensiometer (stretches) ■ Dia-Stron MTT (stretches or compresses) ■ Dia-Stron Dermal Torque Meter (twists) ■ Gas Bearing Electrodynometer (wiggles)

Box 5.4 Instrumental methods for evaluating skin biomechanics

certainly appreciate the distribution of erythema and/or pigmented lesions on the basis of color. Moreover, by evaluating changes in the hue and/or intensity of color over time, they will be able to tell if patients are responding to treatment or not. Although the human eye is very sensitive, especially in detecting very subtle differences in contrast, the evaluation of color is still highly subjective. Color measuring devices offer the advantages of objectivity and quantification on a continuous scale that can be referenced to color standards.

The devices that are currently being employed in experimental dermatology, skin pharmacology, toxicology, and cosmetic science to measure skin color changes fall into two distinct types of instruments as shown in Box 5.3. In one category we have the tristimulus colorimeters, which are based on the three-dimensional $L^*a^*b^*$ color space (CIELAB). $L^*a^*b^*$ allows any color to be mathematically described by its hue (position on the color wheel), value (lightness), and chroma (saturation). These would include the Minolta ChromaMeter and the MicroColor of Dr Bruno Lange GmbH & Co. which have seen widespread use for the quantification of erythema in the study of irritant dermatitis due to exposure to detergents, topical corticoid activity in the vasoconstriction test, and for measuring the percutaneous penetration of vasodilators such as nicotinic acid.

Other types of instruments are the Derma-Spectrophotometer (Cortex Technology) and the Erythema Meter (Dia-Stron Ltd.) which are based on the two wavelength method of Diffey et al. These instruments emit green and red light and measure the reflected light from the skin surface. Because changes in skin redness will greatly affect the absorption of green light but will have very little effect on that of red light, an erythema index can be

calculated. Since increased melanin pigmentation will lead to an increased absorption of both red and green light, a melanin index can be computed in a similar fashion.

Instrumental Methods Related to Tactile Assessments

Dermal firmness/elasticity

Another characteristic change which is well documented in photoaged skin is the loss of firmness and elasticity due to structural changes in collagen and elastin. Over the years, a wide variety of instruments have been developed to objectively measure the biomechanical properties of the skin. Box 5.4 lists some of the more popular devices. Although there are fundamental differences in how they interact with the skin, the basic approach is the same for all of them, i.e. load the skin in a standard fashion and measure the subsequent deformation. These changes in deformation represent a change in skin elasticity and firmness, which can be altered by cosmeceuticals.

Instrumental Methods Based on Physiological Processes

Blood flow

As previously mentioned, increased blood flow generally leads to increased skin surface redness that can be visually, assessed by either the dermatologist or the patient as well as by instrumentally measuring a color change. Blood flow can be analyzed by using laser Doppler velocimetry. This instrument utilizes the Doppler effect to determine the speed of blood flow.

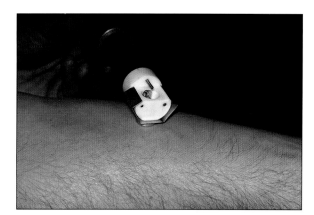

Instrumental methods for measuring skin hydration levels

- IBS Skicon-200 Conductance Meter
- C-K Corneometer CM 825
- Nova Dermal Phase Meter
- DermaLab Moisture Probe

Box 5.5 Instrumental methods for measuring hydration levels based on the electrical properties of the stratum corneum

Fig. 5.3 A collecting chamber with two humidity meters is used to assess cutaneous transepidermal water loss

Transepidermal water loss

Another physiologic process that has been extensively measured with instrumentation, that has no visual or tactile counterparts, is transepidermal water loss. Measurement of transepidermal water loss (TEWL) rates through human skin can be used to noninvasively monitor changes in stratum corneum barrier function (Fig. 5.3). In normal healthy skin, the barrier is quite effective and water loss rates are typically very low. If the barrier is compromised due to pathologic processes or damaged by physical or chemical agents, there will be a corresponding increase in water loss rate that directly relates to the degree of impairment. Conversely, there will be a corresponding decrease in TEWL as the barrier is restored. This means that monitoring changes in TEWL over time not only allows one to evaluate the therapeutic response to different treatments, but also to determine the effectiveness of various prophylactic strategies that might prevent or lessen the injury. Thus, it is not surprising that there is considerable literature dealing with TEWL measurements. Indeed, TEWL measurements were the very first to be reviewed by the Standardization Group of the European Society of Cosmetic Dermatitis.

Instrumental Measurements Based on Physical Properties

Skin hydration

There are many biophysical methods available for measuring the relative hydration state of the stratum corneum. Most, such as those shown in

Box 5.5, are based on the electrical properties of the skin surface. It has been shown most notably by Obata and Tagami that the ability of an alternating current to flow through the stratum corneum is an indirect measure of its water content. Higher water content translates into increased electrical conduction.

High frequency ultrasound

Another useful technique that allows characterization of the physical properties of the skin is high frequency ultrasound images, such as the Dermascan C (Cortex Technology). As sound waves travel through the skin they generate 'echoes' at tissue interfaces where acoustical impedance changes. In the A mode display, the echo information is presented as an amplitude modulated oscilloscope trace versus time of flight. Since only one spatial domain is displayed, the diagnostic information is limited. The B mode display is a two dimensional image of each echo producing interface and thus is equivalent to a radar screen. By using a graphic presentation that shows the intensity of the echoes at each location, it is possible to gain additional insights into skin structure and function without taking a biopsy. This technique allows better visualization of skin tumors. It has also revealed the existence of an echo poor band that seems to be characteristic of photodamaged skin.

Summary and Conclusions

The intent has been to provide a brief introduction to the various instruments that can be used to evaluate effects of various cosmeceuticals on photoaged skin. Over the years, it has been found by our group and others that 'static' measurements of the skin often do not reveal very much about the age-associated changes that certainly must exist. It is only when you ask the skin to respond to a challenge and follow the dynamics of the response that these differences begin to manifest themselves. Although the term 'noninvasive' is in widespread use, a more appropriate term for many of our applications would be 'nonintrusive'. Nonintrusive methods should be convenient and easy to administer. They should also cause little or no discomfort and leave no permanent sequelae such as scars or pigmentary changes, etc.

Further Reading

Barardesca E, Elsner P, Wilhelm K-P et al (eds) 1995 Bioengineering of the skin: methods and instrumentation. CRC Press, Boca Raton

Diffey BL, Oliver RJ, Farr PM 1984 A portable instrument for quantifying erythema induced by ultraviolet radiation. British Journal of Dermatology 111:663–672

Elsner P, Barardesca E, Maibach H (eds) 1994 Bioengineering of the skin: water and the stratum corneum. CRC Press, Boca Raton

Elsner P, Barardesca E, Wilhelm K-P et al (eds) 2002 Bioengineering of the skin: skin biomechanics. CRC Press, Boca Raton

Grove GL 1981 Dermatological applications of the Magiscan image analyzing computer. In: Marks R, Payne PA (eds) Bioengineering and the skin. MTP Press, Lancaster, p. 173–181

Grove GL 1982 Techniques for substantiating skin care product claims. In: Kligman AM, Leyden JJ (eds) Safety and efficacy of topically applied drugs and cosmetics. Grune & Stratton, New York, pp 157–176

Grove GL 1987 Design of studies to measure skin care product performance. Bioengineering and the Skin 3:359–373

Grove GL, Grove MJ 1989 Objective methods for assessing skin surface topography noninvasively. In: Leveque JL (ed) Cutaneous investigation in health and disease. Marcel Dekker, New York, pp 1–31

Grove GL, Grove MJ, Leyden JJ 1989 Optical profilometry: an objective method for quantification of facial wrinkles. Journal of the American Academy of Dermatology 21:631–637

Grove GL, Grove MJ, Leyden JJ et al 1991 Skin replica analysis of photodamaged skin after therapy with tretinoin emollient cream. Journal of the American Academy of Dermatology 25:231–237

Grove G, Zerweck C, Pierce E 2002 Noninvasive instrumental methods for assessing moisturizers. In: Leyden JJ, Rawlings AV (eds) Skin moisturization. Marcel Dekker, New York, pp 499–528

Kollias N, Stamatas N 2002 Optical noninvasive approaches to diagnosis of skin diseases. Journal of Investigative Dermatology Symposium Proceedings 7:64–75

Obata M, Tagami H 1990 A rapid in vitro test to assess skin moisturizers. Journal of the Society of Cosmetic Chemists 41:235–241

Pinnagoda J, Tupker RA, Agner T et al 1990 Guidelines for trans-epidermal water loss (TEWL) measurement. Contact Dermatitis 22:164–178

Serup J, Jemec GBE (eds) 1995 Handbook of noninvasive methods and the skin. CRC Press, Boca Raton

Shriver MD, Parra EJ 2000 Comparison of narrow-band reflectance spectroscopy and tristimulus colorimetry for measurements of skin and hair color in persons of different biological ancestry. American Journal of Physical Anthropology 112:17–27

Part 2

Cosmeceutical Actives

Cosmeceutical actives fall into a variety of categories: vitamins, lipids, moisturizers, botanicals, metals, exfoliants, peptides, antioxidants, growth factors, and sunscreens. The topical cosmeceutical vitamin category overlaps with the nutraceutical category. Nutraceuticals are the oral counterpart of cosmeceuticals, and are also sold over the counter in an unregulated fashion. Many vitamin cosmeceuticals are adapted from their oral counterparts, since substances felt to be safe for oral consumption are also felt to be safe for topical application. This is mostly true, however contact dermatitis is known to occur in sensitized individuals from vitamin and botanical cosmeceuticals. Probably the largest category of cosmeceuticals is moisturizers that can aid in restoration of the skin barrier, delivering sun protection and other active agents. Many times it is a challenge to separate the effects of the moisturizer from the effects of the added novel ingredients. Novel ingredients, such as antioxidants, peptides, and growth factors, are intended to both prevent and reverse the effects of extrinsic and intrinsic aging on the skin. This section of text presents a detailed survey of those cosmeceutical actives that are most important in the current marketplace.

Retinoids

6

John E. Oblong, Donald L. Bissett

Introduction

Traditionally, retinoids have been classified as a class of compounds that have the basic core structure of vitamin A and its oxidized metabolites. More recently, this classification has been broadened to include newer series of synthetic compounds that share similar mechanisms of action as naturally occurring retinoids. The identification of these novel retinoid analogs has been driven in large part by mechanistic understanding of the role of retinoids in molecular biology, gene expression profiling, and basic metabolic research. While current knowledge of vitamin A metabolism and activity profiles can be further grouped into two different delivery routes, oral and topical, this chapter will focus primarily upon pharmacological profiles and metabolic rates as per topical delivery in humans. Also, this chapter will highlight key understandings of current topically used retinoids both in the dermatological field as well as in the over-the-counter (OTC) and cosmetic marketplace.

Molecular Biology of Retinoids

Retinoids are naturally occurring derivatives of beta-carotene and historically labeled as vitamin A and its direct metabolites. Included in this class are retinol, retinaldehyde, retinyl esters, and retinoic acid (Fig. 6.1). These compounds have an essential role in such processes in higher order mammals as development (including ocular), angiogenesis, and dermatological homeostasis. One of the key biological relevant retinoids is retinoic acid, which exists as several isomeric forms (e.g. all-*trans*, 9-*cis* and 13-*cis*) and is essentially an oxidized form of retinol. This molecule has been shown to function at the molecular level by serving as an agonist for a class of nuclear family receptors described as retinoic acid receptors (RAR)

and retinoid X receptors (RXR). In these protein families, there exist three isoforms of respective receptors, described as α, β, and γ. Upon binding of the retinoic acid ligand, RAR and RXR will form a heterodimer that then is capable of interacting with critical DNA sequences located in the promoter regions of select genes. These sequences are described as retinoic acid response elements (RARE). More recently, it has become apparent that the transcription factor AP-1 has a significant effect upon regulating activation of genes through its interactions at the RARE site as well. In summary, retinoic acid can influence the function of a cell by altering gene expression patterns through its facilitated binding to RAREs of a dimerized RAR/RXR complex (Fig. 6.2). This knowledge of the mechanistic role in retinoid regulation of gene expression patterns allowed for the synthesis of novel pharmacological classes of compounds that have a broader structural diversity with varying pharmacological properties than natural retinoids. Additionally, it appears that the majority of biological effects observed from topical delivery of various retinoids are mediated by interaction through the RAR/RXR complex, including in some cases any obligatory metabolic conversion to retinoic acid.

Metabolism of Cutaneously Delivered Retinoids

The metabolic pathways that have been identified as involved in retinoid metabolism in the digestive system have been confirmed in large part as existing in human skin (Fig. 6.3). While much of free retinol is esterified via lecithin:retinol acyltransferase (LRAT) or acyl CoA:retinol acyltransferase (ARAT) to retinyl palmitate for storage, a small percentage is further oxidized to the active acid form. The oxidation of

Retinoid	Structure
retinol	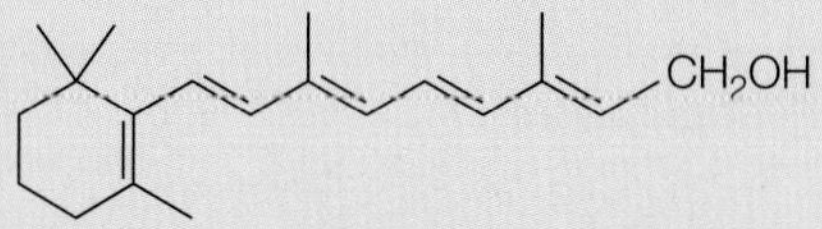
retinaldehyde	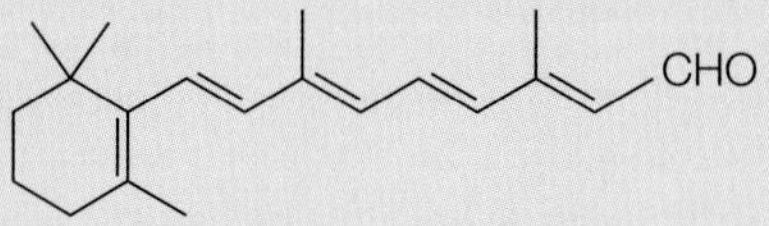
tretinoin	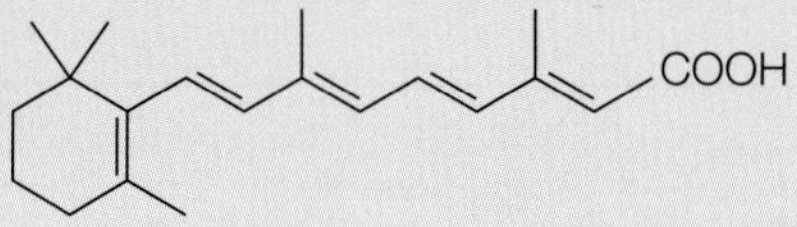
retinyl propionate	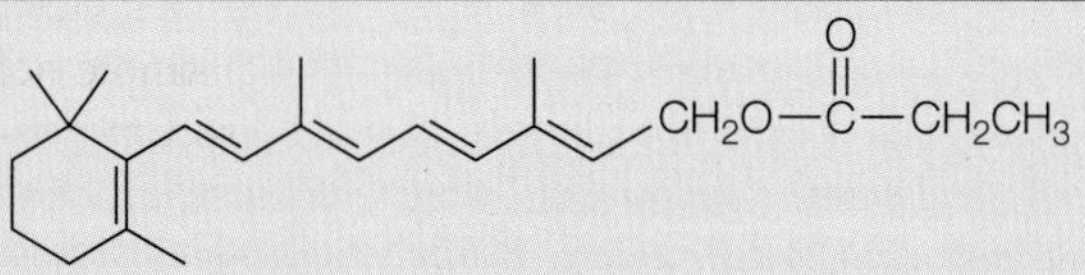
retinyl palmitate	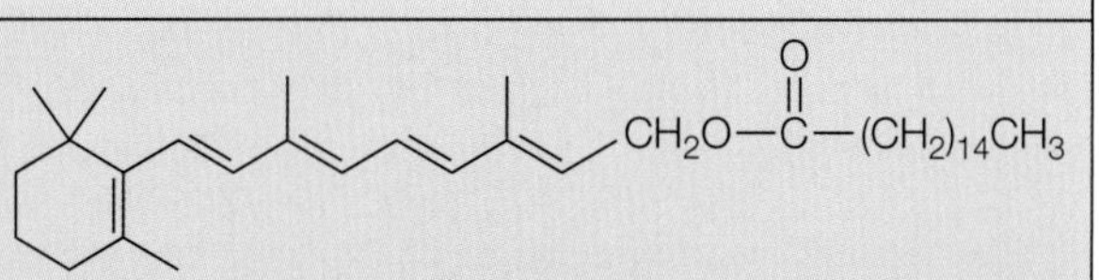
adapalene	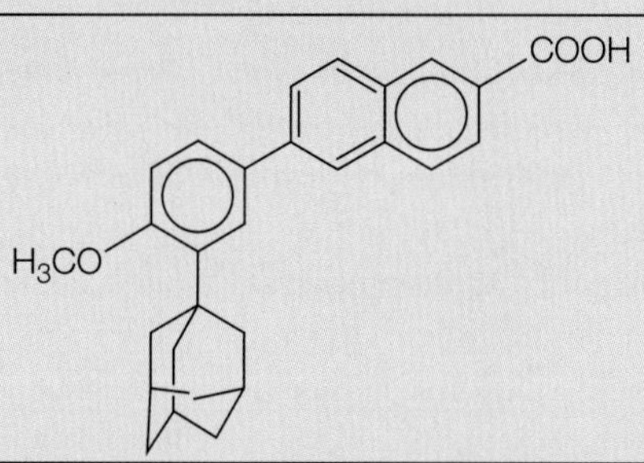
tazarotene	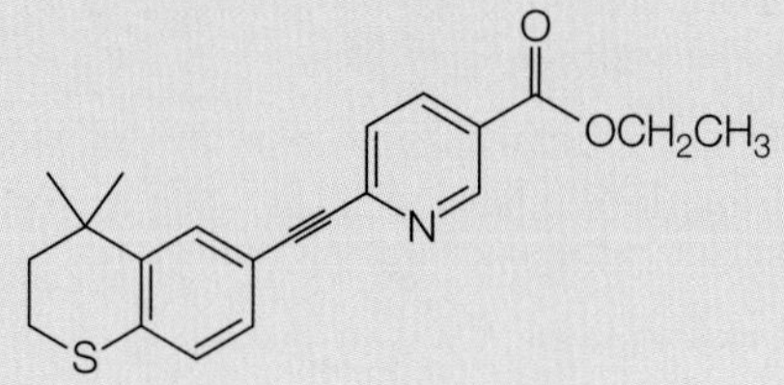

Fig. 6.1 Chemical structures of key retinoids

free retinol to retinoic acid is the limiting step in the generation of active retinoid metabolites within cells. This process is begun when free retinol associates with a specific cytoplasmic retinol-binding protein (CRBP). The retinol–CRBP complex is a substrate for retinol dehydrogenase, a microsomal enzyme uniquely capable of catalyzing the conversion of retinol to retinaldehyde. Retinaldehyde is then rapidly and quantitatively oxidized to retinoic acid by retinaldehyde oxidase. Once converted, retinoic acid regulates gene expression profiles via RAR/RXR for skin keratinocyte growth and differentiation.

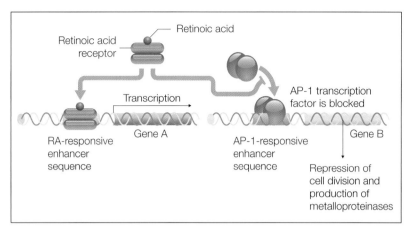

Fig. 6.2 Retinoic acid regulation of gene expression

This multistep processing of retinyl esters serves as a point of regulation to control the level of active retinoid in the skin and may thus contribute to the lower irritation potential of these derivatives. Ultimately, retinoic acid can be metabolized irreversibly via hydroxylation to 4-hydroxy-retinoic acid and 4-oxo-retinoic acid via various cytochrome P450. It is important to note that the majority of retinoid metabolism that occurs is mediated via retinoid bound to cytosolic lipid binding proteins. This family of proteins with high retinoid specificity includes retinol binding protein (CRBP) and retinoic acid binding protein (CRABP), of which there are two isoforms, I and II.

Topical usage of retinoids has shown a high degree of efficacy against acne, photodamage, and psoriasis. These effects can be ascribed on some level as being a normalization of altered skin conditions. However, two of the key negatives associated with topical retinoids are:

- irritation that, in some instances, does not mitigate itself completely even after long-term chronic exposure
- teratogenic effects

Thus, a significant effort has been expended to identify retinoids that are efficacious and have an overall lower irritation profile and lessened teratogenic safety concerns.

To minimize these negatives and yet still alter photodamaged skin, retinoic acid precursors such as retinol, retinaldehyde, and retinyl esters (e.g. retinyl propionate and retinyl palmitate) have been used widely in the skin care industry. It is hypothesized that the acyl chain length of retinyl esters plays a key role in determining the activity and irritation profiles. It may therefore be possible to identify an acyl chain length retinol that provides robust retinoid activity yet has minimal irritation.

Retinol

Retinol (vitamin A) is derived from the hydrolysis of beta-carotene to two molecules of retinol. Retinol serves as a key junction point for retinoid metabolism that allows for either storage in the form of retinyl esters or further oxidation to the pharmacologically potent form, retinoic acid. Historically, retinol has been studied extensively for topical treatment of photodamage and acne, and current cosmetic products contain relatively low levels of retinol, ranging from about 0.08% to much lower. This is due largely in part to intolerance amongst consumers for the irritation side effects. It is hypothesized that any efficacy from topically delivered retinol occurs via its sequential conversion to the intermediate retinaldehyde and finally retinoic acid, the endogenous active form.

There is sufficient evidence to support that some of the fundamental metabolic processes that occur in such tissues as the liver and other cell types exist in epidermal keratinocytes and melanocytes, as well as in dermal fibroblasts. Specifically, basal keratinocytes are supplied with vitamin A from the bloodstream, and although the precise mechanism(s) are not completely understood, retinol gains entry into the

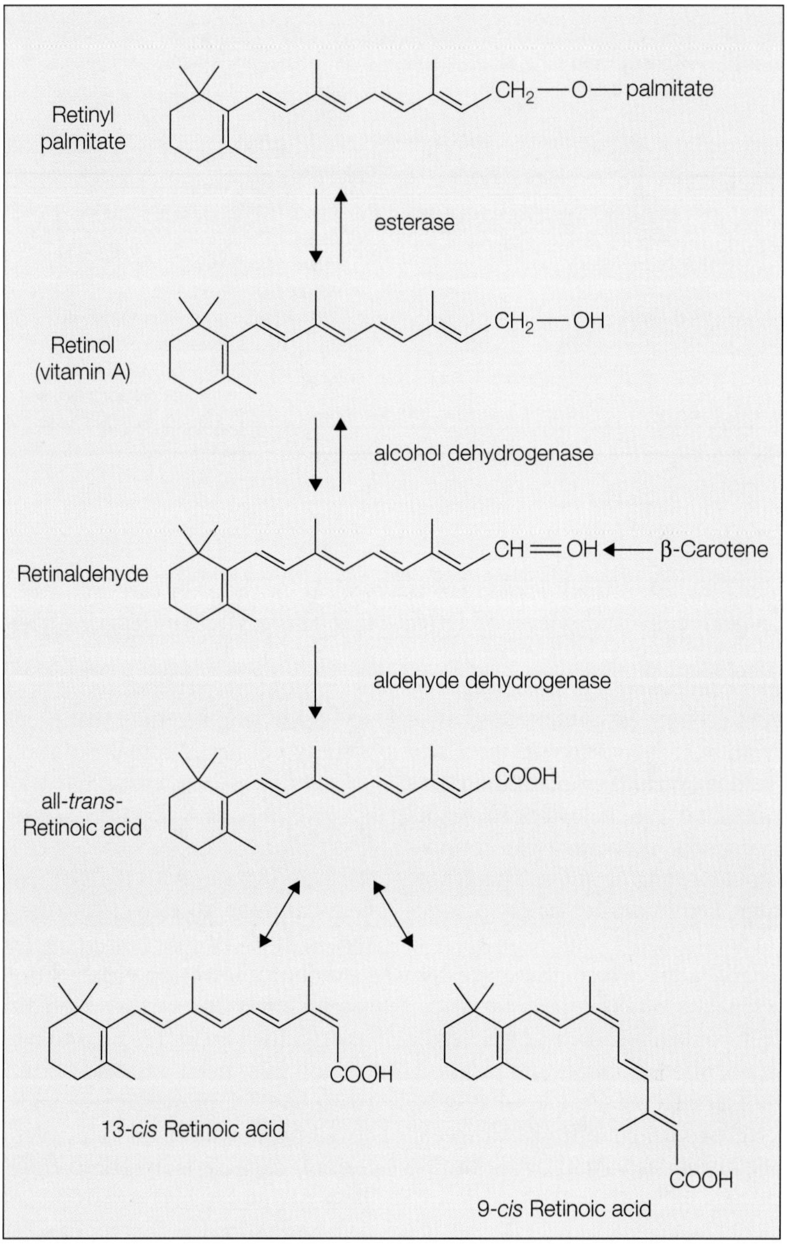

Fig. 6.3 Retinoid metabolism in skin

cells through receptor-dependent and -independent processes. Once inside the cell, retinol may be converted to retinyl palmitate or sequentially oxidized to retinoic acid. This metabolic process also applies to exogenously delivered retinoids via cutaneous delivery routes.

Retinaldehyde

Oxidation of the alcohol group on retinol yields retinaldehyde, which is viewed in large part as an intermediate form during the conversion of retinol to retinoic acid. Topical studies of retinaldehyde have been reported with the conclusions that

Back irritation measures for retinol and its esters				
Topical treatment (oil-in-water emulsions)	Expert Grader cumulative irritation scores	Significance of Expert Grader cumulative scores*	Chromameter 'a' measure (day 21)	Significance of chromameter 'a' measure*
Emulsion control	3.9	a	0.4	a
0.09% Retinyl propionate	24	b	2.7	b
0.086% Retinyl acetate	39	b	3.8	bc
0.18% Retinyl propionate	44	b	4.9	cd
0.172% Retinyl acetate	104	c	5.8	de
0.30% Retinyl propionate	121	cd	6.1	def
0.30% Retinyl acetate	145	cd	7.5	def
0.05% Retinol	147	d	6.5	def
0.075% Retinol	164	d	7.6	f

*Treatments with the same letter codes are not significantly different from each other ($p < 0.05$). The least square mean estimates are from the ANOVA model with terms for subject, side (or application site), and treatment (JE Oblong et al, unpublished results).

Table 6.1 Back irritation measures for retinol and its esters

retinaldehyde has retinoid activity in human skin, is better tolerated than retinoic acid, and can alleviate rosacea symptoms. Outside of some few instances that retinaldehyde is used for Rx indications, it is not commonly used OTC and in few examples in the cosmetic marketplace for topical usage.

Retinyl esters

Retinyl esters serve the primary role of storage of vitamin A in cellular locations, primarily lipids, with retinyl palmitate being the predominant form. The conversion of retinol from retinyl palmitate is believed to occur via retinyl esterase activities residing in a number of subcellular locations and through non-specific esterases, which are abundant in the skin.

Retinyl propionate

Retinyl propionate has been reported to be active in human skin and to have less irritation than other active retinoid options. More recently, it has been observed that this particular ester is capable of eliciting retinoid-like effects in human skin via both histological assessments as well as clinical measures of photodamage changes (Fig. 6.4). Furthermore, retinoid-induced irritation appears to be less evident from retinyl propionate in comparison with retinol or retinyl acetate (Table 6.1). As with the palmitate

ester of retinol, retinyl propionate must be hydrolyzed to free retinol, a process that occurs via skin esterases. Additionally, it has been reported that the propionate ester has an improved stability profile relative to other esters, thereby increasing half-life upon skin during topical delivery.

Retinyl palmitate

The primary role of endogenous retinyl palmitate is to provide a storage form of retinol, thereby serving as a control point. Although topical application of retinyl palmitate may be considered a nonphysiological route of exposure, there is ample evidence to support the view that the skin possesses all of the enzymatic machinery necessary to convert retinyl palmitate to retinol. Accordingly, the small amount of retinyl palmitate that actually penetrates the skin would be expected and has been indirectly demonstrated to enter the normal physiological pathways controlling vitamin A homeostasis. Based on published information and historical cosmetic usage, it is accepted that retinyl palmitate has, at best, an overall weak activity profile and is nonirritating.

Tretinoin

The usage of tretinoin, also known as *trans*-retinoic acid, in the dermatological field has an extensive

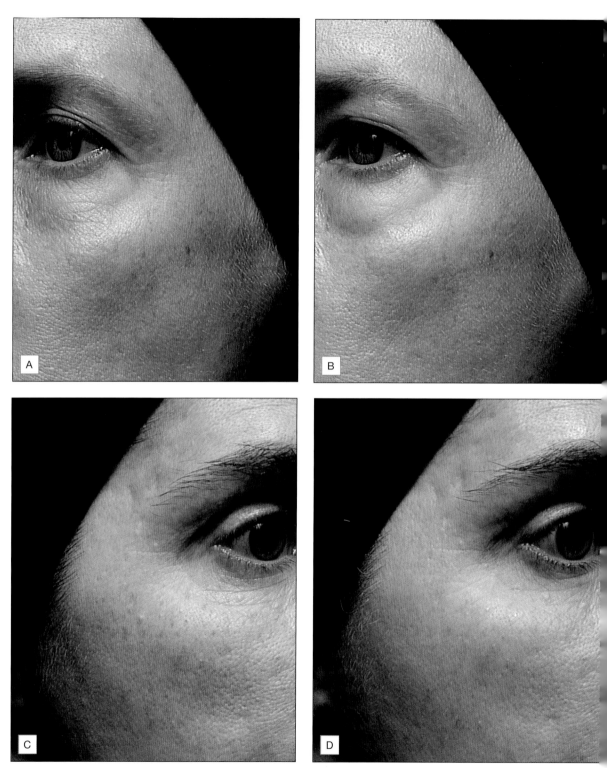

Fig. 6.4 Effect of retinyl propionate upon photodamaged skin. 0.2% retinyl propionate in a stable skin care emulsion system was applied twice daily for 12 weeks. Images were taken at baseline, and weeks 4, 8, and 12. Showing impact upon fine lines/wrinkes (A, baseline image; B, week 12 image) and impact upon hyperpigmented age spots (C, baseline image; D, week 12 image)

history, due in large part to pioneering work to understand the pharmacological and molecular impact of the active upon photodamaged skin, acne lesions as well as its role in cellular differentiation and developmental biology. Topical retinoic acid (Retin A, Renova, Ortho-Neutrogena) is well known for its activity in improving the appearance of the signs of skin photodamage such as fine lines, wrinkles, and pigmentation. However, it has also been found to elicit significant irritation and dryness. Tretinoin (Retin-A) was originally approved up to 0.1% levels for the treatment of acne and was later approved, under the name Renova, at 0.025 and 0.05% to be used for topical treatment of photodamaged skin. Tretinoin is relatively effective against clinical indications of photodamage, including hyperpigmented spots, fine lines, and wrinkles. However, the significant side effects of irritation and presence of a retinoid resistance portion of the population have limited its broad acceptance. Nonetheless, it is viewed as a benchmark agent for topical treatment of dermatological conditions related to aging and UV exposure. The numerous OTC forms previously discussed, including retinol, retinaldehyde, and the retinyl esters, attempt to mimic the effect of tretinoin in cosmeceutical formulations. The ultimate hope is that these tretinoin precursors are ultimately converted to active tretinoin.

Adapalene

A dose of 0.1% adapalene (Differin, Galderma) is a prescription topical gel and cream that is prescribed for the indication of acne vulgaris. Adapalene itself is a synthetic retinoid analog that mimics tretinoin in its efficacy potential, with reported reduced irritation when compared with tretinoin. However, adapalene has not been well-studied as a cosmeceutical retinoid valuable in photoaging. Early studies that have been completed suggest it may have some ability to reverse photoaging, but a comparison to tretinoin has not yet been performed. At present, adapalene is only approved for topical acne therapy.

Tazarotene

Much like adapalene, tazarotene is a synthetic retinoic analog. It is currently available in prescription form for the treatment of plaque psoriasis and acne at 0.05 and 0.1% levels under the name Tazorac (US,

Allergan) and Zorac (outside of US, Allergan). It has also been reported to be effective for treatment of skin photodamage, where it is known by the trade name Avage (Allergan). While it has established efficacy it also still has side effects of retinoid-induced irritation from topical exposure. It is generally felt to be more irritating than both adapalene and tretinoin. The main advantage of tazarotene is extremely rapid retinization of the face, with early improvement perceived in facial fine wrinkling. The patient must be carefully counseled during the early weeks of tazarotene use, as the dryness and peeling can be pronounced and require supplemental low potency topical corticosteroids to avoid intense irritation. Early studies indicate that the forte of tazarotene may be rapid improvement in resistant dyspigmentation from melasma or post-inflammatory hyperpigmentation.

Conclusion

Retinoids are a broad family of molecules whose primary function is to serve as agonists for members of the RAR and RXR nuclear receptor family. In turn, this denotes their role in regulating gene expression profiles via RAR/RXR binding to RAREs. In dermatology, retinoids have been shown to have beneficial effects upon acne, psoriasis, actinic keratosis, and photodamaged/aging skin attributes. The ability of synthetic retinoid analogs to mimic the effects of endogenous ligands such as retinoic acid is based in part on similar mechanism of action but with variant pharmacokinetic properties that renders them as more functional for specific purposes, based on the disease state being targeted. Future research directions in better understanding the connections between efficacy and retinoid-induced irritation should allow for the identification of analogs or optimized therapies that decouple these two phenomena.

Further Reading

Bailey JS, Siu CH. Purification and partial characterization of a novel binding protein for retinoic acid from neonatal rat. Journal of Biological Chemistry 1988; 263(19): 9326–9332.

Boehnlein J, Sakr A, Lichtin JL, Bronaugh RL. Characterization of esterase and alcohol dehydrogenase activity in skin. Metabolism of retinyl palmitate to retinol (vitamin A) during percutaneous absorption. Pharmacy Research 1994; 11: 1155–1159.

Creidi P, Humbert P. Clinical use of topical retinaldehyde on photoaged skin. Dermatology 1999; 199(Suppl 1): 49–52.

Duell EA, Kang S, Voorhees JJ. Unoccluded retinol penetrates human skin in vivo more effectively than unoccluded retinyl palmitate or retinoic acid. Journal of Investigations in Dermatology 1997; 109(3): 301–305.

Effendy I, Kwangsukstith C, Lee JY, Maibach HI. Functional changes in human stratum corneum induced by topical glycolic acid: comparison with all-trans retinoic acid. Acta Dermatologica Venereologica 1995; 75(6): 455–458.

Fluhr JW, Vienne MP, Lauze C, Dupuy P, Gehring W, Gloor M. Tolerance profile of retinol, retinaldehyde and retinoic acid under maximized and long-term clinical conditions. Dermatology 1999; 199(Suppl 1): 57–60.

Galvin SA, Gilbert R, Baker M, Guibal F, Tuley MR. Comparative tolerance of adapalene 0.1% gel and six different tretinoin formulations. British Journal of Dermatology 1998; 139(Suppl 52): 34–40.

Goodman DS. Retinoid-binding proteins. Journal of American Academy of Dermatology 1982; 6 (4 Pt 2 Suppl): 583–590.

Green C, Orchard G, Cerio R, Hawk JLM. A clinicopathological study of the effects of topical retinyl propionate cream in skin photoageing. Clinics in Experimental Dermatology 1998; 23: 162–167.

Harrison EH. Enzymes catalyzing the hydrolysis of retinyl esters. Biochimica Biophysica Acta 1993; 1170 (2): 99–108.

Kang S, Duell EA, Fisher GJ, Datta SC, Wang ZQ, Reddy AP, Tavakkol A, Yi JY, Griffiths CE, Elder JT, Voorhees JJ. Application of retinol to human skin in vivo induces epidermal hyperplasia and cellular retinoid binding proteins characteristic of retinoic acid but without measurable retinoic acid levels of irritation. Journal of Investigations in Dermatology 1995; 105: 549–556.

Kang S, Leyden JJ, Lowe NJ, Ortonne JP, Phillips TJ, Weinstein GD, Bhawan J, Lew-Kaya DA, Matsumoto RM, Sefton J, Walker PS, Gibson JR. Tazarotene cream for the treatment of facial photodamage: a multicenter, investigator-masked, randomized, vehicle-controlled, parallel comparison of 0.01%, 0.025%, 0.05%, and 0.1% tazarotene creams with 0.05% tretinoin emollient cream applied once daily for 24 weeks. Archives of Dermatology 2001; 137(12): 1597–1604.

Kligman AM, Grove GL, Hirose R, Leyden JJ. Topical tretinoin for photoaged skin. Journal of American Academy of Dermatology 1986; 15: 836–859.

Kurlandsky SB, Duell EA, Kang S, Voorhes JJ, Fisher GJ. Auto-regulation of retinoic acid biosynthesis through regulation of retinol esterification in human keratinocytes. Journal of Biological Chemistry 1996; 271: 15346–15352.

Kurlandsky SB, Xiao J-H, Duell EA, Voorhees JJ, Fisher GJ. Biological activity of all-trans retinol requires metabolic conversion to all-trans-retinoic acid and is mediated through activation of nuclear retinoid receptors in human keratinocytes. Journal of Biological Chemistry 1994; 269: 32821–32827.

Navarro JM, Casatorres J, Jorcano JL. Elements controlling the expression and induction of the skin hyperproliferation-associated keratin K6. Journal of Biological Chemistry 1995; 270(36): 21362–21367.

Phillips TJ, Gottlieb AB, Leyden JJ, Lowe NJ, Lew-Kaya DA, Sefton J, Walker PS, Gibson JR. Tazarotene Cream Photodamage Clinical Study Group. Efficacy of 0.1% tazarotene cream for the treatment of photodamage: a 12-month multicenter, randomized trial. Archives of Dermatology 2002; 138(11): 1486–1493.

Randolph, RK, Simon M. Characterization of retinol metabolism in cultured human epidermal keratinocytes. Journal of Biological Chemistry 1993; 268: 9198–9205.

Ridge BD, Batt MD, Palmer HE, Jarrett A. The dansyl chloride technique for stratum corneum renewal as an indicator of changes in epidermal mitotic activity following topical treatment. British Journal of Dermatology 1988; 118: 167–174.

Sachsenberg-Studer EM. Tolerance of topical retinaldehyde in humans. Dermatology 1999; 199(Suppl 1): 61–63.

Sefton J, Kligman AM, Kopper SC, Lue JC, Gibson JR. Photodamage pilot study: a double-blind, vehicle-controlled study to assess the efficacy and safety of tazarotene 0.1% gel. Journal of American Academy of Dermatology 2000; 43(4): 656–663.

Semenzato A, Bovenga L, Faiferri L, Austria R, Bettero A. Stability of vitamin A propionate in cosmetic formulations. SÖFW Journal 1997; 123: 151–154.

Verschoore M, Poncet M, Czernielewski J, Sorba V, Clucas A. Adapalene 0.1% gel has low skin-irritation potential. Journal of American Academy of Dermatology 1997; 36(6 Pt 2): S104–109.

Vienne MP, Ochando N, Borrel MT, Gall Y, Lauze C, Dupuy P. Retinaldehyde alleviates rosacea. Dermatology 1999; 199(Suppl 1): 53–56.

Weiss JS, Ellis CN, Headington JT, Tincoff T, Hamilton TA, Voorhees JJ. Topical tretinoin improves photoaged skin. A double-blind vehicle-controlled study. Journal of American Medical Association 1988; 259: 527–532.

7

Cosmeceutical Vitamins: Vitamin E

Jens J. Thiele, Swarna Ekanayake-Mudiyanselage,
Sherry N. Hsieh

Introduction

While some cosmeceutical antioxidants, such as glutathione or ubiquinol-10, can be synthesized by humans, vitamin E is supplied to the body solely by oral intake. The main natural sources of vitamin E are fresh vegetables, vegetable oils, cereals, and nuts. Recent studies suggest that the majority of men and women in the United States fail to meet the current recommendations for vitamin E intake. The aim of this chapter is to review the biological activity of vitamin E in human skin with special emphasis on its cosmeceutical antioxidative and photoprotective properties.

Terminology and Definitions

Vitamin E is an important cosmeceutical since it functions as the major lipophilic antioxidant in plasma, membranes, and tissues. The term 'vitamin E' collectively refers to the eight naturally occurring molecules (four tocopherols and four tocotrienols) which exhibit vitamin E activity. Tocotrienols differ from tocopherols in that they have an isoprenoid instead of a phytyl side chain; the four forms of tocopherols and tocotrienols differ in the number of methyl groups on the chromanol nucleus (α- has three, β- and γ- have two, and δ- has one; Fig. 7.1). In humans, α-tocopherol is the most abundant

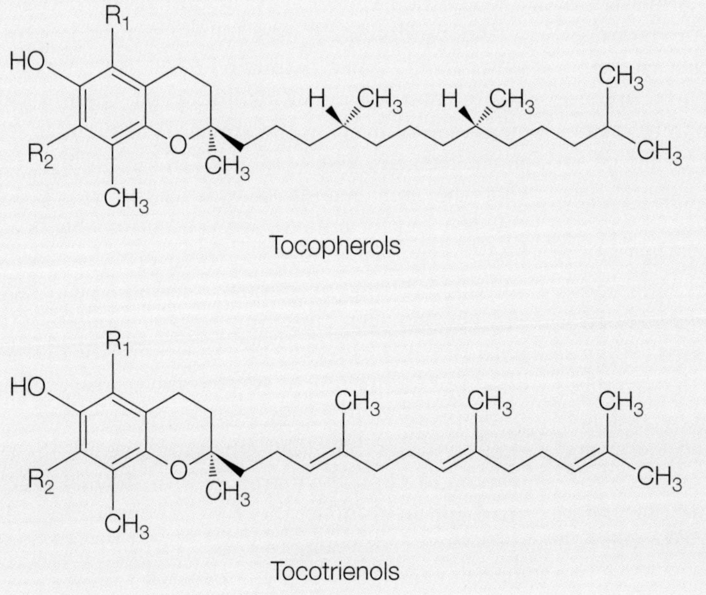

Fig. 7.1 Chemical structure of tocopherols and tocotrienols. **Tocopherols** (α: $R_1 = R_2 = CH_3$, 430.7 g/mol; β: $R_1 = CH_3$, $R_2 = H$, 416.7 g/mol; γ: $R_1 = H$, $R_2 = CH_3$, 416.7 g/mol; δ: $R_1 = R_2 = H$, 402.7 g/mol); **Tocotrienols** (α: $R_1 = R_2 = CH_3$, 424.7 g/mol; β: $R_1 = CH_3$, $R_2 = H$, 410.6 g/mol; γ: $R_1 = H$, $R_2 = CH_3$, 410.6 g/mol; δ: $R_1 = R_2 = H$, 396.6 g/mol)

vitamin E homologue, followed by γ-tocopherol. To compare the potency of different vitamin E derivates, their biologic activities are measured and compared to RRR-α-tocopherol. The potency is expressed as international units (IU) α-tocopherol equivalents (a-TE) and was developed for oral supplemation.

Indications and Biological Activity

After more then half a century of research there is still little convincing evidence of vitamin E's effectiveness in treating specific dermatologic disorders. In trials and case reports, oral vitamin E supplementation is recommended in the therapy of yellow nail syndrome, vibration disease, epidermolysis bullosa, cancer prevention, claudication, cutaneous ulcers, and collagen synthesis and wound healing. Clearly, with vitamin E not being a pharmaceutical, there is a lack of placebo controlled studies for the treatment of these conditions. However, in the field of skin care, which includes cosmeceuticals, there is a large body of experimental evidence pointing to, in particular, photoprotective effects (for review see Table 7.1). Moreover, recent studies indicate that vitamin E may reveal dermatologic cosmeceutical benefits.

Recently, Tsoureli-Nikita et al performed a clinical single blind, placebo controlled study in which 96 atopic dermatitis patients were treated with either placebo or oral vitamin E (400 IU/day) for 8 months. They found an improvement and near remission of atopic dermatitis and a 62% decrease in serum IgE levels based on initial conditions in the vitamin E treated group. The correlation between α-tocopherol intake, IgE levels, and the clinical manifestations of atopy indicates that oral vitamin E could be an excellent therapeutic adjunct for atopic dermatitis. Other multiclinical double blinded study revealed a significant improvement of chloasma and pigmented contact dermatitis lesions using topical vitamins E and C, with the combination clearly proving superior to the single vitamin treatment groups. Topical formulations used for depigmentation that contain, besides the commonly used hydroquinone and sunscreen, vitamins C and E, appear to be safe and efficient. Further research in well designed controlled trials is needed to clarify the role of vitamin E and its derivates in the above mentioned and further skin disorders.

Mechanisms of Action

Vitamin E is among the early recognized cosmeceutical antioxidants, and its redox and free radical chemistry are well documented. The major antioxidant role of vitamin E is generally considered to be the arrest of chain propagation by scavenging lipid peroxyl radicals. The initial oxidation product of tocopherol is the metastable tocopheroxyl radical, which can be either reduced to tocopherol by co-antioxidants, or reacts with another lipid peroxyl radical, yielding tocopherol-quinone. Thus, one molecule of tocopherol has the ability to scavenge two peroxyl radical molecules. Since the physiologic molar ratio of tocopherols to polyunsaturated phospholipids, first-line targets of oxidative attack, is less than about $1:1000$ in most biological membranes, regeneration of tocopherol is essential for its high antioxidant efficacy in vivo. Several hydrophilic co-antioxidants, such as ascorbate and glutathione, can regenerate vitamin E from the tocopheroxyl radical and thus enhance the antioxidant capacity of vitamin E. Furthermore, there is some in vitro evidence that ubiquinol-10 ('co-enzyme Q') protects α-tocopherol from photo-oxidation by recycling mechanisms. Hence, the lack of such 'co-antioxidants' from the antioxidant network may diminish the antioxidant properties of vitamin E and result in limited antioxidant protection of lipid bilayers or other lipophilic domains. A series of studies investigating nonenzymatic stratum corneum antioxidants have demonstrated that, in human skin, vitamin E is the predominant physiologic antioxidant of the skin barrier. When compared to nucleated epidermal layers, there is a lack of important co-antioxidants such as vitamin C in the stratum corneum as well as in the dermis. Taken together, these findings suggest that the skin barrier as well as the upper dermis reveal a lack of antioxidant protection. Accordingly, upon solar UV exposure, these are the cutaneous sites exhibiting the most pronounced oxidative protein damage. Thus, antioxidant supplementation with vitamin E as well as synergistically active co-antioxidants, such as vitamin C, may enhance photoprotective strategies using sunscreens. While single studies have demonstrated significant penetration of topical vitamin E into dermal layers in vitro and in animals, there is still controversy about the efficacy of such strategies for dermal targets in human skin.

Photoprotective effects of topically applied vitamin E (α-tocopherol) and derivatives *in vivo*

Compound(s)	Species	Endpoint(s)	Efficacy	Remarks	Author, year, reference
Vitamin E Vitamin E acetate	Rabbit	Erythema (MED)	Vitamin E protective; vitamin E acetate not protective	BHT also protective; Vitamin E also protective when applied after UVR exposure	Roshchupkin et al 1979
Vitamin E	Human	Mechanoelectrical properties of skin	Protection against UVR and PUVA induced damage		Potapenko et al 1983
Vitamin E Vitamin E derivatives with shorter hydrocarbon chains Vitamin E acetate	Human, rabbit	PUVA induced erythema and changes in mechanoelectrical properties of skin	Vitamin E and derivatives with shorter hydrocarbon chain protective; vitamin E acetate not protective	No protection of vitamin E and derivatives when applied after UVR exposure	Potapenko et al 1984
Vitamin E	Mouse	Lipid peroxidation	Protective	Vitamin A, BHT, and β-carotene also protective	Khettab et al 1988
Vitamin E	Mouse	Skin wrinkling, skin tumor incidence, and histology	Protective		Bissett et al 1989
Vitamin E	Human	Erythema (MED)	Protective	SPF determination	Möller et al 1989
Vitamin E Trolox Vitamin E acetate Vitamin E succinate Vitamin E linoleate Vitamin E nicotinate	Mouse	Skin wrinkling and sagging, skin tumor incidence, and histology	Vitamin E esters not as protective as vitamin E or vitamin E analog Trolox; no protection against UVA induced skin sagging	Glutathione, β-carotene, BHT, and mannitol not protective	Bissett et al 1990
Vitamin E	Mouse	Skin tumor incidence and immunosuppression	Protective	Prolonged pre-treatment	Gensler et al 1991
Vitamin E Vitamin E acetate	Rat	UVA induced binding of 8-MOP and CPZ to epidermal biomacromolecules	Vitamin E protective after single application; vitamin E acetate only protective after prolonged application	Limited conversion of vitamin E acetate into vitamin E after single application	Schoonderwoerd et al 1991
Vitamin E acetate	Mouse	Lipid peroxidation and DNA synthesis rate	Protective		Record et al 1991

BHT = butylated hydroxytoluene, CPZ = chlorpromazine, MED = minimal erythema dose, 8-MOP = 8-methoxypsoralen, PUVA = 8-methoxpsoralen and UVA treatment, SPF = sun protection factor

Continued

Table 7.1 Photoprotective effects of topically applied vitamin E (α-tocopherol) and derivatives *in vivo*

Photoprotective effects of topically applied vitamin E (α-tocopherol) and derivatives *in vivo*—cont'd

Compound(s)	Species	Endpoint(s)	Efficacy	Remarks	Author, year, reference
Vitamin E	Mouse	Skin wrinkling, skin tumor incidence, and histology	Protective	Additive protection in combination with anti-inflammatory agents	Bissett et al 1992
Vitamin E acetate	Mouse	Erythema, edema, and skin sensitivity	Protective	Treatment immediately after UVR exposure	Trevithick et al 1992
Vitamin E acetate	Mouse	Edema and histology	Protective	Delayed treatment after UVR exposure; increased skin vitamin E concentration	Trevithick et al 1993
Vitamin E Vitamin E acetate Vitamin E sorbate	Mouse	Skin wrinkling	Vitamin E and sorbate ester protective; vitamin E acetate ester only modestly protective	Sorbate ester more protective than free vitamin E	Jurkiewicz et al 1995
Vitamin E Vitamin E acetate	Human	Erythema (skin color)	Moderate protection of vitamin E and vitamin E acetate when applied occlusively after UVR exposure	No protection when applied occlusively before UVR exposure	Montenegro et al 1995
Vitamin E Vitamin E acetate	Rat	UVA induced binding of 8-MOP to epidermal biomacromolecules	Vitamin E protective; vitamin E acetate only protective after prolonged application	Conversion of vitamin E acetate into vitamin E slow	Beijersbergen van Henegouwen et al 1995
Vitamin E acetate Vitamin E succinate	Mouse	Skin tumor incidence and immunosuppression	No protection		Gensler et al 1996
Vitamin E	Yorkshire pig	Sunburn cell formation	Protection against UVR induced damage	Minimal protection in reducing PUVA induced damage	Darr et al 1996
Vitamin E	Mouse	Immunosuppression and lipid peroxidation	Protective	No protection when applied after UVR exposure	Yuen et al 1997
Vitamin E	Mouse	Histology (sunburn cell formation and skin thickness)	Protective		Ritter et al 1997

Vitamin E Vitamin E acetate Vitamin E methyl ether	Mouse	Formation of DNA photoadducts	Vitamin E derivatives less protective than vitamin E	Sunscreening properties of vitamin E	McVean et al 1997
Vitamin E	Mouse	Chemiluminescence after UVA exposure	Protective	β-Carotene also protective	Evelson et al 1997
Vitamin E	Mouse	Formation of DNA photoadducts in epidermal p53 gene	Protective		Chen et al 1997
Vitamin E	Mouse	Lipid peroxidation	Protective	Skin's enzymatic and non-enzymatic antioxidant capacity investigated	Lopez-Torres et al 1998
Vitamin E	Human	Erythema (skin color and skin blood flow)	Moderate protection	No protection when applied after UVR exposure; SPF (determined in vitro) = 1	Dreher et al 1998
Vitamin E γ–Tocopherol δ–Tocopherol Vitamin E acetate Vitamin E methyl ether	Mouse	Formation of DNA photoadducts	Vitamin E, γ-tocopherol and δ-tocopherol protective; vitamin E acetate and vitamin E methyl ether not protective	Application as dispersion in cream	McVean et al 1999
Vitamin E Vitamin E succinate	Mouse	Erythema, pigmentation, skin tumor incidence	Protective after prolonged application	No sign of toxicity observed for vitamin E and vitamin E succinate	Burke et al 2000

BHT = butylated hydroxytoluene, CPZ = chlorpromazine, MED = minimal erythema dose, 8-MOP = 8-methoxypsoralen, PUVA = 8-methoxypsoralen and UVA treatment, SPF = sun protection factor

Table 7.1 Photoprotective effects of topically applied vitamin E (α-tocopherol) and derivatives *in vivo*

Photoprotection by vitamin E

The largest body of scientific evidence for a beneficial cosmeceutical role of topical vitamin E exists for photoprotection (summarized in Table 7.1). Numerous topical studies demonstrated significantly reduced acute skin responses when vitamin E was applied before UVR exposure, such as erythema and edema, sunburn cell formation, lipid peroxidation, DNA-adduct formation, immuno-suppression, as well as chemiluminescence. Chronic skin reactions due to prolonged UVR exposure, such as skin wrinkling and skin tumor incidence, were also diminished by topical vitamin E formulations. Vitamin E esters, particularly vitamin E acetate, were also shown to be promising agents in reducing UVR induced skin damage. However, their photo-protective effects appeared to be less pronounced as compared to vitamin E; moreover, some studies failed to detect photoprotection provided by vitamin E esters. Since the free aromatic hydroxyl group is responsible for the antioxidant properties of vitamin E, vitamin E esters need to be hydrolyzed during skin absorption to show activity.

Vitamin E acetate was shown to be absorbed and penetrate skin. A skin bioavailability study demon-strated that vitamin E and vitamin E acetate behave similarly with regard to penetration of rat epidermis. The difference between physicochemical parameters determining skin transport for vitamin E and its esters seems negligible. Notably, the bioconversion of vitamin E acetate to its active antioxidative form, α-tocopherol, was found to be slow and to occur only to a minor extent in vivo. As demonstrated in recent studies with viable micro-Yucatan pig skin or viable human skin ex vivo, vitamin E acetate was not found to be hydrolyzed in the skin penetration limiting layer, the stratum corneum. In the nucleated epidermis, however, the bioconversion of vitamin E acetate into vitamin E occurs, but seems to be dependent on formulation. Some evidence exists, however, that the bioconversion of vitamin E acetate into vitamin E might be enhanced due to UVR exposure. UVB exposure was demonstrated to cause an increase in esterase activity in murine epidermis.

Dosage and Practical Usage Regimens

Topical supplementation

Vitamin E is one of the most frequently used cosme-ceutical ingredients. While products with concen-trations of less than 0.1% and up to 20 have been developed and marketed in Europe and the United States, there is a surprising lack of published data on dose–response studies defining the optimal dosage of vitamin E. In addition to the relative lack of efficacy control requirements for over-the-counter (OTC) products, this might also be attributed to ill defined endpoints as well as to the difficulty of measuring oxidative stress in vivo. Recent advances in biophysical (e.g. ultraweak photon emission; near-infrared/Raman spectroscopy; electron paramagnetic resonance) and biochemical research (e.g. the recent identification of highly sensitive and specific skin surface lipid photo-oxidation products/SqmOOH) have led to the development of noninvasive assays (e.g. the 'sebum photo-oxidation test') that will help to better define relevant dose–response curves of antioxidants such as vitamin E.

Using this approach, we have recently demon-strated that even the use of rinse-off products containing α-tocopherol in concentrations of less than 0.5% leads to significantly increased levels of vitamin E in the stratum corneum of human skin. Therefore, if the product claim is improved anti-oxidant protection of the skin barrier, topical formulations with α-tocopherol at concentrations ranging from 0.1 to 1%, but not vitamin E esters, are very likely to be efficient. According to the anti-oxidant network theory outlined earlier, combina-tions with co-antioxidants such as vitamin C may help to improve antioxidant effects and the stability of vitamin E.

Systemic/dietary supplementation

While topical vitamin E has been studied exten-sively, little is known on the oral bioavailability of this antioxidant in skin. Ongoing studies by our labo-ratory indicate that a daily intake of as low as 400 IU vitamin E functions to increase cutaneous vitamin E levels. Conflicting results published on this issue are due to the fact that differing analytical methods and compartments of the skin have been investigated. While earlier studies have investigated full skin thickness, recent research efforts have focused on vitamin E delivery via sebaceous gland secretion, which would primarily lead to increased vitamin E levels in skin surface lipids and the upper epidermis/stratum corneum. Our recent results indicate that:

1. Sebaceous gland secretion is a major mechanism leading to site-specific differences in vitamin E increases.

2. The bioavailability of 400 mg RRR-α-tocopheryl acetate (derived from natural vitamin E) or 400 mg all-rac-α-tocopheryl acetate (derived from synthetic vitamin E) is comparable.
3. Possible protective effects in the skin require a supplementation period of 2–3 weeks.

These results are important in that they suggest that no improvement of antioxidant protection of skin barrier lipids and proteins can be obtained in the first 2 weeks of oral vitamin E supplementation.

Cautions, Contraindications, and Adverse Effects

Although vitamin E is widely used in many topical cosmetic products, reports of side effects such as allergic or irritant skin reactions are rare. Nevertheless, clinical side effects have been described after topical application of vitamin E containing products, for example local and generalized contact dermatitis, contact urticaria, and erythema-multiforme-like eruptions. In 1992, an 'epidemic outbreak' of about 1000 cases of allergic papular and follicular contact dermatitis caused by α-tocopherol linoleate in a cosmetic line was reported in Switzerland. The authors found that this compound was easily oxidized under the storage conditions used. Therefore, secondary or tertiary oxidation products of α-tocopherol linoleate, rather than the reduced vitamin E ester, are likely to have caused irritation or even the oxidation of proteins and subsequent hapten formation. Furthermore, positive patch test reactions were reported in several cases after application of α-tocopherol acetate, a widely used water soluble derivate of α-tocopherol.

In conclusion, reported positive patch test results due to α-tocopherol are rare and need to be critically reviewed. Investigators used the oil of vitamin E capsules for patch testing without further evaluating the tocopherol derivates, source or further components of these capsules. However, it could not be excluded in many cases that the symptoms were caused by soybean oil, glycerin, or gelatin, all of which were also present in the topically applied vitamin E capsules.

Doses of 50 IU up to 1000 IU α-tocopherol per day have been tolerated in humans with no or minimal side effects. Vitamin E supplements for pregnancy usually contain smaller doses of vitamin E, but adverse effects have not been observed even with higher doses. Theoretically, however, due to the involvement of the cytochrome P450 system in the metabolism of orally supplemented *RRR*-α-tocopherol, drug interactions have to be taken into account when supranutritional dosages of vitamin E are provided. Since tocopherols and their oxidation products are able to inhibit platelet aggregation, simultaneous supplementation of anticoagulants and vitamin E is not recommended.

Current Research and Possible Future Applications

As indicated above, topical strategies alone may not be sufficient to bolster the skin's antioxidative defense in the dermis and thus to prevent or lessen photoaging in this skin compartment. Therefore, current research on vitamin E focuses on systemic delivery of vitamin E to the various compartments of human skin. It was recently discovered that human sebum contains high amounts of α-tocopherol and that sebaceous gland secretion is a relevant physiologic route of α-tocopherol delivery to skin regions rich in sebaceous glands, such as facial skin. Similarly, orally administered drugs have been reported to be transported to the skin surface and the stratum corneum by the sebaceous gland secretion route. Ongoing studies investigate the relevance and time course of this delivery pathway for increasing the levels of vitamin E in human skin. A further ongoing study focuses on the relevance of this mechanism for the physiologic vitamin E levels in skin surface lipids at different age groups. The outcome of these studies will certainly have implications for conditions of sebostatic, dry skin (for example, as in atopic dermatitis), as well as for the skin of prepubertal children, who have a low activity of sebaceous glands. Vitamin E remains an important cosmeceutical in the dermatologic armamentarium.

Further Reading

Baschong W, Artmann C, Hueglin D, Roeding J 2001 Direct evidence for bioconversion of vitamin E acetate into vitamin E: an ex vivo study in viable human skin. Journal of Cosmetic Science 52: 155–161
Brigelius-Flohe R, Kelly FJ, et al 2002 The European perspective on vitamin E: current knowledge and future research. American Journal of Clinical Nutrition 76: 703–716
Burke K E, Clive J, Combs GF, et al 2000 Effects of topical and oral vitamin E on pigmentation and skin cancer induced by ultraviolet irradiation in Skh: 2 hairless mice. Nutrition Cancer 38: 87–97
Ekanayake-Mudiyanselage S, Hamburger M, Elsner P, Thiele JJ 2003 Ultraviolet a induces generation of squalene monohydroperoxide isomers in human sebum and skin surface lipids in vitro and in vivo. Journal of Investigative Dermatology 120: 915–922

Ekanayake-Mudiyanselage S, Kraemer K, Thiele JJ 2004 Oral supplementation with all-rac- and RRR-alpha-tocopherol increases vitamin E levels in human sebum after a latency period of 14–21 days in: Vitamin and Health Annals of the New York Academy of Science 1031: (in press)

Fuchs J, Groth N, Herrling T 2002 In vivo measurement of oxidative stress status in human skin. Methods in Enzymology 352:333–339

Harris BD, Taylor JS 1997 Contact allergy to vitamin E capsules: false negative patch tests to vitamin E. Contact Dermatitis 36: 273

Sander CS, Chang H, Salzmann S, et al 2002 Photoaging is associated with protein oxidation in human skin in vivo. Journal of Investigative Dermatology 118: 618–625

Thiele JJ, Weber SU, Packer L 1999 Sebaceous gland secretion is a major physiologic route of vitamin E delivery to skin. Journal of Investigative Dermatology 113: 1006–1010

Thiele JJ, Schroeter C, Hsieh SN, Podda M, Packer L 2001 The antioxidant network of the stratum corneum. Current Problems in Dermatology 29: 26–42

Tsoureli-Nikita E, Hercogova J, Lotti T, Menchini G 2002 Evaluation of dietary intake of vitamin E in the treatment of atopic dermatitis: a study of the clinical course and evaluation of the immunoglobulin E serum levels. International Journal of Dermatology 41: 146–150

Cosmeceutical Vitamins: Vitamin C

8

Patricia K. Farris

Introduction

Vitamin C is a naturally occurring antioxidant incorporated into cosmeceuticals for the purpose of preventing and treating sun damaged skin. Most plants and animals have the capacity to synthesize vitamin C. In humans, however, vitamin C cannot be synthesized because of loss of the ability to produce L-glucono-gamma-lactone oxidase, the enzyme necessary for its production. Vitamin C must instead be obtained from dietary sources such as citrus fruits and leafy green vegetables (Fig. 8.1). Interestingly, oral supplementation with vitamin C produces only a limited increase in skin concentration. This is because even with ingestion of massive doses, the absorption of vitamin C is limited by active transport mechanisms in the gut. Therefore, vitamin C has become a popular topically applied cosmeceutical.

Three forms of vitamin C are found in cosmeceuticals marketed as creams, serums, and patches. The first form is the active form of vitamin C, L-ascorbic acid. Early formulations of L-ascorbic acid often turned yellow due to the oxidation byproduct dehydroascorbic acid produced upon exposure to air. For this reason, many cosmetic chemists turned to more stable esterified derivatives, such as ascorbyl-6-palmitate and magnesium ascorbyl phosphate. Stability studies comparing all three compounds have demonstrated that magnesium ascorbyl phosphate is the most stable in solution and emulsion followed by ascorbyl-6-palmitate, while L-ascorbic acid is least stable. In spite of these finding, cosmeceuticals containing all forms of vitamin C can be purchased in the marketplace today.

Oxidative Stress, Aging Skin, and Vitamin C

Antiaging research has elucidated the role of reactive oxygen species in the pathogenesis of photoaging. Reactive oxygen species (ROS) including superoxide anion, peroxide and singlet oxygen are generated when human skin is exposed to ultraviolet light. These ROS mediate their deleterious effects by causing direct chemical alterations of DNA, cell membranes, and proteins including collagen.

Oxidative stress can also activate certain cellular events mediated by transcription factors. ROS upregulate transcription factor activator protein-1 (AP-1). AP-1 increases metalloproteinase (MMP) production resulting in collagen breakdown. Nuclear transcription factor kappa-B (NF-κB) is also induced by oxidative stress and produces a number of inflammatory mediators that contribute to skin aging. Additionally, ROS increases elastin mRNA levels in dermal fibroblasts which may provide an explanation for the elastotic changes found in the photoaged dermis.

The skin relies on a complex system of enzymatic and nonenzymatic antioxidants to protect itself from harmful ROS. L-ascorbic acid is the most plentiful antioxidant in human skin. This water soluble vitamin functions in the aqueous compartment of the cell. Vitamin C sequentially donates electrons,

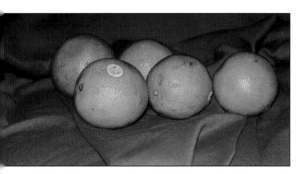

Fig. 8.1 Citrus fruits, such as oranges, are a rich dietary source of vitamin C

neutralizes free radicals, and protects intracellular structures from oxidative stress. Following the donation of the first electron, a more stable ascorbate free radical is formed and after the second electron is donated, dehydroascorbic acid remains. Dehydroascobic acid can be converted back to L-ascorbic acid by dehydroascorbic acid reductase or may be broken down as the lactone ring opens. Vitamin C also helps regenerate the oxidative form of vitamin E, a potent lipid soluble antioxidant. In this regard, these two vitamin antioxidants appear to function synergistically within the cell.

In a compounding manner, while ultraviolet light increases production of intracellular ROS, it is at the same time impairing the skin's ability to neutralize them. UVB exposure depletes skin of many key antioxidants, including vitamin C. It is known that exposure to ultraviolet light depletes the skin reservoir of vitamin C in a dose dependent manner. Even minimal exposure to 1.6 MED (minimal erythema dose) can decrease vitamin C levels to 70% of normal while exposing murine skin to 10 times MED further increases depletion to 54% of normal. In addition, ozone depletes stores of vitamin C and E in epidermal cells. Thus environmental exposure impairs the skin's natural defense mechanisms against oxidative stress.

Vitamin C: Effects on Collagen and Elastin Synthesis

Vitamin C is essential for collagen biosynthesis. Ascorbate serves as a cofactor for prolyl and lysyl hydroxylase, the enzymes responsible for stabilizing and cross-linking collagen. Ascorbate can also stimulate collagen synthesis directly by activating its transcription and stabilizing procollagen mRNA. Scurvy serves as prototype for the physiologic changes that occur when vitamin C is lacking and collagen biosynthesis is impaired.

In view of this, it is no surprise that topically applied vitamin C has been shown to enhance collagen production in human skin. Skin biopsies taken from postmenopausal women who applied 5% L-ascorbic acid to one forearm and vehicle to the other showed an increase in mRNA levels of collagen I and III. Additionally, levels of tissue inhibitor of MMP 1 were also increased, suggesting that topical vitamin C may mitigate collagen breakdown. Interestingly, mRNA levels of elastin, fibrillin and tissue inhibitor of MMP 2 remained unchanged.

The authors note that those most affected by topical vitamin C had low dietary intake of the vitamin C and conclude that the functional activity of dermal cells can be improved by topically applied vitamin C.

L-ascorbic acid also appears to influence elastin biosynthesis. In vitro studies suggest elastin biosynthesis by fibroblasts may be inhibited by ascorbate. This may be helpful in reducing the elastin accumulation that is characteristic of photoaged skin.

Photoprotection by Vitamin C

While sunscreens remain the mainstay for protecting skin against UV-induced changes, topical antioxidants are gaining favor. Recent studies suggest that while sunscreens reduce UV-induced erythema and thymine dimer formation, they do little to protect skin from free radicals. Sunscreens, even when applied properly, block only 55% of free radicals produced by UVA exposure. This is important in that UVA is believed to be important in the pathogenesis of skin aging and possibly melanoma formation. These data suggest that in order to optimize UV protection sunscreens should be used in conjunction with topical antioxidants.

L-ascorbic acid is known to have photoprotective effects on skin. Vitamin C does not act as a sunscreen per se as it does not absorb sunlight in the UV spectrum. Topical L-ascorbic acid has been shown to protect porcine skin from UVB-induced erythema and sunburn cell formation. Topical application of 10% vitamin C was shown to decrease UVB induced erythema by 52% and the number of sunburn cells by 40–60%. Pre-treatment with topical vitamin C prior to PUVA mitigated phototoxic injury as measured by sunburn cells and resulted in a normal histology devoid of the usual PUVA associated findings.

While vitamin C alone can confer photoprotection, it appears to function optimally in conjunction with vitamin E. In studies designed to evaluate this synergy, vitamin C and E were applied alone or in combination for 4 days to pig skin and then irradiated with a solar simulator (295 nm). On day 5, antioxidant protection factor was measured including erythema, sunburn cells, and thymine dimers. The combination of 15% L-ascorbic acid and 1% alpha-tocopherol provided superior photoprotective effects (fourfold) that were progressive over the 4 day period. Both antioxidants conferred photoprotection when applied alone but to a lesser degree than when used in combination.

It is important to note that topically applied antioxidants must be applied prior to UV exposure in order to photoprotect. In a randomized, double blinded, placebo controlled human study, the short term photoprotective effects of a variety of antioxidants was evaluated when applied after UV irradiation. Melatonin, vitamin C, and vitamin E were applied alone and in combination 30 minutes, 1 hour, and 2 hours after UV irradiation. No photoprotective effects were observed when these antioxidants were applied after UV irradiation.

Vitamin C as an Anti-Inflammatory

Vitamin C is known to have anti-inflammatory activity and has been used by dermatologists to treat a variety of inflammatory dermatoses. Cultured human cells loaded with vitamin C show a significantly decreased activation of the transcription factor nuclear factor kappa B (NF-κB). NF-κB is the transcription factor responsible for the production of a number of pro-inflammatory cytokines such as tumor necrosis factor alpha (TNF-α), IL-1, IL-6, and IL-8. It is believed that this downregulation of NF-κB by vitamin C occurs by blocking TNF-α induced activation of NF-κB. This mechanism provides an explanation for the anti-inflammatory properties that are observed with vitamin C.

Delivery and Metabolism of L-Ascorbic Acid and Derivatives

While some believe that the ester derivatives are preferable in formulation, others remain committed to the use of L-ascorbic acid. Studies performed by Pinnell et al suggest that topical L-ascorbic acid can be formulated in a manner that ensures stabilization and enhances permeation. These studies demonstrated that L-ascorbic acid can be delivered across the stratum corneum as long as the ionic charge on the molecule is removed. This is achieved only at a pH of less than 3.5. The maximal concentration of L-ascorbic acid for percutaneous absorption was 20% and, curiously, higher levels failed to increase absorption. Daily application of 15% L-ascorbic acid at a pH of 3.2 increased skin L-ascorbic acid levels 20-fold and tissue levels were saturated after 3 days. The half life of L-ascorbic acid after tissue saturation was approximately 4 days. By contrast, topical 13%

magnesium ascorbyl phosphate and 10% ascorbyl-6-palmitate failed to increase skin levels of L-ascorbic acid according to this study.

A recent study provides insight into the mechanisms involved in delivery of L-ascorbic acid and magnesium ascorbyl phosphate (MAP) across the stratum corneum. In vitro studies utilizing nude mice assessed the ability of lasers and microdermabrasion to enhance and control skin permeation and deposition of L-ascorbic acid and MAP. At baseline, L-ascorbic acid possessed very low passive permeability while MAP appeared to be more readily transported into the dermis where it was converted to L-ascorbic acid. This difference in permeability is likely due to the fact that L-ascorbic acid is hydrophilic whereas MAP is lipophilic. These studies demonstrated that microdermabrasion, erbium, and carbon dioxide lasers enhanced skin permeation of topically applied L-ascorbic acid, while there was no improvement in permeation of magnesium ascorbyl phosphate by these treatments. This data suggests that the rate determining step for topical delivery of MAP is not permeation across the skin, since it appears to traverse the stratum corneum readily, but instead diffusion from the vehicle. By contrast, L-ascorbic acid permeation was improved by treatments that disrupt the stratum corneum thus breaking the barrier for its absorption. Studies such as these further elucidate biochemical difference between vitamin C and its derivatives as they relate to biologic activity.

Ascorbyl-6-palmitate

Ascorbyl palmitate is a fat soluble analog of L-ascorbic acid with a palmitic acid chain attached at the sixth position. This molecule when hydrolyzed yields ascorbic acid and palmitic acid. Because it is fat soluble, ascorbyl palmitate is easily transported into cells where it functions as an antioxidant.

Perricone has published extensively on the use of ascorbyl-6-palmitate. His studies have demonstrated that ascorbyl-6-palmitate has physiologic activity that is not dependent on its breakdown to ascorbic acid. Ascorbyl-6-palmitate is a free radical scavenger in and of itself. Because it is nonirritating at a neutral pH, it is ideal for topical application and has a shelf-life of two years

Clinical studies performed by Perricone indicate that 15% ascorbyl-6-palmitate is effective for reducing UVB induced erythema. Ascorbyl palmitate applied after UV burning reduced redness 50% quicker than in areas left untreated. These effects are likely the result of anti-inflammatory activity. Topical ascorbyl palmitate also proved thirty times more effective than ascorbic acid as a tumor inhibitor in mice.

Perricone has also demonstrated that ascorbyl palmitate is useful for treating inflammatory dermatoses. He suggests that conditions such as psoriasis and asteatotic eczema may be improved by topical application of ascorbyl palmitate. Formal clinical trials confirming these observations have not been reported.

Magnesium ascorbyl phosphate

Magnesium ascorbyl phosophate (MAP) is found commonly in cosmetics and is stable at neutral pH. MAP is known to be a free radical scavenger and stimulant of collagen production. Studies have demonstrated that MAP protects against UVB induced lipid peroxidation in hairless mice and confirmed that it crosses the epidermis and is converted to ascorbic acid.

In vitro studies utilizing human fibroblasts demonstrated magnesium ascorbyl phosophate is equivalent to ascorbic acid in its ability to stimulate collagen synthesis. These findings were confirmed by additional studies that demonstrated enhanced collagen synthesis and cell growth of cultured fibroblasts treated with MAP. Finally, in vitro studies demonstrated that MAP phosphate regulates type I collagen production.

Clinical Studies Regarding Topical Vitamin C

Clinical studies have investigated the cosmeceutical effect of products containing L-ascorbic acid. A 3 month double blind, randomized, vehicle controlled study was performed on 19 patients between 36 and 72 years with moderately photodamaged facial skin. Patients applied topical ascorbic acid 10% (Cellex-C high-potency serum, Cellex-C International, Toronto, Ontario) or vehicle serum to half the face for 3 months. Optical profilometry image analysis demonstrated a statistically significant improvement in the vitamin C treated side when compared to control. Clinical assessment showed significant improvement in fine wrinkling, tactile roughness, coarse rhytids, skin laxity/tone, sallowness/yellowing, and overall features on the side treated with active. Photographic assessment showed a 57.9% improvement in

the vitamin C treated group compared to control. The patients shown in Figures 8.2 and 8.3 demonstrate the type of clinical improvement that can be expected with continued use of topical L-ascorbic acid. The patient in Figure 8.2 shows vastly improved periorbital wrinkles while the patient in Figure 8.3 demonstrates a significant lightening of actinically induced mottled hyperpigmentation.

More recently, Humbert et al reported a 6 month double blind, vehicle controlled study of moderately photoaged patients applying 5% vitamin C cream to the neck and forearms. A highly significant decrease in deep furrows was observed and substantiated with silicon replicas on the vitamin C treated side. Histology demonstrated ultrastructural evidence of elastic tissue repair. The authors suggest that topical vitamin C had a positive influence on all parameters of actinically damaged skin.

Fitzpatrick and Rostan reported a double blind, half face study of ten patients treated with a new formulation containing 10% L-acorbic acid and 7% tetrahexyldecyl ascorbate in an anhydrous polysilicone gel base. The inactive polysilicone gel base served as a control on the opposite side. Clinical evaluations were performed at 4, 8, and 12 weeks and punch biopsies were performed. There was overall improvement on the vitamin C treated side that was statistically significant when compared to vehicle at 12 weeks. The vitamin C treated side showed a decrease in photoaging score on the cheeks and perioral area. The periorbital areas improved on both sides, which the authors contribute to improved hydration. Skin biopsies after vitamin C showed an increase in grenz zone collagen and increased staining for mRNA for type I collagen.

In addition to improving wrinkles, vitamin C may also be helpful for lightening hyperpigmentation. Studies conducted by Kameyama et al demonstrated that magnesium-L-ascorbyl-2-phosphate suppressed melanin formation by tyrosinase and melanoma cells. Additionally, topically applied 10% magnesium-L-ascorbyl-2-phosphate cream when applied to human skin caused a significant lightening of melasma and lentigenes in 19 of 34 patients.

It has been suggested that topical vitamin C may be helpful in treating acne due to its anti-inflammatory properties. Sodium L-ascorbyl-2-phosphate (APS), a less frequently used derivative, has been shown to have beneficial effects on acne and acne scarring when used in conjunction with glycolic acid peels.

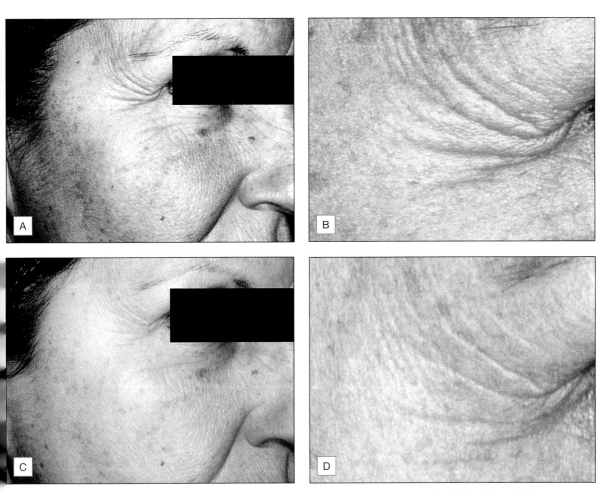

Fig. 8.2 A patient with moderate photoaging. (**A**) Before with enlarged area (**B**) showing periorbital wrinkling. (**C**) One year after treatment, with enlarged area (**D**) showing a significant improvement in periorbital wrinkles. (Courtesy of Sheldon R Pinnell, MD)

Patients applied 5% sodium L-ascorbyl-2-phosphate or vehicle twice daily after 50% glycolic acid peels. The peels were applied between one and three times monthly at 10 day intervals. Seventy-nine percent of patients applying APS showed moderate to excellent improvement compared to 44% in the control group. The investigators conclude that topical sodium L-ascorbyl-2-phosphate may improve outcomes in patients treated for acne scarring. There are anecdotal reports that topical vitamin C may improve inflammatory forms of rosacea but objective clinical studies are lacking to date.

An innovative use for topical L-ascorbic was described by Alster and West who evaluated its efficacy for treating post-CO_2 laser resurfacing erythema. Split face studies showed a significant decrease in post-CO_2 laser resurfacing erythema by the eighth postoperative week in patients treated with an aqueous solution containing topical 10% L-ascorbic acid, 2% zinc sulphate, and 0.5% tyrosine. Interestingly, the same formulation in a cream base did not improve post-laser erythema.

Conclusion

Topically applied vitamins continue to be a mainstay of our antiaging armamentarium. There is now significant data confirming the benefits of topically applied vitamin C and supporting its use as a cosmeceutical. Its diverse biologic activity in the skin makes vitamin C a valuable agent for the practicing dermatologist.

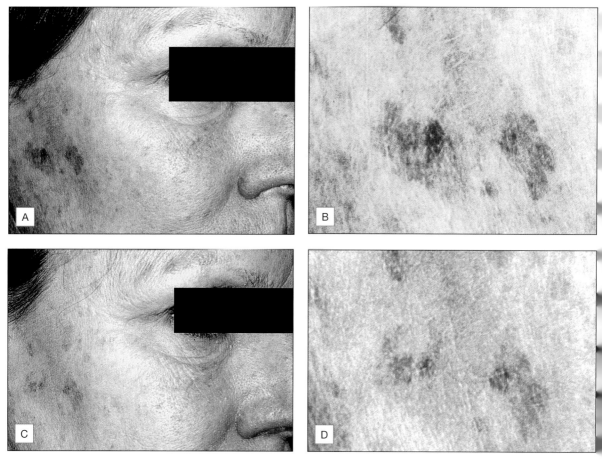

Fig. 8.3 A patient with actinically induced mottled hyperpigmentation. (**A**) Before with enlarged area (**B**) showing hyperpigmentation. (**C**) One year after treatment, with enlarged area (**D**) showing an improvement in sun induced hyperpigmentation. (Courtesy of Sheldon R Pinnell, MD)

Further Reading

Austria R, Semenzato A, Bettero A 1997 Stability of vitamin C derivatives in solution and topical formulations. Journal of Pharmaceutical and Biomedical Analysis 15:795–801

Carcamo JM, Pedraza A, Borquez-Ojeda O, Golde DS 2002 Vitamin C suppresses TNF alpha-induced NF kappa B activation by inhibiting I Kappa B alpha phosphorylation. 41:12995–30002

Darr D, Combs S, Dunston S, Manning T, Pinnell S 1992 Topical vitamin C protects porcine skin from ultraviolet radiation-induced damage. British Journal of Dermatology 127:247–253

Fisher GJ, Kang S, Varani J, et al 2002 Mechanisms of photoaging and chronological skin aging. Archives of Dermatology 138:1462–1470

Haywood R, Wardman P, Sanders R, Linge C 2003 Sunscreens inadequately protect against ultraviolet A-induced free radicals in skin: Implications for skin aging and melanoma? Journal of Investigative Dermatology 121:862–868

Humbert PG, Haftek M, Creidi P, et al 2003 Topical ascorbic acid on photoaged skin. Clinical, topographical and ultrastructural evaluation: double-blind study vs. placebo. Experimental Dermatology 12:237–244

Lin JY, Selim MA, Shea CR, et al 2003 UV photoprotection by combination topical antioxidants vitamin C and vitamin E. Journal of the American Academy of Dermatology 48:866–867

Perricone NV 1997 Topical vitamin C ester (ascorbyl palmitate). Journal of Geriatric Dermatology 5:162–170

Pinnell SR, Yang HS, Omar M, et al 2001 Topical L-ascorbic acid percutaneous absorption studies. Dermatologic Surgery 27:137–142

Pinnell SR 2003 Cutaneous photodamage, oxidative stress and topical antioxidant protection. Journal of the American Academy of Dermatology 48:1–19

Shindo Y, Witt E, Hans D, et al. Enzymic and nonenzymic antioxidants in epidermis and dermis of human skin. Journal of Investigative Dermatology 1994; 102:122–124

Cosmeceutical Vitamins: Vitamin B

9

Donald L. Bissett, John E. Oblong

Introduction

The nutritional value of the B vitamins has long been known, and in recent years the utility of topical vitamin B3 (also known as niacinamide) and pro-vitamin B5 (also known as panthenol) is being increasingly recognized. There are several reports of topical niacinamide and panthenol providing dermatologic effects (e.g. treatment of acne and wounds), and they have been used therapeutically for such effects. More recently, both of these B vitamins have been utilized in topical cosmetic products to provide beneficial effects for a wide array of more common skin problems such as those associated with aging and photoaging (e.g. dryness, red blotchiness, hyperpigmentation, and texture problems). In those applications, these B vitamins have been found to be well tolerated by the skin and can thus be used broadly across skin types.

The likely mechanisms involved in these effects have not been completely elucidated. However, since both of these B vitamins are precursors to important co-factors in metabolism, a general mechanism involving this precursor function can be invoked. For niacinamide, its physiologic role is as a precursor to the important co-factors nicotinamide adenine dinucleotide (NAD), its phosphate derivative (NADP), and their reduced forms (NADH and NADPH). For panthenol, it is converted to pantothenic acid (vitamin B5), a component of the co-enzyme A complex.

This chapter will overview the topical effects and mechanisms of these B vitamins, with primary focus on their cosmeceutical benefits. Since there is a considerable literature on both materials, this chapter will discuss those aspects of the B vitamins relevant to dermatology.

Niacinamide

Material

Vitamin B3 encompasses a family of structurally similar compounds. The focus of this review is on niacinamide which is also known as nicotinamide and in older literature as vitamin PP (for pellagra preventing). Niacinamide is a water soluble, stable, and low molecular weight substance which readily penetrates the stratum corneum.

Topical therapeutic effects

Niacinamide has been used topically in the prevention of photoimmunosuppression and photo-carcinogenesis, reduction in acne severity, and improvement in bullous pemphigoid. The specific mechanisms for these effects have not been clarified. However, niacinamide is a precursor to NAD(P) and their reduced forms NAD(P)H, co-factors which are important in many cellular metabolic enzyme reactions, so it has potential to impact many tissue functions. Also since the reduced forms of these co-factors are potent anti-oxidants, a redox regulation mechanism is a strong possibility at least for some of the observed cosmeceutical effects.

Topical cosmeceutical effects

Topical niacinamide is extremely well tolerated by the skin, i.e. it does not induce skin irritation responses (redness, dryness, burn, sting, or itch responses). The mildness, and the broad use potential noted above, have triggered several recent controlled cosmeceutical clinical studies. These studies have

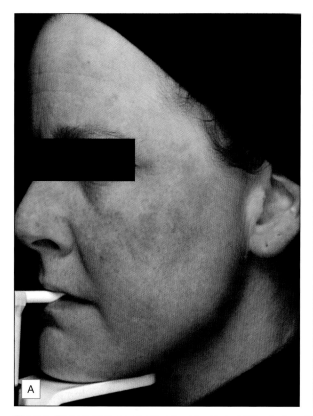
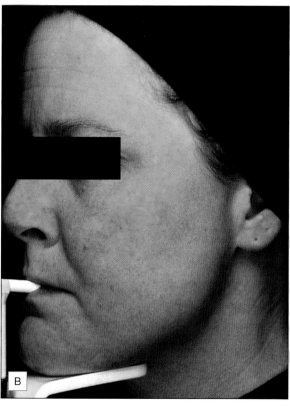

Fig. 9.1 Red blotchiness improvement by topical 5% niacinamide in Caucasian facial skin: (**A**) baseline; (**B**) 8 weeks

revealed cutaneous effects of chronic topical niacinamide in aging skin, such as improved barrier function, decreased appearance of signs of facial photoaging (texture, hyperpigmented spots, irritation/red blotchiness), and reduced sebum production. Some mechanistic effects were also noted in those and related studies to suggest how niacinamide functions as a cosmeceutical.

Barrier and irritation

For example, in forearm testing, topical niacinamide led to a reduction in transepidermal water loss (TEWL) indicating improved barrier function. The treated skin was then found to be significantly more resistant to damage by barrier destructive agents such as the surfactant sodium lauryl sulfate (SLS). Thus, skin pretreated with niacinamide will be less prone to damage from insults that are encountered in the environment, such as detergents. That will likely translate into less irritation and redness and thus contribute to a visible color benefit (Fig. 9.1).

In fact, in facial clinical testing, irritation as assessed by facial red blotchiness was found to be reduced by daily use of topical niacinamide.

The mechanism by which this barrier improvement effect occurs is likely due to niacinamide induced increase in skin barrier layer lipids such as ceramides and barrier layer proteins such as keratin, involucrin, and filaggrin. Such increases in these primary structural components would be expected to have a significant effect on building the barrier.

Hyperpigmented spots

In addition to decreased facial erythema chronic topical niacinamide may have an effect on facial hyperpigmentation. From clinical testing on both Caucasian and Asian facial skin, reduced facial dyspigmentation was observed. The mechanism of this pigmentation reduction has been investigated in vitro and found to involve inhibition of melanosome transfer from melanocytes to the keratinocytes. With transfer inhibited, the melanocytes stop producing

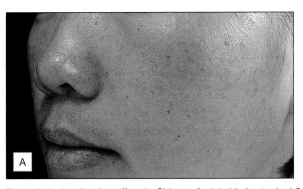 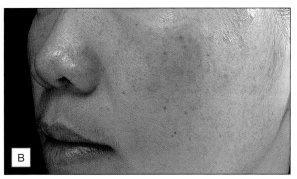

Fig. 9.2 Anti-yellowing effect in Chinese facial skin by topical 3.5% niacinamide: (A) baseline; (B) 4 weeks

melanin, resulting in a reduction in melanin content in hyperpigmented skin.

Yellowing (sallowness)

A third color benefit of chronic topical niacinamide is reduction in skin sallowness or yellowing. In facial testing, cutaneous yellowing was reduced (Figs 9.2, 9.3). The mechanism by which this effect occurs may involve an antioxidant mechanism via NAD(P)H, specifically prevention of protein glycation. Glycation (Maillard reaction) is a spontaneous oxidative reaction between protein and sugar, resulting in cross-linked proteins (Amedori products) that are yellow-brown in color. These products can accumulate in matrix components such as collagen that have long half-lives. An 'experiment of nature' that illustrates the impact of glycation on the appearance of skin is diabetes, where sugar levels are elevated. This leads to increased glycation and visibly more yellow appearance. There is thus potential for glycation to have a significant role in the aging induced changes in normal skin appearance (e.g. yellowing or sallowness). Niacinamide has been reported to have antiglycation properties.

Texture

The poor texture of older skin in the cheek area encompasses two factors: enlarged pore size and 'pebbly, rippled' appearance. Topical niacinamide has been observed to improve skin texture with chronic usage. The underlying cause of poor skin texture is not defined. However, since enlarged pore size is a component, the observed niacinamide induced reduction in sebum production (in particular the di-

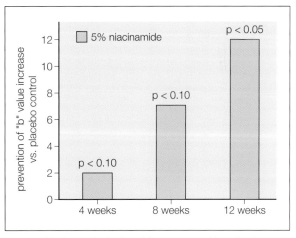

Fig. 9.3 Topical 5% niacinamide prevents skin yellowing ('b' value analysis from images)

and triglyceride fractions) may lead to reduction in pore size and thus smoother texture.

Wrinkles

Chronic topical niacinamide treatment (Fig. 9.4) may reduce facial wrinkles. There are two mechanisms which have been explored regarding this wrinkle reduction. The first is increased dermal collagen production by niacinamide. The second is decrease in excess dermal GAG (glycosaminoglycan) production. While a low level of GAG is required for normal structure and function of the dermal matrix, excess levels are associated with poor visible appearance of skin, for example, the wrinkled skin of Shar Pei dogs is the result of excess dermal GAG. Both increased dermal collagen and decreased excess dermal GAG

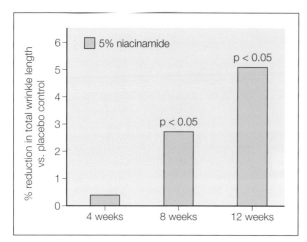

Fig. 9.4 Topical 5% niacinamide reduces facial skin wrinkles (total wrinkle line length reduction from quantitative computer image analysis)

are associated with the wrinkle improvement effect of therapeutic approaches such as topical *trans*-retinoic acid and chemical peel.

Panthenol

Material

Panthenol or pro-vitamin B5 is also known as pantothenol and pantothenyl alcohol. The D optical isomer of panthenol is termed dexpanthenol. Panthenol is a water soluble, stable, and low molecular weight cosmeceutical that readily penetrates into the stratum corneum.

Topical therapeutic effects

Panthenol has been used topically in the treatment of wounds, bruises, scars, pressure and dermal ulcers, thermal burns, postoperative incisions, and dermatoses such as radiation dermatitis. The specific mechanisms for these effects have not been clarified. However, dexpanthenol is a precursor to pantothenic acid (vitamin B5). Pantothenic acid is a component of co-enzyme A which serves a critical role in cellular metabolism, for example in acyl group transfer during fatty acid biosynthesis and gluconeogenesis. By increasing skin lipid synthesis, an improved barrier would result, and improved barrier is expected to be beneficial to damaged skin such as from wounding. Additionally, panthenol has been shown to promote fibroblast prolifera-

tion and epidermal re-epithelializaion, effects that would promote wound healing. In addition, panthenol has also found utility for skin penetration enhancement.

Topical cosmeceutical effects

Topical panthenol is extremely well tolerated by the skin, not inducing skin irritation responses (redness, dryness, burn, sting, or itch responses). That mildness has led to wide topical use of this material and many reported skin benefits which have been reviewed previously. Among those are moisturization or hydration of the stratum corneum and the associated improvement in roughness, scaling, and epidermal elasticity; protection against skin irritation and SLS-induced damage; anti-inflammatory and antipruritic effects, for example on UV-induced erythema; and skin soothing.

Hydration

Panthenol's hydration effect likely derives from its hygroscopic properties. Panthenol has been shown to be an effective moisturizer of the stratum corneum, and to be even more effective when combined with the widely used moisturizing agent glycerol. In addition to its utility for increasing hydration of normal skin, it also has been shown to improve the dryness, roughness, scaling, pruritus, and erythema associated with a wide variety of skin problems such as atopic dermatitis, ichthyosis, psoriasis, and contact dermatitis. It also reduces the cutaneous side effects associated with retinoid therapy. This hydration effect has further led to its use in hair care, promoting improved elasticity, softening, and easier combing.

Barrier and irritation

For skin care, in addition to hydration, an important mechanism likely involved for this diversity of benefits is protection against irritation via improvement in and repair of skin barrier function. As illustration of the barrier enhancement effect, topical pretreatment with panthenol was observed to increase skin's resistance to subsequent exposure to the surfactant SLS as measured by resistance to visible irritation (Table 9.1). Since panthenol is the precursor to pantothenic acid which is a co-factor in barrier layer lipid biosynthesis, this could account

Prevention of SLS-induced erythema by topical panthenol		
Time point post SLS treatment	**Erythema score (0–6 scale) for skin treated with**	
	SLS	**Panthenol then SLS**
2 days	4.0	2.4
3 days	3.4	1.7
4 days	2.7	1.4

Table 9.1 Prevention of SLS-induced erythema by topical panthenol

Reduction in negative kinesthetic effects of formulation containing panthenol	
Visible or kinesthetic attribute	**Reduction in attribute by panthenol (0–6 scale)**
Redness	−1.4
Burning	−2.4
Tingling	−5.7
Stinging	−4.9
Itching	−4.9
Warming	−5.7

Table 9.2 Reduction in negative kinesthetic effects of formulation containing panthenol

for the noted barrier layer improvement. This barrier lipid impact is reminiscent of the effect noted above for niacinamide.

In addition to visible irritation (e.g. erythema), some patients are sensitive to specific components (e.g. certain preservatives, fragrances, sunscreen actives, etc.) in cosmetic formulations, leading to the induction of negative kinesthetic irritation effects such as burn, sting, itch, and tingling. Topical panthenol incorporated into such formulations can reduce those negative effects (Table 9.2). While the mechanism for this is not known, it could well be related to the reported soothing or anti-inflammatory effect of panthenol.

Discussion

Topical vitamin B3 and pro-vitamin B5 provide a variety of cosmeceutical skin effects. Their cosmeceutical effects encompass barrier enhancement, moisturization, and for the aging skin improvement in the appearance of texture, wrinkles, hyperpigmentation, red blotchiness, and yellowing. While there is still room to better understand their specific mechanisms in each of these benefit areas, there is currently a solid foundation of mechanistic learning that points the way for future experimentation. In topical use, these water soluble agents are non-irritating to facial skin, easily formulated, chemically stable, and compatible with other formulation components. They are thus ideal cosmeceuticals.

Further Reading

Biro K, Thaci D, Ochsendorf FR, Kaufmann R, Boehncke WH 2003 Efficacy of dexpanthenol in skin protection against irritation: a double-blind, placebo-controlled study. Contact Dermatitis 49:80–84

Bissett DL 2002 Topical niacinamide and barrier enhancement. Cutis 70S:8–12

Bissett DL, Mrowczynski E, Hicks S 2004 Retinyl propionate and niacinamide: reduction in excess dermal GAGs as a mechanism for their effects in improving the appearance of aging skin. Journal of the American Academy of Dermatology 50:S26

Bissett DL, Oblong JE, Saud A, Berge CA, Trejo AV, Biedermann KA 2003 Topical niacinamide provides skin aging appearance benefits while enhancing barrier function. Journal of Clinical Dermatology 32:S9–S18

Dunstan RW, Kennis RA 1994 Selected heritable diseases of domesticated animals. In: Sundberg JP (ed) Handbook of mouse mutations with skin and hair abnormalities. CRC Press, Boca Raton, pp 509–532

Dyer DG, Dunn JA, Thorpe SR, et al 1993 Accumulation of maillard reaction products in skin collagen in diabetes and aging. Journal of Clinical Investigation 91:2463–2469

Ebner F, Heller A, Rippke F, Tausch I 2002 Topical use of dexpanthenol in skin disorders. American Journal of Clinical Dermatology 3:427–433

Gloor M, Senger B, Gehring W 2002 Do dexpanthenol/glycerin combinations achieve better skin hydration than either component alone? Aktuelle Dermatologie 28:402–405

Gonzalez S, Moran M, Kochevar IE 1999 Chronic photodamage in skin of mast cell-deficient mice. Photochemistry and Photobiology 70:248–253

Hakozaki T, Minwalla L, Zhuang J, et al 2002 The effect of niacinamide on reducing cutaneous pigmentation and suppression of melanosome transfer. British Journal of Dermatology 147:22–33

Huntley AC 1993 Cutaneous manifestations of diabetes mellitus. Diabetes Metabolism Reviews 9:161–176

Kligman AM, Baker TJ, Gordan HL 1975 Long-term histologic follow-up of phenol face peels. Plastic and Reconstructive Surgery 75:652–659

Matts PJ, Oblong JE, Bissett DL 2002 A review of the range of effects of niacinamide in human skin. International Federation of the Society of Cosmetic Chemists Journal 5:285–289

Nozaki S, Sueki H, Fujisawa R, Aoki K, Kuroiwa Y 1988 Glycosylated proteins of stratum corneum, nail, and hair in diabetes mellitus: correlation with cutaneous manifestations. Journal of Dermatology 15:320–324

Odetti P, Pronzato MA, Noberasco G, et al 1994 Relationships between glycation and oxidation related fluorescence in rat collagen during aging. Laboratory Investigation 70:61–67

Proksch E, Nissen, HP 2002 Dexpanthenol enhances skin barrier repair and reduces inflammation after sodium lauryl sulphate-induced irritation. Journal of Dermatologic Treatment 13:173–178

Reber F, Geffarth R, Kasper M, et al 2003 Graded sensitiveness of the various retinal neuron populations on the glyoxal-mediated formation of advanced glycation end products and ways of protection. Graefes Archive for Clinical and Experimental Ophthalmology 241:213–225

Romiti R, Romiti N 2002 Dexpanthenol cream significantly improves mucocutaneous side effects associated with isotretinoin therapy. Pediatric Dermatology 19:368

Sauberlich HE 1980 Pantothenic acid. In: Goodhart RS, Shils ME (eds) Modern nutrition in health and disease. Lea and Febiger, Philadelphia, pp 209–216

Schwartz E, Kligman LH 1995 Topical tretinoin increases the tropoelastin and fibronectin content of photoaged hairless mouse skin. Journal of Investigative Dermatology 104:518–522

Shindo Y, Witt E, Han D, Epstein W, Packer L 1994 Enzymic and nonenzymic antioxidants in epidermis and dermis of human skin. Journal of Investigative Dermatology 102:122–124

Thornalley PJ 2002 Glycation in diabetic neuropathy: characteristics, consequences, causes, and therapeutic options. International Review of Neurobiology 50:37–57

Wozniacka A, Sysa-Jedrzejowska A, Adamus J, Gebicki J 2003 Topical application of NADH for the treatment of rosacea and contact dermatitis. Clinical and Experimental Dermatology 28:61–63

10

Physiological Lipids for Barrier Repair in Dermatology

Peter M. Elias

Introduction

Although the stratum corneum (SC) serves many defensive functions (Table 10.1), none is as important as its ability to prevent excess loss of fluids and electrolytes; i.e. the permeability barrier. Permeability barrier function is mediated by the organization of the extracellular lipids of the SC into a series of parallel lamellar membranes, which mediate not only permeability barrier function, but also additional, key protective functions of the epidermis (Fig. 10.1). The functions of the SC can be further localized to either the cellular (corneocyte) compartment or extracellular matrix (Table 10.1).

Dynamics of Barrier Recovery

The skin barrier is assaulted frequently in daily life by hot water, detergents, solvents, mechanical trauma, and occupation-related chemicals. If these insults are frequently repeatedly and/or insufficiently repaired, they threaten the organism with desiccation due to accelerated transepidermal water loss (TEWL). To avoid this outcome, the underlying epidermis mounts a coordinated metabolic response, ranging from increased lipid synthesis to accelerated lipid secretion, aimed at rapidly restoring normal function. This response is elicited by any type of barrier insult (e.g. organic solvents, detergents, tape stripping), that depletes the SC of its complement of lipids. Although the total time required for barrier recovery varies according to age, there is an initial, rapid recovery phase that leads to 50–60% recovery in young humans in about 12 hours, with full recovery requiring about 3 days (Fig. 10.2). But in aged humans (> 75 years), complete recovery from comparable insults is prolonged to about 1 week. Restoration of barrier function is accompanied by reaccumulation of lipids, visible with either oil red O staining or Nile

Protective functions of mammalian stratum corneum	
Function	**Localization**
Permeability barrier*	Extracellular
Initiation of inflammation (cytokine activation)*	Corneocyte (and granular cell)
Cohesion (Integrity) → Desquamation*	Extracellular
Antimicrobial barrier (innate immunity)*	Extracellular
Mechanical (impact and shear resistance)	Corneocyte
Toxic chemical/antigen exclusion	Extracellular
Selective absorption	Extracellular
Hydration	Corneocyte
UV barrier	Corneocyte
Psychosensory interface	Unknown
Thermal barrier	Unknown
*Regulated by SC pH.	

Table 10.1 Protective functions of mammalian stratum corneum

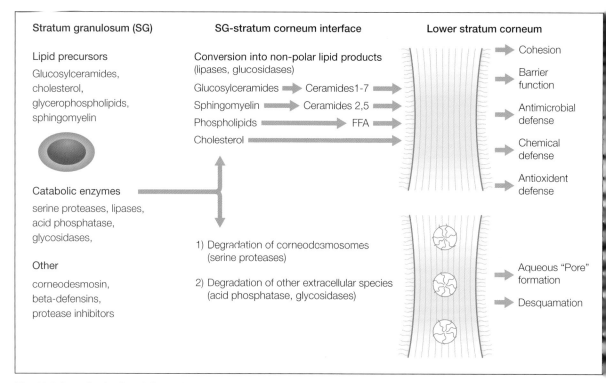

Fig. 10.1 Lamellar bodies deliver lipids and enzymes that mediate several key protective functions

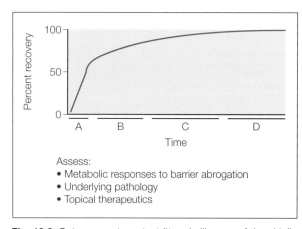

Assess:
• Metabolic responses to barrier abrogation
• Underlying pathology
• Topical therapeutics

Fig. 10.2 Cutaneous stress test ('treadmill exam of the skin') demonstrates the dynamic response of the epidermis to barrier disruption

red fluorescence, and by the reappearance of membrane structures within the SC interstices, as early as 2 hours after acute disruption. Because artificial restoration of the barrier with vapor-impermeable membranes inhibits barrier recovery, as well as all of the metabolic process linked to it, the entire

metabolic response represents a response that is aimed specifically at restoring normal permeability barrier homeostasis.

Clinical Applications of the Cutaneous Stress Test

The kinetics of barrier recovery after acute perturbations (also called the 'cutaneous stress test') can discern abnormal function or underlying pathology, even when basal parameters are normal (Fig. 10.2), analogous to the cardiac treadmill exam. Indeed, the cutaneous stress test reveals deficient barrier function both in aged and in neonatal skin, despite deceptively normal function in both age groups under basal conditions. Further, it amplifies differences between other 'normal' groups (Fig. 10.3):

■ testosterone-replete versus testosterone-deficient individuals
■ skin exposed to humid versus dry environments
■ individuals with type 5–6 versus 1–2 pigmentation

Finally, individuals subjected to increased psychologic stress reveal a defect in barrier recovery,

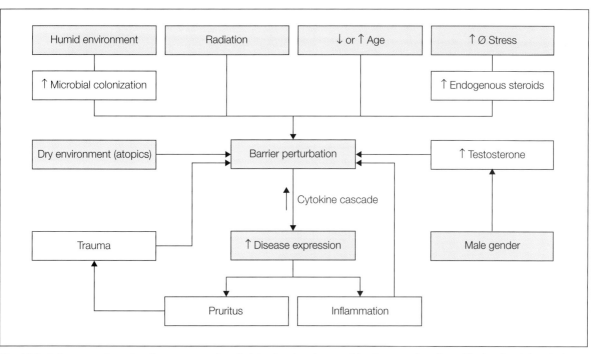

Fig. 10.3 Cutaneous stress test has uncovered underlying barrier abnormalities in several settings. The barrier defect in these instances could exacerbate inflammatory skin diseases via amplification of the cytokine cascade

explaining the propensity for these factors to exacerbate inflammatory dermatoses, such as psoriasis and atopic dermatitis, which already display barrier abnormalities. We have proposed that these factors further amplify the cytokine cascade that characterizes these disorders (Fig. 10.3).

Lipid Composition of Lamellar Membranes

The extracellular lipids in the SC derive primarily from the secreted contents of epidermal lamellar bodies (LB), which are enriched in cholesterol, glucosylceramide, phospholipids, as well as their respective hydrolytic enzymes (Fig. 10.1). These lipid-processing enzymes catalyze the extracellular degradation of sphingomyelin and glucosylceramides to ceramides (Cer), and phospholipids to free fatty acids (FFA), that along with cholesterol (Chol), form the lamellar membranes required for permeability barrier function. Thus, the SC lamellar membrane comprises unique biological membranes that mediate the barrier because:

- they lack phospholipids
- they are extremely hydrophobic

- their total lipid weight percentage in SC (= number of lamellae in the extracellular spaces)
- their presence in an equimolar mixture
- the presence of certain lipids, such as acylceramides, bearing linoleic acid.

Together, these characteristics largely explain the barrier properties of the SC.

Lipid Synthesis and Requirements for the Barrier

The formation of epidermal LB requires a coordinated synthesis of the major lipid components of LB; i.e. cholesterol, glucosylceramides, and phospholipids. Although the epidermis is a very active site of lipid synthesis even under basal conditions, permeability barrier disruption stimulates a further, marked increase in the synthesis of Chol, Cer, and FFA, which provides the pool of lipids that is required for the formation of new LB. However, synthesis of these lipids is not only **regulated** by barrier requirements, but it is also **required** for normal function. Using specific inhibitors of key lipid synthetic enzymes, we demonstrated an individual

Barrier recovery after various topical treatments				
	Recovery (%)			
Treatment (after acute perturbations)	**45 minutes**	**2 hours**	**4 hours**	**8 hours**
Air exposure or vehicle	15	25	35	55
Physiologic lipids* (incomplete)	15	20	25	35
Physiologic lipids (optimal)	10	55	75	90
Physiologic lipids (equimolar)	15	25	35	55
Petrolatum	50	50	50	40
Physiologic lipids* + petrolatum*	55	70	90	95

*Optimal
Optimal molar ratio: 3:1:1 (ceramides:free sterols:free fatty acids).
Equimolar ratio: 1:1:1.

Table 10.2 Barrier recovery after various topical treatments

requirement for Chol, FA, Cer, and glucosylceramide synthesis for barrier formation. In fact, blockade of these enzymes always produces a similar result: decreased LB, as well as a paucity of extracellular lamellar membranes. Thus, each of the three key lipids is required individually for permeability barrier function.

Equimolar distribution of the three key SC lipids

Whereas the above-described studies clearly demonstrate the **individual** requirement for Chol, FFA, and Cer for the permeability barrier, when these lipids are applied topically, they must be supplied in approximately equimolar proportions for normal barrier recovery to occur (Table 10.2). For example, topical applications of any one or two of the three key lipids to acutely perturbed skin actually delays barrier recovery (Table 10.2). Both incomplete and complete mixtures of the three key lipids rapidly traverse the SC, internalize within the granular cell layer, targeting the trans-Golgi network, where LB are formed (Fig. 10.4). Exogenous and endogenous lipids mix within nascent LB, producing normal or abnormal LB contents and derived lamellar membrane structures, depending on the molar distribution of the applied lipids. Barrier recovery can be further accelerated by increasing the proportion of any one of the three key lipids to a 3:1:1 ratio (Table 10.2 and Fig. 10.5). Thus, physiologic mixtures of topical lipids influence barrier function, not by partially occluding the SC, as do nonphysiologic

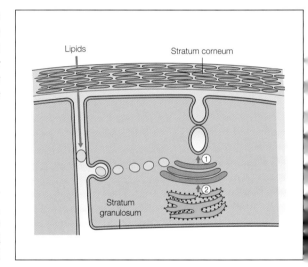

Fig. 10.4 Physiologic lipids traverse the stratum corneum, enter the nucleated cell layers, targeting the lamellar body secretory system

lipids (see below), but rather by contributing to the epidermal lipid pool that is delivered to the SC interstices.

Nonphysiologic Lipids: Mechanism of Action

In contrast to physiologic lipids, classic nonphysiologic lipids, such as petrolatum, do not enter the lipid-secretory pathway of the granular cell, and, in fact, they do not penetrate beneath the SC. They do, however, fully infiltrate the extracellular domains of the SC, where they form a hydrophobic,

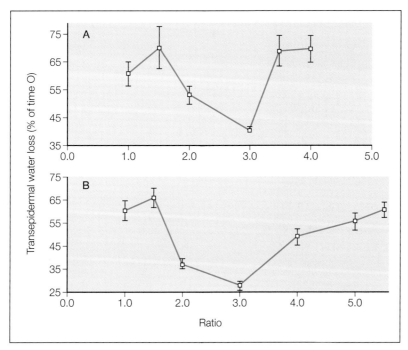

Fig. 10.5 Barrier repair accelerates (towards a '0' abnormality), as the proportion of any one of the three key lipids increases towards (but not beyond) 3:1:1. A: cholesterol; B: ceramides (from Man et al 1996)

nonlamellar phase that largely displaces the lamellar bilayers. These lipids, which include not only petrolatum, but also agents such as beeswax, lanolin, squalane, and a variety of other hydrocarbons, function largely as a vapor-permeable membrane; i.e. they reduce water loss immediately (Table 10.2) but not completely. In contrast, physiologic lipids display a lag time that reflects the time necessary for SC transport, endocytosis, secretion, and lamellar membrane formation (Table 10.2 – compare petrolatum to physiologic lipids; Fig. 10.4). Nonphysiologic lipids have the further advantage that they do not discriminate among types of barrier abnormalities, and the same degree of correction is achieved, regardless of the nature of the barrier disturbances. Further, it should be noted that the nonphysiologic lipids, though not components of the lamellar membranes, in some cases display a host of other, potentially beneficial properties, including anti-inflammatory, hydrating, waterproofing, and insulating characteristics. Because of the fundamental differences in their mechanisms, the two classes of molecules are complementary in improving barrier function (e.g. Table 10.2 – nonphysiologic plus physiologic).

Rationale for Barrier Repair Therapy

The contrasting features of nonphysiologic and physiologic lipids further dictate the clinical settings where each should be uniquely useful. While nonphysiologic lipids, like petrolatum, function like vapor-permeable membranes at the surface of the SC, physiologic lipids augment or supplement the epidermis's own lipid biosynthetic machinery. As noted above, many skin diseases are associated with barrier abnormalities, and other pathophysiologic insults, such as psychological stress or aging, can further aggravate these processes (Fig. 10.3). In some of these cases, e.g. psychological stress or glucocorticoid therapy, there is an equivalent, global reduction in lipid production. In others, e.g. aging and atopic dermatitis, the global reduction is aggravated by a further reduction in one of the three key species (see below).

Logically then, in these studies, bolstering epidermal barrier status should decrease susceptibility not only to these skin diseases, but also to others that are triggered, sustained, or exacerbated by external perturbations, most notably contact

Logical barrier repair strategies – clinical indications*	
Repair strategy	**Clinical indication**
Dressings Vapor-permeable Vapor-impermeable	Healing wounds Keloids
Nonphysiologic lipids (NPL) Petrolatum or Lanolin	Radiation dermattis or severe sunburn Premature infants (aged <34 weeks)
Physiologic lipids (PL):Optimal molar ratio Cholesterol-dominant Ceramide-dominant Free fatty acid-dominant Cholesterol-, ceramide-, or free fatty acid-dominant	Aging or photoaging Atopic dermatitis Neonatal skin, including psoriasis, diaper dermatitis (with added NPL) Irritant contact dermatitis (with added NPL) Glucocorticoid-treated (vehicle), psychological stress

Modified from Elias and Feingold (2001).

Table 10.3 Logical barrier repair strategies – clinical indications

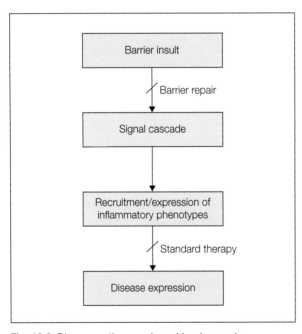

Fig. 10.6 Disease pathogenesis and barrier repair

Deployment of Barrier Repair Therapy

The recent emergence of 'barrier repair' therapy represents a set of pathophysiologically based strategies that should decrease the susceptibility to these and other disorders, characterized by barrier abnormalities. These repair approaches can be classified into three subcategories (Table 10.3):

- Optimized mixtures of the three **physiologic lipids** (ceramides, cholesterol, and free fatty acids) in appropriate molar ratios that correct underlying biochemical abnormalities in the targeted disease
- One or **more nonphysiologic** lipids (e.g. petrolatum, lanolin), which restore function transiently without correcting specific abnormalities.
- **Dressings**, either **vapor-permeable**, which allow metabolic (repair) processes to continue in the underlying epidermis, or **vapor-impermeable**, which shut down metabolic responses in the underlying epidermis.

Nevertheless, all of these strategies have their appropriate use and clinical indications. In fact, we can now choose an appropriate barrier strategy for a specific clinical indication based upon knowledge of disease pathogenesis (Table 10.3). For example atopic dermatitis (AD) is characterized by a global decrease in SC lipids with a steep reduction in ceramides attributable to increased sphingomyelin, glucosylceramide deacylase activity in affected

dermatitis and psoriasis (Fig. 10.6). In fact, in all skin disorders characterized by a barrier abnormality, the extent of the barrier abnormality parallels the extent of clinical severity, a further indication of the importance of the barrier abnormality for disease pathogenesis.

Effects of physiologic lipid mixtures on barrier recovery in young versus aged human skin		
Physiologic lipids	**Young**	**Aged**
Single lipid	Delays	Accelerates (cholesterol only)
Triple lipids (equimolar)	No change	Accelerates
Triple lipids (optimized):		
Fatty acid-dominant	Accelerates	Delays
Ceramide-dominant	Accelerates	Not studied
Cholesterol-dominant	Accelerates	Accelerates

Physiologic lipids = free fatty acids, cholesterol, ceramides (modified from Zettersten et al 1997).

Table 10.4 Effects of physiologic lipid mixtures on barrier recovery in young versus aged human skin

epidermis. Hence, the logic, and recent apparent success, of a ceramide-dominant mixture of the three physiologic lipids as ancillary therapy in AD. In contrast, aged and photoaged epidermis exhibits a global reduction in SC lipids, with a further decrease in cholesterol synthesis. Hence, the success of a cholesterol-dominant mixture of physiological lipids in this setting. So critical is choice of proper formulation that substitution of an FFA-dominant mixture for the cholesterol-dominant version drastically delays barrier recovery in aged skin (Table 10.4). Yet, there are several clinical situations where physiologic lipids might not be effective, if deployed alone, due to an impaired LB secretory system. These examples include: radiation dermatitis (both UV-B and x-irradiation), very premature infants (i.e. < 33 weeks), and perhaps the initial stages of wound healing. In such situations, nonphysiologic lipids or vapor-permeable dressing alone, with or without added physiologic lipids, would become the most logical choice.

This chapter has addressed some of the new understandings regarding barrier function and the role of ceramides. The ideas are nicely summarized in Table 10.4 where the effects of physiologic lipid mixtures on barrier recovery in young versus aged skin are compared. Note that the relationship between the components of the intercellular lipids, consisting of fatty acids, ceramides, and cholesterol, may affect the ability of the skin to effect barrier repair. In contrast, ceramide containing lipid mixtures represent an interesting cosmeceutical that may have an important role in atopic dermatisis (Table 10.3).

Further Reading

Altemus M, Rao B, Dhabhar FS, Ding W, Granstein RD 2001 Stress-induced changes in skin barrier function in healthy women. Journal of Investigative Dermatology 117:309–317

Behne MJ, Barry NP, Hanson KM, Aronchik I, Clegg RW, Gratton E, Feingold K, Holleran WM, Elias PM, Mauro TM 2003 Neonatal development of the stratum corneum pH gradient: localization and mechanisms leading to emergence of optimal barrier function. Journal of Investigative Dermatology 120:998–1006

Chamlin SL, Kao J, Frieden IJ, Sheu MY, Fowler AJ, Fluhr JW, Williams ML, Elias PM 2002 Ceramide-dominant barrier repair lipids alleviate childhood atopic dermatitis: changes in barrier function provide a sensitive indicator of disease activity. Journal of American Academy of Dermatology 47:198–208

Denda M, Sato J, Masuda Y, Tsuchiya T, Koyama J, Kuramoto M, Elias PM, Feingold KR 1998 Exposure to a dry environment enhances epidermal permeability barrier function. Journal of Investigative Dermatology 111:858–863

Elias PM, Feingold KR 2001 Does the tail wag the dog? Role of the barrier in the pathogenesis of inflammatory dermatoses and therapeutic implications. Archives of Dermatology 137:1079–1081

Elias PM, Feingold KR 2003 Skin as an organ of protection In: Freedberg I. et al, editors. Fitzpatrick's Dermatology in General Medicine. Philadelphia: McGraw-Hill, pp.164–174

Elias PM, Menon GK 1991 Structural and lipid biochemical correlates of the epidermal permeability barrier. Advances in Lipid Research 24:1–26

Elias PM, Wood LC, Feingold KR 1999 Epidermal pathogenesis of inflammatory dermatoses. American Journal of Contact Dermatitis 10:119–126

Feingold KR 1991 The regulation and role of epidermal lipid synthesis. Advances in Lipid Research 24:57–82

Garg A, Chren MM, Sands LP, Matsui MS, Marenus KD, Feingold KR, Elias PM 2001 Psychological stress perturbs epidermal permeability barrier homeostasis: implications for the pathogenesis of stress-associated skin disorders. Archives of Dermatology 137:53–59

Ghadially R, Brown BE, Sequeira-Martin SM, Feingold KR, Elias PM 1995 The aged epidermal permeability barrier. Structural, functional, and lipid biochemical abnormalities in humans and a senescent murine model. Journal of Clinical Investigations 95:2281–2290

Ghadially R, Halkier-Sorensen L, Elias PM 1992 Effects of petrolatum on stratum corneum structure and function. Journal of American Academy of Dermatology 26:387–396

Ghadially R, Reed JT, Elias PM 1996 Stratum corneum structure and function correlates with phenotype in psoriasis. Journal of Investigative Dermatology 107:558–564

Grubauer G, Elias PM, Feingold KR 1989 Transepidermal water loss: the signal for recovery of barrier structure and function. Journal of Lipid Research 30:323–333

Halkier-Sorensen L, Menon GK, Elias PM, Thestrup-Pedersen K, Feingold KR 1995 Cutaneous barrier function after cold exposure in hairless mice: a model to demonstrate how cold interferes with barrier homeostasis among workers in the fish-processing industry. British Journal of Dermatology 132:391–401

Hara J, Higuchi K, Okamoto R, Kawashima M, Imokawa G 2000 High-expression of sphingomyelin deacylase is an important determinant of ceramide deficiency leading to barrier disruption in atopic dermatitis. Journal of Investigative Dermatology 115:406–413

Holleran WM, Uchida Y, Halkier-Sorensen L, Haratake A, Hara M, Epstein JH, Elias PM 1997 Structural and biochemical basis for the UVB-induced alterations in epidermal barrier function. Photodermatology Photoimmunology Photomedicine 13:117–128

Imokawa G, Abe A, Jin K, Higaki Y, Kawashima M, Hidano A 1991 Decreased level of ceramides in stratum corneum of atopic dermatitis: an etiologic factor in atopic dry skin? Journal of Investigative Dermatology 96:523–526

Kao JS, Garg A, Mao-Qiang M, Crumrine D, Ghadially R, Feingold KR, Elias PM 2001 Testosterone perturbs epidermal permeability barrier homeostasis. Journal of Investigative Dermatology 116:443–451

Man MQ, Feingold KR, Elias PM 1993 Exogenous lipids influence permeability barrier recovery in acetone-treated murine skin. Archives of Dermatology 129:728–738

Man MM, Feingold KR, Thornfeldt CR, Elias PM 1996 Optimization of physiological lipid mixtures for barrier repair. Journal of Investigations in Dermatology 106:1096–1101

Mao-Qiang M, Brown BE, Wu-Pong S, Feingold KR, Elias PM 1995 Exogenous nonphysiologic versus physiologic lipids. Divergent mechanisms for correction of permeability barrier dysfunction. Archives of Dermatology 131:809–816

Proksch E, Jensen JM, Elias PM 2003 Skin lipids and epidermal differentiation in atopic dermatitis. Clinics in Dermatology 21:134–144

Reed JT, Ghadially R, Elias PM 1995 Skin type, but neither race nor gender, influence epidermal permeability barrier function. Archives of Dermatology 131:1134–1138

Schmuth M, Sztankay A, Weinlich G, Linder DM, Wimmer MA, Fritsch PO, Fritsch E 2001 Permeability barrier function of skin exposed to ionizing radiation. Archives of Dermatology 137:1019–1023

Sugarman JL, Fluhr JW, Fowler AJ, Bruckner T, Diepgen TL, Williams ML 2003 The objective severity assessment of atopic dermatitis score: an objective measure using peermeability barrier function and stratum corneum hydration with computer-assisted estimates for extent of disease. Archives of Dermatology 139:1417–1422

Williams ML, Elias PM 2003 Enlightened therapy of the disorders of cornification. Clinics in Dermatology 21:269–273

Zettersten EM, Ghadially R, Feingold KR, Crumrine D, Elias PM 1997 Optimal ratios of topical stratum corneum lipids improve barrier recovery in chronologically aged skin. Journal of American Academy of Dermatology 37:403–408

Cosmeceutical Botanicals: Part 1

11

Zoe Diana Draelos

Introduction

Botanicals form the largest category of cosmeceutical additives found in the marketplace today. They are plant extracts from leaves, roots, fruits, berries, stems, twigs, barks, and flowers. Crushing, grinding, boiling, distilling, pressing, and drying can prepare the extracts. They can be easily added to cleansers, moisturizers, astringents, treatment creams, colored cosmetics, and face masks. Their popularity as cosmeceutical additives can be attributed to the fact that they are an unregulated category of ingredients that fit nicely into over-the-counter products. Botanical additives for topical application are considered safe by the United States Food and Drug Administration, thus allowing the products to be marketed without obtaining drug status or being restricted by monographed ingredients.

Historically, botanicals formed the basis of all medical treatments at the time European settlers were first coming to America. These Europeans learned that the American Indians had an extensive pharmacopeia, based on native plants, that was passed from generation to generation through the wisdom of the medicine man in each community. These plant concoctions were mastered by the settlers, transported back to England, and incorporated into some of the earliest books on medical treatment. When the new English settlers were learning about North American plant extracts, a large body of knowledge utilizing plants from the Orient was also being developed. The richness of plant material in the tropical Orient led to different plant extracts of great diversity that were used in Oriental medicine and religious practices. Today cosmetic formulators have access to plant materials worldwide for incorporation into cosmeceuticals.

Botanical Additive Manufacture

The popularity of botanicals is largely due to the aura of natural products. Products derived from plants are felt to be free of synthetic chemicals, somehow providing benefits above and beyond active agents that are created in a laboratory. It may come as a surprise to many that botanicals must undergo a significant amount of chemical processing prior to incorporation into a cosmeceutical and this processing greatly affects the biologic effect of the botanical on the skin surface. Box 11.1 summarizes some of these considerations, which are discussed next.

The most important factor contributing to the biological activity of botanical cosmeceuticals is the source of the plant material. The chemical constituents of the leaves, berries, stems, roots, and

---

Botanical formulation considerations

Plant source
Leaves, roots, fruits, berries, stems, twigs, barks, flowers

Growing conditions
Soil composition, amount of available water, climate variations, plant stress

Harvesting conditions
Time from harvest to transport, care of plant materials during shipping, storage conditions prior to manufacture

Preparation method
Crushing, grinding, boiling, distilling, pressing, drying

Final extract status
Liquid, powder, paste, syrup, crystal

Concentration
Sufficient amount of activity to produce biological effect

Box 11.1 Botanical formulation considerations

Botanical cosmeceutical categories	
Category	**Botanical additive**
Antioxidant	Soy, curcumin, silymarin, pycnogenol
Anti-inflammatory	*Gingko biloba*, green tea
Soothing agent	Prickly pear, aloe vera, allantoin, witch hazel, papaya

Table 11.1 Botanical cosmeceutical categories

Nutritionally derived botanical cosmeceutical antioxidants	
Common botanical name	**Chemical class**
Rutin (apples, blueberries)	Flavone
Quercetin (apples, blueberries)	Flavone
Hesperedin (lemons, oranges)	Flavone
Diosmin (lemons, oranges)	Flavone
Mangiferin (mango plant)	Xanthone
Mangostin (bilberry plant)	Xanthone
Astaxanthin (tomatoes)	Carotenoid
Lutein (tomatoes)	Carotenoid
Lycopene (tomatoes)	Carotenoid
Rosmarinic acid (rosemary)	Polyphenol
Hypericin (St John's wort)	Polyphenol
Ellagic acid (pomegranate fruit)	Polyphenol
Chlorogenic acid (blueberry leaf)	Polyphenol
Oleuropein (olive leaf)	Polyphenol

Table 11.2 Nutritionally derived botanical cosmeceutical antioxidants

flowers may be different, each containing over 200 different individual chemical constituents. Furthermore, the season in which the plant material was gathered may also greatly influence its composition. Certain actives are present only in the fall when the leaves are shedding while other actives are only present in early spring when immature leaves are present on the branches.

It is also important to consider the processing that a plant-derived material must undergo before it can be placed in a skin care product. Raw crushed leaves added to a moisturizer will not provide an esthetically pleasing result. Usually, the plant material is heated or processed to obtain essential oils or other distillates that can be easily added to a cosmetic formulation, however heating may destroy some of the active chemicals providing skin benefits.

Lastly, the amount of the active in the botanical extract is important in determining efficacy. Sometimes the botanical active is added in small amounts providing more marketing benefit than skin benefit, however many botanicals are only required in low concentrations to provide the desired effect. In an attempt to obtain some standardization of botanical fractions, many raw material manufacturers procure the actual plant materials and determine which fraction produces the desired effect. This fraction, which may be a particular turpene, for example, is analyzed carefully to isolate its chemical composition. Once the mass spectrophotometry is completed, a synthetic copy can be created. In some ways these synthetic copies are better since they eliminate some of the variability associated with plant materials grown in various environments at various times of year. It is also possible to concentrate the active agent. However, there are some that feel plant materials can never be accurately duplicated by organic chemistry.

Botanical Additives

Botanical pharmacopoeias contain thousands of plants with anecdotal purported skin benefits lacking scientific validation. It is not possible to cover all currently existing extracts in this text, yet there are some botanicals that are currently widely used in the cosmeceutical marketplace. These botanicals can be characterized as antioxidants, anti-inflammatories, and skin-soothing agents (Table 11.1).

Botanical Antioxidants

There are many botanical antioxidants, since all plants must protect themselves from oxidation following UV exposure in the outdoor environment in which they grow. These protective mechanisms have evolved over many years providing interesting chemicals for extraction and incorporation into cosmeceuticals. Antioxidant botanicals quench singlet oxygen and reactive oxygen species, such as superoxide anions, hydroxyl radicals, fatty peroxy radicals, and hydroperoxides. Most botanical antioxidants can be classified as flavonoids, carotenoids, and polyphenols. Flavonoids and polyphenols possess a polyphenolic structure accounting for their antioxidant effect while carotenoids are derivatives of vitamin A. The largest source of botanical antioxidants is foods, such as those listed in Table 11.2. These extracts can be used topically, as well as consumed.

Botanical cosmeceutical antioxidant agents		
Antioxidant	**Chemical classification of antioxidant fraction**	**Cosmeceutical active**
Soy	Flavonoids	Genistein, daidzein
Curcumin	Polyphenol	Tetrahydrocurcumin
Silymarin	Flavonoids	Silybin, silydianin, silychristine
Pycnogenol	Phenols, phenolic acids	Phenolic constituents: taxifolin, catechin, procyanidins Phenolic acids: *p*-hydroxybenzoic, protocatechuic, gallic, vanillic, *p*-couric, caffeic, ferulic acids

Table 11.3 Botanical cosmeceutical antioxidant agents

Other popular botanical antioxidants include soy, curcumin, silymarin, and pycnogenol (Table 11.3).

Soy (Fig. 11.1)

Soybeans are a rich source of antioxidant flavonoids, known as genistein and daidzein. These substances have also been classified as phytoestrogens, since they are plant derivatives with a chemical structure similar to human estrogen. Topical estrogens have been shown to function as cosmeceuticals by increasing skin thickness and promoting collagen synthesis. It is interesting to note that genistein increases collagen gene expression in cell culture, however there are no published reports of this collagen-stimulating effect in topical human trials. Genestein is a popular cosmeceutical topically functioning as a potent antioxidant scavenging peroxyl radicals and protecting against lipid peroxidation in vivo.

Curcumin (Fig. 11.2)

Curcumin is a polyphenol antioxidant derived from the turmeric root. Turmeric is a popular natural yellow food coloring sometimes used to color cosmeceuticals claiming to be free of artificial ingredients. Curcumin is consumed orally as an Asian spice, frequently found in rice dishes to color the otherwise white rice yellow. However, this yellow color is sometimes undesirable in cosmetic preparations, since yellowing of products is typically associated with oxidative spoilage. Tetrahydrocurcumin, a hydrogenated form of curcumin, is off-white in color and can be added to skin care products not

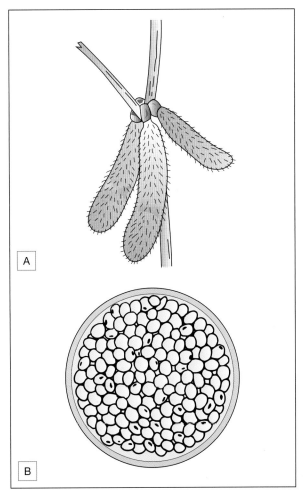

Fig. 11.1 Soybeans

Botanical cosmeceutical anti-inflammatory agents		
Anti-inflammatory	**Chemical classification of anti-inflammatory**	**Cosmeceutical active**
Gingko biloba	Polyphenol fraction Flavonoids fraction	Ginkgolides, bilobalides Quercetin, kaempferol, sciadopitysin, ginkgetin, isoginkgetin
Green tea	Polyphenols	Epigallocatechin, epigallocatechin-3-gallate

Table 11.4 Botanical cosmeceutical anti-inflammatory agents

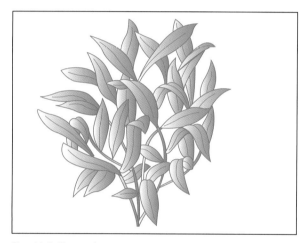

Fig. 11.2 Curcumin

only to function as a skin antioxidant, but also to prevent the lipids in the moisturizer from becoming rancid. The antioxidant effect of tetrahydrocurcumin is said to be greater than vitamin E by cosmetic chemists. Resveratrol, a chemical related to curcumin, is found in red wine accounting for the antioxidant effect of this beverage. Thus, curcumin is a multifunctional ingredient providing cosmeceutical antioxidant benefits and also functioning as an antioxidant preservative.

Silymarin

Silymarin is an extract of the milk thistle plant, botanically known as *Silbum marianum*. It belongs to the aster family of plants, which includes daisies, thistles, and artichokes. The extract consists of three flavonoids derived from the fruit, seeds, and leaves of the plant. These flavonoids are silybin, silydianin, and silychristine. Silymarin is a strong antioxidant preventing lipid peroxidation by scavenging free

radical species. A 92% reduction in UVB-induced skin tumors in topical silymarin-treated hairless mice has been demonstrated. The mechanism for this decrease in tumor production is unknown, but topical silymarin has been shown to decrease the formation of pyrimidine dimers in a mouse model.

Pycnogenol

Pycnogenol is a botanical cosmeceutical antioxidant derived from an extract of French marine pine bark. It is botanically known as *Pinus pinaster* and is a water-soluble liquid that contains several phenolic constituents, including taxifolin, catechin, and procyanidins. It also contains several phenolic acids, including *p*-hydroxybenzoic, protocatechuic, gallic, vanillic, *p*-couric, caffeic, and ferulic acids. It is a potent free radical scavenger that can reduce the vitamin C radical, returning the vitamin C to its active form. The active vitamin C in turn regenerates vitamin E to its active form maintaining the natural oxygen scavenging mechanisms of the skin intact.

Botanical Anti-inflammatories

Botanical anti-inflammatory additives are used in many different cosmeceuticals, since aging is in part the end result of chronic inflammation. Commonly used botanical anti-inflammatories include: *Ginkgo biloba* and green tea (Table 11.4).

Ginkgo biloba (Fig. 11.3)

Ginkgo biloba is a plant with numerous purported benefits that is a common part of homeopathic medicine in the Orient. The plant leaves are said to contain unique polyphenols such as terpenoids (ginkgolides, bilobalides), flavonoids, and flavonol

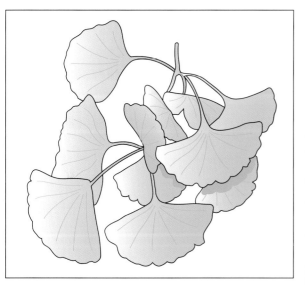

Fig. 11.3 Ginkgo biloba

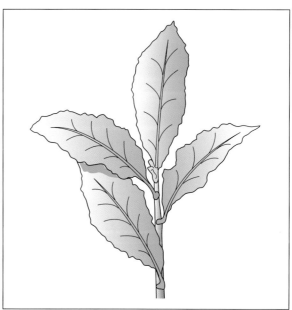

Fig. 11.4 Green tea

glycosides that have anti-inflammatory effects. These anti-inflammatory effects have been linked to antiradical and antilipoperoxidant effects in experimental fibroblast models. *Ginkgo* flavonoid fractions containing quercetin, kaempferol, sciadopitysin, ginkgetin, and isoginkgetin have been demonstrated to induce human skin fibroblast proliferation in vitro. Increased collagen and extracellular fibronectin were also demonstrated by radioisotope assay. Various unknown *Ginkgo* fractions are added to skin moisturizers for anti-aging benefits, even though no controlled trials exist regarding cutaneous benefits.

Green tea (Fig. 11.4)

Green tea is a botanical popular in the Orient for both topical application and oral ingestion. Orally, green tea is said to contain beneficial flavonoids that act as potent endogenous antioxidants. A study by Katiyar et al demonstrated the anti-inflammatory effect of topical green tea application with C3H mice. A topically applied green tea extract containing the polyphenol epigallocatechin-3-gallate was found to reduce UVB-induced inflammation. This has been validated by measuring skin fold thickness before and after UVB exposure, which correlates with tissue edema, a sign of inflammation. Even though this is the cosmeceutical industry standard for assessing inflammation, it is a difficult test to replicate and may not directly correlate with a human response. At present, green tea remains a

nutritional supplement and not an approved sun protective agent.

Botanical Skin-Soothing Agents

Botanical cosmeceuticals can also be used for the purpose of skin soothing. While this is a somewhat nebulous term, skin-soothing agents claim to calm, normalize, replenish, or relax the skin. Botanicals with these properties include prickly pear, aloe vera, allantoin, witch hazel, and papaya (Table 11.5). These plants have been selected for discussion due to their current novelty and popularity.

Prickly pear (Fig. 11.5)

Prickly pear, a plant native to the southwestern desert, is also known as cactus pear, Indian pear, or tuna fig. It was imported to Europe in the sixteenth century and became a part of a salve designed to soothe cutaneous wounds and burns. The fleshy pad of the prickly pear contains 83% water and 10% sucrose with small amounts of tartaric acid, citric acid, and other mucopolysaccharides. American Indians would rub the mucilage from the broken pad over the skin surface to act as a sunscreen and moisturizer.

Mucilages in general have a soothing cooling effect on the skin, due to evaporation of water, when the

Botanical cosmeceutical skin soothing agents		
Skin soothing agent	**Chemical classification of skin soothing agent**	**Cosmeceutical active**
Prickly pear	Mucilage containing 83% water and 10% sucrose	Tartaric acid, citric acid, and mucopolysaccharides
Aloe vera	Muclilage containing 99.5% water and a mixture of mucopolysaccharides, amino acids, hydroxy quinone glycosides, and minerals	Aloin, aloe emodin, aletinic acid, choline, and choline salicylate
Allantoin	Comfrey root	Alkaline oxidation of uric acid in a cold environment
Witch hazel	Leaf, stem distillate	Tannins
Papaya	Proteolytic enzyme	Papain

Table 11.5 Botanical cosmeceutical skin soothing agents

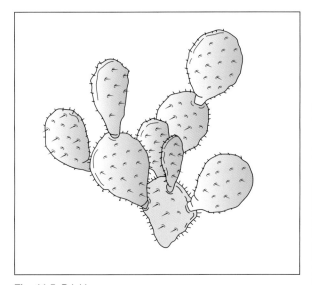

Fig. 11.5 Prickly pear

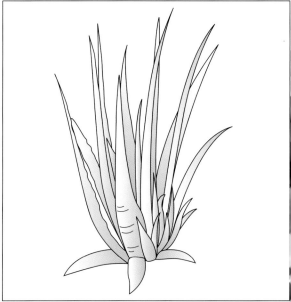

Fig. 11.6 Aloe vera

plant juice is rubbed over the skin. Additionally, the mucopolysaccharides dry to form a protective coating over wounded or dermatitic skin. An extract of prickly pear is found in some moisturizer formulations. However, the extract is added as a dried powder and not as a mucilage which defeats the skin-soothing benefits for the most part. Nevertheless, prickly pear juice is found in a variety of skin care products.

Aloe vera (Fig. 11.6)

Probably the most widely used botanical additive to soothe the skin is aloe vera. The mucilage is released from the plant leaves as a colorless gel and contains 99.5% water and a complex mixture of mucopolysaccharides, amino acids, hydroxy quinone glycosides, and minerals. Compounds isolated from aloe vera juice include aloin, aloe emodin, aletinic acid, choline, and choline salicylate. The reported cutaneous effects of aloe vera include increased blood flow, reduced inflammation, decreased skin bacterial colonization, and enhanced wound healing.

In most skin preparations, aloe vera is added as a powder, not as a mucilage. The composition of aloe vera powder may not be the same as aloe vera juice

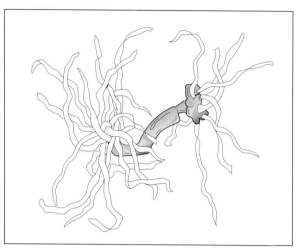

Fig. 11.7 Witch hazel

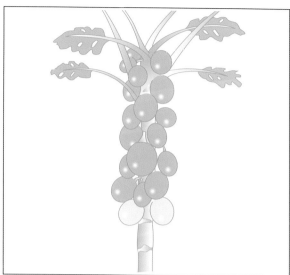

Fig. 11.8 Papaya

that oozes from the freshly broken plant leaf. Aloe vera extract is found in soaps, hair shampoos, hand lotions, body moisturizers, etc. It is estimated that aloe vera must be present at a concentration of 10% to have a moisturizing effect in products designed to remain on the skin for extended periods of time.

Allantoin

Allantoin is a currently popular botanical extract that is obtained from the comfrey root. It is the active ingredient upon which sensitive skin claims are made for a number of facial moisturizers. Interestingly, the source of allantoin in the current cosmeceutical market is not botanically derived, but rather manufactured by the alkaline oxidation of uric acid in a cold environment. It is a white crystalline powder that is readily soluble in hot water, making it easy to formulate in a variety of products. Allantoin is felt to induce cell proliferation.

Witch hazel (Fig. 11.7)

Witch hazel is a botanical extract most commonly used as an astringent in persons with oily skin. The plant was originally discovered by the Indians of the New England area of the United States. The extract is prepared by boiling the twigs and leaves of the plant, which grows as a low bush. The leaves can also be crushed and applied to the skin as a paste. The astringent action of witch hazel is probably due to the high tannin content of the plant.

Many cosmeceutical vein treatments contain witch hazel extract, since the tannins of the plant

function as venous vasoconstrictors. Whether vasoconstriction can be achieved through topical application remains unknown. Witch hazel ointments, known as *Hamamelis* ointments, are used as acne cosmeceuticals.

Papaya (Fig. 11.8)

Latex from the unripened fruit of the papaya plant, also known as the paw paw plant, is rich in papain. Papain is a proteolytic enzyme that is used in cosmeceutical wound healing and scar creams. It is also present in creams designed to speed the resolution of bruises.

Summary

Botanical cosmeceuticals provide endless opportunities to add new marketing interest to traditional cleansers and moisturizers. Some botanicals actually contain substances that may provide skin benefits, while others are of questionable value. It is the knowledge base of the dermatologist that will ultimately determine those which are of patient value.

Further Reading

Chatterjee L, Agarwal R, Mukhtar H 1996 Ultraviolet B radiation-induced DNA lesions in mouse epidermis: an assessment using a novel ^{32}P-postlabeling technique. Biochemical and Biophysical Research Communications 229:590–595

Cossins E, Lee R, Packer L 1998 ESR studies of vitamin C regeneration, order of reactivity of natural source phytochemical preparations. Biochemistry and Molecular Bioliogy International 45:583–598

Devaraj S, Vega-Lopez S, Kaul N, Schonlau F, Rohdewald P, Jialal I 2002 Supplementation with a pine bark extract rich in polyphenols increases plasma antioxidant capacity and alters the plasma lipoprotein profile. Lipids 37:931–934

Glazier MG, Bowman MA 2001 A review of the evidence for the use of phytoestrogens as a replacement for traditional estrogen replacement therapy. Archives of Internal Medicine 161:1161–1172

Joyeux M, Lobstein A, Anton R, Mortier F 1995 Comparative antilipoperoxidant, antinecrotic and scavenging properties of terpenes and biflavones from Ginkgo and some flavonoids. Plant Medicine 61:126–129

Katiyar SK, Elmets CA, Agarwal R, et al 1995 Protection against ultraviolet-B radiation-induced local and systemic suppression of contact hypersensitivity and edema responses in C3H/HeN mice by green tea polyphenols. Photochemistry and Photobiology 62:855–861

Katiyar SK, Korman NJ, Mukhtar H, Agarwal R 1997 Protective effects of silymarin against photocarcinogenesis in a mouse skin model. Journal of the National Cancer Institute 89:556–566

Kim SJ, Lim MH, Chun IK, Won YH 1997 Effects of flavonoids of Ginkgo biloba on proliferation of human skin fibroblast. Skin Pharmacology 10:200–205

McKeown E 1987 Aloe vera. Cosmetics and Toiletries 102:64–65

Maheux R, Naud F, Rioux M, et al 1994 A randomized, double-blind, placebo-controlled study on the effect of conjugated estrogens on skin thickness. American Journal of Obstetrics and Gynecology 170:642–649

Schonlau F 2002 The cosmetic Pycnogenol. Journal of Applied Cosmetology 20:241–246

Waller T 1992 Aloe vera. Cosmetics and Toiletries 107:53–54

Wiseman H, O'Reilly JD, Adlercreutz H, et al 2000 Isoflavone phytoestrogens consumed in soy decrease F-2-isoprostane concentrations and increase resistance of low-density lipoprotein to oxidation in humans. Am J Clin Nutr 72:395–400

12

Cosmeceutical Botanicals: Part 2

Carl R. Thornfeldt

Introduction

The dawning of this new century has seen sales of consumer products based on single botanicals grow to over $4 billion per annum. Now over 60 different botanicals are integral components of cosmeceutical products. Botanical product growth has burgeoned to 25% of all health and lifestyle related products in dollar value. Thus dermatologists must have a working knowledge of these botanicals to optimally provide medical care and answer patient's questions.

Botanicals used for medicinals, flavorings, or fragrances are known as herbs. These are the historic foundation of pharmacologic medicine. An understanding of the significant science underlying the function of the botanical base is usually lacking. Specific issues include: (i) complete characterization of the huge number of active compounds in a single plant source; (ii) documenting the activity and interaction of each of these compounds and their many metabolites; (iii) understanding the therapeutic synergy of these active components within the single plant and between multiple plants; and (iv) discovering how the potential toxicity of specific compounds is modified by using an entire plant or an anatomic structure of the plant. For example, the castor bean is the source of ricin, one of the most poisonous compounds known to man, and azelaic acid, a nontoxic prescription dermatologic medicine.

Several botanical treatments for cutaneous diseases have stood the test of time for their effectiveness, as documented by modern scientific evidence. Podophyllotoxin is a prescription product for the treatment of condyloma/verruca that is extracted from the mayapple (*Podophyllum peltatum*). Capsaicin is a nonprescription therapy for pruritis and pain extracted from cayenne peppers (*Capsicum annuum*).

In the USA, botanical remedies are considered dietary supplements or food additives by federal regulators so there are no standards for potency of the components and efficacy of the products. In 2003, the Food and Drug Administration removed ephedra or ma huang (*Ephedra sinica*) from the market due to 155 deaths. The German E Commission regulates botanical products based on usage, clinical efficacy, and the quality of this evidence. It then developed standardization of botanical products which permeated throughout Europe. Such regulation is more important with botanicals because the time of harvest, preparation of the herb, and final product, as well as specific combinations of herbs, can substantially alter solubility, stability, pharmacokinetics, pharmacologic activity, and toxicity.

Most of the 50% of the US population who use alternative botanical products believe all natural products are safe. Yet topical applications can give rise to severe reactions, such as Stevens–Johnson syndrome, lupus erythematosus, Sweet's syndrome, and exfoliative erythroderma, although very rarely. These reactions are usually reported with unadulterated botanical products.

The methods of topical application of botanicals include: (i) water based cream and lotion; (ii) oil and wax based ointment; (iii) powder and paste; (iv) poultice of freshly cut herb; (v) fomentation or compress of warmed moistened herb; and (vi) juice, tea, tincture, elixir, decoction, and infusion.

The botanicals of known and potential dermatologic significance are divided into therapeutic categories and specific indications in Tables 12.1–12.8. Many botanicals have excellent functionality in several different categories. The major botanicals discussed below are based on descending order of domestic sales.

Botanical therapeutic categories	
Category	**Indications**
Aging	Photoaging Skin cancer prevention
Alopecia	Areata Androgenic Antiandrogen
Infections	Bacterial Condyloma/warts Herpes Scabies Tinea/onychomycosis/yeast
Inflammation	Acne Dermatitis Psoriasis In vitro anti-inflammatory
Injury	Atrophy Bruising Burns/wounds/ulcers
Relief	Soothing Anesthetic/counter irritants Pruritis
Systemic	Chronic venous insufficiency Immunostimulatory

Table 12.1 Botanical therapeutic categories

Aging	
Indication	**Botanical**
Photoaging	EUOL tea (*Eucommia ulmoides oliver*) Soy (*Glycine soja*) Grape Seed (*Vitis vinifera*) Pomegranate (*Punica granatum*) Green and black teas (*Camellia sinensis*) Echinacea (*Echinacea purpurea*, *pallida* and *angustifolia*) Avocado (*Persea americana*) Garlic (*Allium sativa*)
Skin cancer prevention	Rosemary (*Rosmarinus officinalis*) Ginseng (*Panax ginseng*) Silymarin (*Silybum marinuum*) Green, black, oolong, white teas (*Camellia sinensis*) Garlic (*Allium sativa*) Spearmint (*Mentae spica*) Ginger (*Zingiber officinale*) Pomegranate (*Punica granatum*)

Table12.2 Aging

Alopecia	
Indication	**Botanical**
Areata	Essential oil mixture of thyme, rosemary, lavender, cedarwood, grapeseed, and jojoba
Androgenic	Dabao (10 Chinese herbs) Apple (*Malus domestica*)
Antiandrogen/antiestrogen	Saw palmetto (*Serenoa repens*)

Table 12.3 Alopecia

Infections	
Indication	**Botanical**
Bacterial	Arnica (*Arnica montana*) St John's Wort (*Hypericum perforatum*) Tea tree (*Melaleuca alternifolia*) Chamomile (*Matricaria recutita*) Bittersweet nightshade (*Solanum dulcamara*) Burdock (*Arctium lappa*) Yellow dock (*Rumex crispus*) Alder (*Alnus serrulata*) Garlic (*Allium sativum*) Oregon grape root (*Berberis aquafolium*) Echinacea (*Echinacea purpurea*, *pallida* and *angustifolia*)
Condyloma/verruca	Podophyllotoxin (*Podophyllum peltatum*) Bittersweet nightshade (*Solanum dulcamara*) Calatropis (*Calotropic procera*) Celandrine (*Chelidonium majus*) Oat straw (*Avena sativa*) Garlic (*Allium sativum*) White willow (*Salix* species)
Herpes	Lemon balm (*Melissa officinalis*) Echinacea (*Echinacea purpurea*, *pallida* and *angustifolia*) Sweet marjoram (*Origanum marjorana*) Peppermint (*Mentha piperita*) Licorice (*Glycyrrhiza glabra* and *uralensis*) Hibiscus (*Hibiscus sabdariffa*) Marigold (*Calendula officinalis*) Grape seed (*Vitis vinifera*) Lavender (*Lavandula officinalis*) Capsaicin (*Capsicum annuum*)
Scabies	Anise (*Pimpinella anisum*) Neem plus turmeric
Tinea/onychomycosis/yeast	Tea tree (*Melaleuca alternifolia*) Garlic (*Allium sativum*) Goldenseal (*Hydrastis canadensis*) Chamomile (*Matricaria recutita*) Lavender (*Lavandula officinalis*) Aloe vera (*Aloe barbadensis*)

Table 12.4 Infections

Inflammation	
Indication	**Botanical**
Acne	White willow (*Salix* species) Tea tree (*Melaleuca alternifolia*) Witch hazel (*Hamamelis virginiana*) Vitex (*Vitex agnus-castus*) Bittersweet nightshade (*Solanum dulcamara*) Duckweed (*Lemma minor*) Oak (*Quercus robur*) Walnut (*Juglans regia*) Fruit hydroxyacids Blue flag rhizome (*Iris versicolor*) Lavender (*Lavandula angustifolia*) Chamomile (*Matricaria recutita*)
Dermatitis	Witch hazel (*Hamamelis virginiana*) Aloe vera (*Aloe barbadensis*) Chamomile (*Matricaria recutita*) Evening primrose (*Oenothera biennis*) Oolong and green tea (*Camellia sinensis*) Zemophyte (10 Chinese herbs) Arnica (*Arnica montana*) Burdock (*Arctium lappa*) Yellow dock (*Rumex crispus*) Stillingia (*Stillingia sylvatica*) Sarsaparilla rhizome (*Smilax ornata*) Lavender (*Lavandula officinalis*) Borage (*Borago officinalis*) Grape seed (*Vitis vinifera*) Saw palmetto (*Serenoa repens*) St John's wort (*Hypericum perforatum*)
Psoriasis	Capsaicin (*Capsicum annuum*) Burdock (*Arctium lappa*) Aloe vera (*Aloe barbadensis*) *Angelica dahuricae* (Radix) *Comptotheca acuminata decne* Arnica (*Arnica montana*) Stillingia (*Stillingia sylvatica*) Sarsaparilla rhizome (*Smilax ornata*) Zemophyte (10 Chinese herbs) Avocado (*Persea americana*) Echinacea (*Echinacea purpurea*, *pallida* and *angustifolia*) White willow (*Salix* species) Lavender (*Lavandula officinalis*)
In vitro anti-inflammatory	Nettle (*Urtica urens*) Apis mellifica Belladonna (*Atropa belladonna*) Pasque (*Pulsatilla*) Flower pollen

Table 12.5 Inflammation

Injury	
Indication	**Botanical**
Atrophy	EUOL (*Eucommia ulmoides oliver*)
	Horsetail (*Equisetum arvense*)
Bruising	Capsaicin (*Capsicum annuum*)
	Comfrey (*Symphytam officinale*)
	Arnica (*Arnica montana*)
Burns/wounds/ulcers	Aloe vera (*Aloe barbadensis*)
	Marigold (*Calendula officinalis*)
	Chamomile (*Matricaria recutita*)
	Echinacea (*Echinacea purpurea*, *pallida* and *angustifolia*)
	Goldenseal (*Hydrastis canadensis*)
	Comfrey (*Symphytam officinale*)
	Arnica (*Arnica montana*)
	Neem (*Azadirachta indica*)
	Turmeric (*Curcuma domestica*)
	Gotu kola (*Centella asiatica*)
	Elder (*Sambucus canadensis*)
	Yellow dock (*Rumex crispus*)
	Stillingia (*Stillingia sylvatica*)
	St John's wort (*Hypericum perforatum*)
	Lavender (*Lavandula officinalis*)

Table 12.6 Injury

Relief	
Indication	**Botanical**
Soothing	Oat straw (*Avena sativa*)
	Flax (*Linum usitatissium*)
	Heartsease (*Viola tricolor*)
	English plantain (*Plantago lanceolala*)
	Fenugreek (*Trigorella foenum-gaecum*)
	Marshmallow (*Althanea officinalis*)
	Mullein (*Verbascum densiflorum*)
	Slippery elm (*Ulmus fulva*)
Anesthetic/counter irritants	Wintergreen (*Gaultheria procumbens*)
	Echinacea (*Echinacea purpurea*, *pallida* and *angustifolia*)
	Chamomile (*Matricaria recutita*)
Pruritis	Capsaicin (*Capsicum annuum*)
	Chamomile (*Matricaria recutita*)
	Chickweed (*Stellaria media*)
	Oat straw (*Avena sativa*)

Table 12.7 Relief

Systemic	
Indication	**Botanical**
Chronic venous insufficiency	Horse chestnut (*Aesculus hippocastanum*) Grape seed (*Vitis vinifera*) Butcher's broom (*Ruscus acerteatus*) Sweet clove (*Melilotus officinalis*) *Ginkgo biloba* Witch hazel (*Hamamelis virginiana*) Marigold (*Calendula officinalis*)
Immunostimulatory	Garlic (*Allium sativum*) Goldenseal (*Hydrastis canadensis*) Echinacea (*Echinacea purpurea*, *pallida* and *angustifolia*)

Table 12.8 Systemic

Echinacea (Fig. 12.1)

Echinacea is the largest selling herb in the US market with nearly $190 million sales in 2003. The three echinacea species are *Echinacea angustifolia*, *E. purpurea*, and *E. pallida*. *E. angustifolia* was originally used by the Sioux Native Americans for the treatment of snake bites and war wounds because of its antiseptic and analgesic properties.

E. purpurea contains the immunostimulating polysaccharides and glycoproteins, flavonoids, caffeic and ferulic acid derivatives, volatile oils, alkamides, polyenes, and pyrrolizidine alkaloids. *E. pallida* and *E. angustifolia* lack glycoproteins and pyrrolizidine alkaloids.

All three *Echinacea* species stimulate immunity, protect collagen, and have antioxidant activity. They are also cytotoxic to multiple bacteria and viruses.

E. purpurea is approved by the German E Commission for the treatment of stomatitis, wounds, burns, and to prevent infection. *E. angustifolia* in Native American medicine was used for insect and snake bites, gonorrhea, measles, poorly healing wounds, abscesses, and ulcers. Modern research has documented echinacea's effectiveness in treating burns, infected inflammatory lesions, psoriasis, decubitus and vascular ulcers, poorly healing wounds, herpes simplex, and photoaging (Tables 12.4–12.6, 12.8).

Garlic

Garlic (*Allium sativum*) activity is primarily due to alkylcysteine sulfoxides, specifically alliin which is oxidized to allicin, the major sulfur containing com-

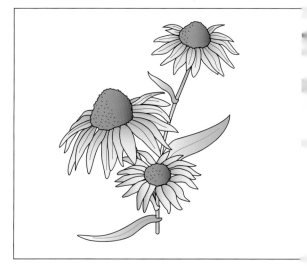

Fig. 12.1 Topical and oral echinacea is an antioxidant. Echinacea is rich in caffeic and ferulic acids

pound responsible for therapeutic activity and the unique odor. Other components include polysaccharides, saponins, and vitamins A, B_2 and C. It has potent antimicrobial and antioxidant activity and stimulates immunity.

Garlic's antibacterial activity is documented against gram positive and gram negative bacteria with potency comparable to many antibiotics. Its anti-yeast activity is comparable to nystatin while its activity against dermatolophytes is superior to seven marketed antifungals. Garlic inhibits herpes hominis I. In folk medicine garlic effectively treats warts, corns and calluses, otitis, and stomatitis. It may be beneficial in treating premature aging (Tables 12.2, 12.4, 12.8).

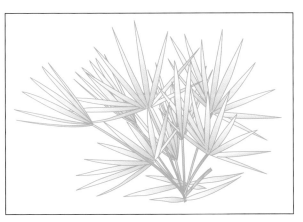

Fig. 12.2 Saw palmetto is used orally for patients with androgenetic alopecia and it possesses antiandrogen and antiestrogen effects

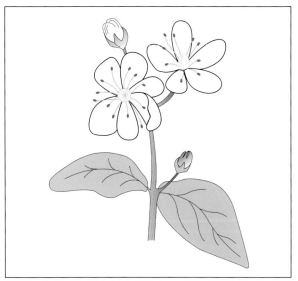

Fig. 12.4 St John's wort contains the anti-inflammatory quercetin. It is used to enhance wound healing

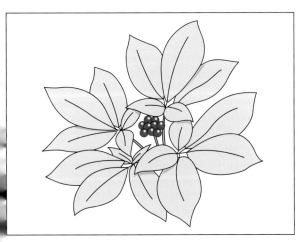

Fig. 12.3 Ginseng contains ginsenosides and it is a topical cosmeceutical antioxidant

Panax ginseng is used in more products and *Panax quinquefolius* is the American indigenous variety. The main active components of ginsengs are steroidal saponins known as ginsenosides. Polysaccharides and polyynes are also present in all species. Lignans, coumarins, steroids, and caffeic acids are only present in *Eleutherococcus senticosus*.

Ginseng enhances immunity and protein synthesis as well as tumor cytotoxicity. This herb has antioxidant and antiviral activity. Ginseng applied topically inhibited tumors in mice. Cases of vaginal bleeding from a topical face cream are very rarely reported (Tables 12.2, 12.8).

Saw Palmetto (Fig. 12.2)

The major components of saw palmetto (*Serenoa repens*) include sitosterols and their glucosides, flavonoids, free fatty acids, and polysaccharides. This botanical has documented antiandrogenic, antiestrogenic, anti-inflammatory, and antiexudative effects. It is a remedy for dermatitis in folk medicine, yet it has been introduced in cosmeceuticals for photoaging (Tables 12.3, 12.5).

Ginseng (Fig. 12.3)

There are three species of ginseng. The most potent is Siberian ginseng (*Eleutherococcus senticosus*). But

St John's Wort (Fig. 12.4)

St John's wort (*Hypericum perforatum*) is a useful wound healing agent due to its proven antistaphylococcal and anti-inflammatory activity with T lymphocyte stimulation. Russian trials support its wound healing effectiveness.

In folk medicine, St John's wort was used to treat infected wounds and dermatitis.

This herb contains 3% flavonoids, including quercetin and over 10% oligomeric procyanidines (OPC). Other components include xanthones, anthracenes including hypericin, acylophloroglucinols, volatile oils, and caffeic acid derivatives (Tables 12.4–12.6).

Teas: Black, White, Oolong

All true teas are derived from *Camellia sinensis*. Black tea is the most fermented with white tea being the least. White tea is more effective than green tea in inhibiting dysplasia.

Black tea has one sixth the content of catechins than green tea, but a higher content of other flavonoids such as quercetin. Black tea inhibits cutaneous photodamage, carcinogenesis, and inflammation. Oral administration of black and oolong teas, like green tea, have been found to suppress both type I and IV hypersensitivity reactions. Oolong tea improved atopic dermatitis within a month in one clinical trial (Tables 12.2, 12.5).

Tea Tree

This essential oil from *Melaleuca alternifolia* is being used throughout American society to treat and prevent a variety of mucocutaneous conditions. Tea tree oil (TTO) consists primarily of terpenes including terpinen, the major sensitizer. TTO does not have antioxidant activity.

Multiple double blinded clinical trials suggest TTO effectively treats acne and onychomycosis. Its antimicrobial spectrum includes gram positive and gram negative bacteria, herpes simplex, *Candida albicans*, and *Trichophyton dermatophytes*. Comparing 100% TTO with 1% clotrimizole solution for onychomycosis therapy for 6 months provided cure rates of 18% for TTO and 11% for clotrimizole. Although 5% TTO did not work as quickly as 5% benzoyl peroxide after 3 months of acne therapy, both produced a significant reduction in lesions. The incidence of irritation for TTO was much lower. Terpene alcohols reduced type I hypersensitivity reactions. TTO failed to effectively treat atopic dermatitis, tinea pedis, and chronic venous insufficiency. TTO is cytotoxic to epithelial cells and fibroblasts, and thus should not be used to treat burns. Photodamaged TTO is a strong sensitizer, indicating caution with the use of these products on sun exposed skin (Tables 12.4, 12.5).

Grape Seed

Grape (*Vitis vinifera*) seed extract primarily consists of polyphenols including flavonoids, tannins, and stilbenes such as resveratrol. The most plentiful and most potent antioxidants are procyandins, also known as proanthocyanidins, leucocyanidins, and condensed tannins. These dimers and oligomers of catechin, epicatechin, and their gallic acid esters are known as oligomeric proanthocyanidins (OPC) which comprise 65% of grape polyphenols. OPC consist mainly of 2–4 units of catechin and epicatechin with smaller amounts of the 5–7 unit oligomers. These larger oligomers dominate in pycnogenol, now specified as the extract of maritime pine (*Pinus maritima*). Originally pycnogenol was the term used for all botanically derived procyanidins. Fruit acids and phenylacrylic acids are components of grape but not of pycnogenol which contains phenolic acids and glycosyl moieties that are not present in grape.

OPCs are potent antioxidant, anti-inflammatory, antihistaminic, and anticarcinogenic agents that also enhance vision, hair growth, wound healing, and ultraviolet protection. OPCs also stabilize elastin, collagen, and ground substance. Grape seed has more antioxidant activity than vitamins C and E. This extract improves photoaged skin, reduces postoperative edema, treats varicosities and vascular insufficiency. Indian medicine claims grape seed effectively treats scabies, dermatitis, gonorrhea, and hemorrhoids.

Chamomile

German chamomile (*Matricaria recutita*) has antiallergic, antimicrobial against staphylococcus and candida, anti-inflammatory, antioxidant, antineoplastic, analgesic, and wound healing activities. The major components of chamomile include bisabolol volatile oils such as levomenol and chamazulene, flavonoids including apigenin, rutin, and quercetin, as well as hydroxycoumarins and mucilages.

Lavender (Fig. 12.5)

Lavandula angustifolia aromatic essential oil contains 70% linalool and linoyl acetate in the volatile phase and 13% tannins. Hydroxycoumarins and caffeic acids also are present. This herb has anti-inflammatory and antimicrobial activity and it inhibits mast cells.

Lavender oil is therapeutic for bites, burns, wounds, lacerations, acne, psoriasis, herpes, and fungal infections. A double blinded clinical trial treating alopecia areata with a mixture of five other botanical oils produced a significant improvement in hair regrowth after 7 months (Tables 12.3, 12.5).

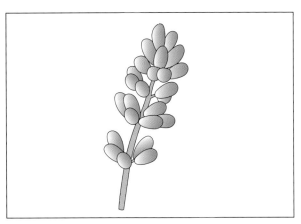

Fig. 12.5 Lavender contains a high concentration of linalool

Pomegranate

Pomegranate (*Punica granatum*) may be a more potent antioxidant than grape seed extract, red wine, or green tea. The major constituents are about 25% tannin polyphenols such as ellagic acid. Ascorbic acid, niacin, and piperidine alkaloids are also present.

This herb's antimicrobial effects include inhibition of gram negative bacteria, fungus, parasites, and viruses. Topical and oral pomegranate products are photoprotective. Pomegranate is used to treat hemorrhoids and sore throat (Table 12.2).

White Willow

There are several willow species but white willow (*Salix*) is the best known because it is the most potent natural source of salicylates including aspirin. This herb is a rich source of tannins and flavonoids which also contribute to its anti-inflammatory, antipyretic, and keratolytic activity. Salicin, the precursor of salicylic acid, comprises about 1% of white willow while other glycosides comprise about 12%.

A 10% willow bark product was superior to 1% salicylic acid in inhibiting inflammation but was less irritating. This herb is a folk medicine used to treat acne and psoriasis.

Summary

This chapter has discussed some of those cosmeceutical botanicals that are dermatologically relevant. These botanical ingredients are incorporated into moisturizers, cleansers, toners, cosmetics, and hair care products to add increased consumer interest and benefits.

Further Reading

Auerbach PS 2001 Wilderness medicine, 4th edn. Mosby, St Louis, MO: pp 411, 1133, 1170, 1176, 1177
Baumann LS 2002 Cosmeceutical critique: tea tree oil. Skin and Allergy News November:14
Baumann LS 2003 Cosmeceutical critique: chamomile. Skin and Allergy News July: 43
Baumann LS 2003 Cosmeceutical critique: lavender. Skin and Allergy News September:33
Baumann LS 2003 Cosmeceutical critique: grape seed extract. Skin and Allergy News November: 26
Baumann LS 2004 Cosmeceutical critique: pomegranate. Skin and Allergy News January: 42
Bedi MK, Shenefelt PD 2002 Herbal therapy in dermatology. Archives of Dermatology 138:232–242
Blake J 2002 Tea for you. Life section. In: The Idaho Statesman February 22: 1
Levin C, Maibach H 2002 Exploration of 'alternative' and 'natural' drugs in dermatology. Archives of Dermatology 138:207–211
Norman R, Nelson D 2000 Do alternative and complementary therapies work for common dermatologic conditions? Skin and Aging 2:28–33
PDR for herbal medicines, 2nd edn 2000 Thomson PDR, Montvale, NJ: pp 261, 277, 327, 331, 346, 362, 605, 629, 664, 757, 807
PDR for nutritional supplements 2001 Thomson PDR, Montvale, NJ: 200
Winston D, Dattner A 1999 The American system of medicine. Clinics in Dermatology 17:53–55
Yarnell E, Absacal K, Hooper CG 2002 Clinical botanical medicine. Larchmont, NY: Mary Ann Liebert, pp 223–242

Cosmeceutical Metals

13 James R. Schwartz

Introduction

Are certain topically applied metal ions simply innocuous treatments or do they provide real technical benefit? Their use goes back to the earliest recorded medical text (~1500 BC), the Ebers papyrus of ancient Egypt. For example, calamine (a natural material containing zinc oxide) was described for treating many skin and eye ailments; green copper-based minerals (likely malachite) were used for burn wounds and itching. Many of these applications have withstood the ensuing 3500 years of history, providing a first clue of real technical merit. For example, zinc is still the first choice to sooth a crying baby's bottom.

This anecdotal support for the importance of metal ions is substantiated by more rigorous investigations, such as those that describe the impact of nutritional deficiencies. A deficiency of zinc can occur either by diet or as a result of a genetic condition that blocks the intestinal uptake of zinc, resulting in acrodermatitis enteropathica (AE). AE manifests itself as severe dermatitis in the vicinity of the mouth, nose, ears, and anal areas (orifices), and on the skin and nails of the fingers and toes (acra). Likewise, a disease resulting in copper deficiency, Menke's syndrome, causes defective keratinization in skin and hair growth, manifested by the formation of kinky hair.

While ancient empiricism, practical utility and clinical manifestations of deficiency support the conclusion that metal ions are important to skin health, a deeper level of understanding is required to confirm this. The molecular basis for these empirical and clinical observations is beginning to emerge that provides strong reinforcement of the links between metal ions and skin condition.

This review will focus specifically on four metals—zinc, copper, selenium, and strontium—which are currently used in cosmeceuticals. Each metal will be covered sequentially, reviewing commonly used materials followed by clinical and scientific data supporting their use. Searching the literature (Medline, 1966 to present) for these individual metals in skin-related articles yields the following hits: zinc, 653; copper, 249; selenium, 130; strontium, 19. Thus, it can be determined immediately that (i) there is far more literature for some of these metals than can be reviewed here, and (ii) there is a wide range in scientific pedigree on the knowledge surrounding the utility of these various materials.

Zinc in Cosmeceutical Products

Materials

There are 55 different zinc-containing materials listed in the International Cosmetic Ingredient (INCI) Dictionary and Handbook (a tabulation of all materials used in cosmetic and personal care products). Of those, seven have been approved by the FDA for OTC usage as safe and effective for a range of benefits, including skin protection, antimicrobial activity, and astringency (Table 13.1). The skin protective benefits of these zinc materials find applications in treating various inflammatory dermatitis conditions such as poison ivy and diaper rash. The wide range of zinc materials approved by the FDA provides a strong indication of the general utility of zinc as a useful treatment.

In most of these materials, zinc ion itself appears to be the primary source of the benefit. All of these materials utilize zinc in its ionic form (Zn^{2+}) with different counterions that result in an electrically neutral compound. These counterions can modulate the solubility and bioavailability of the zinc species

Zinc salt		Therapeutic basis	Application(s)
Name	**Structure**	**Therapeutic basis**	**Application(s)**
Bacitracin zinc		Antibiotic	Topical first aid antibiotic
Zinc sulfate	$ZnSO_4$	Astringent	Ophthalmic care
Zinc carbonate	$ZnCO_3$	Skin protectant	Rhus dermatitis (poison ivy)
Zinc acetate		Skin protectant	Rhus dermatitis (poison ivy)
Zinc oxide (calamine)	ZnO	Astringent / Skin protectant / Skin protectant / Skin protectant / Sunscreen	Hemorrhoid / Dermatitis / Diaper rash / Rhus dermatitis / Sun protection
Zinc undecylenate		Antifungal / Antifungal / Antifungal	Tinea pedis / Tinea cruris / Tinea corporis
Pyrithione zinc		Antifungal / Antifungal	Dandruff / Seborrheic dermatitis

Table caption: Zinc materials approved for use by the FDA for OTC use

Table 13.1 Zinc materials approved for use by the FDA for OTC use

itself. For example, zinc sulfate is water soluble whereas zinc oxide is only sparingly soluble. Zinc sulfate would be expected to be highly available initially with rapid depletion whereas zinc oxide tends to have a lower level of initial activity, but sustained for a long time. By choice of the specific material, the cosmeceutical formulator can tailor the physical properties and activity to the product function. The other zinc containing materials utilized in cosmeceuticals, but not specifically accepted by the FDA for OTC drugs, can likewise be expected to have the *potential* to deliver zinc-based benefits. However, since the use of these materials is not as widespread, the product formulator must exhibit greater pharmacologic expertise with the use of these materials to assure the intended benefits are delivered; bioavailability becomes a complex interaction of material interacting with the product matrix.

Basis for use of zinc materials
Clinical perspective

Damaged skin repairs itself in a very complex process. In the case where the damage is physical and a wound results, a well defined process ensues: inflammation, re-epithelialization, granulation tissue formation, wound contraction, and tissue remodeling. During wound healing, the requirement for zinc increases dramatically. In rat wound models, local zinc levels are seen to increase after wounding, demonstrating the physiologic need for this metal in the repair process. Topically applied zinc compounds have been shown to speed repair, for example in leg ulcers; the rate of delivery of zinc to the damaged site may be initially rate limiting in the repair process. The rate of re-epithelialization was increased with topical zinc in a pig model; the nature (bioavailability) of the zinc material was found to be important—sparingly soluble zinc oxide was superior to soluble zinc forms. An indirect measure of local zinc ion activity at a wound repair site comes from monitoring metallothionein (MT), which is responsible for the storage and delivery of zinc to other proteins and enzymes requiring zinc for their function. MT upregulation can be found in vivo by exposure to zinc; treatment of keratinocytes in vitro with a material that selectively binds zinc inhibits the upregulation of MT and slows cellular proliferation.

Where the damage to skin has more of a 'chemical' nature, the dominant manifestation is inflammation. There is a growing body of evidence that zinc has anti-inflammatory activity. Zinc reduces the irritancy caused by surfactants in the oral cavity. This effect has been observed in vitro as well in skin cultures by monitoring interleukin-1α production and demonstrating pyrithione zinc inhibits surfactant-induced IL-1α release. The inflammatory conditions bullous pemphigoid and decubitus ulcers are accompanied (caused?) by low serum zinc levels. The anti-inflammatory benefits of zinc most likely also play a role in the wound healing process discussed above.

In addition to facilitating repair processes, zinc appears to confer a protective function via providing antioxidant activity. Zinc has been shown to reduce the cellular and genetic damage caused by exposure to UV light and enhance resistance of skin fibroblasts to oxidative stress. For this reason, microfine zinc oxide is used as a broad spectrum physical photoprotectant in sunscreens for its ability to scatter and reflect both UVB and UVA radiation. Zinc oxide paste is found in ointments formulated to improve diaper dermatitis for its barrier and anti-inflammatory capabilities. Zinc pyrithione is another commonly used zinc molecule found in antidandruff shampoos for its ability to act as a potent antifungal.

Scientific foundation

An average human contains 2.5 g of zinc and requires 15 mg/day to remain healthy (this is exceeded only by iron for trace elements). The vast majority of the zinc is present in metalloenzymes and proteins. This field was opened in 1940 with the discovery that carbonic anhydrase, a ubiquitous enzyme required for maintaining physiologic pH, was zinc-containing and that the zinc was required for catalytic activity. Since that time, over 300 enzymes requiring zinc for activity have been structurally characterized. Even more impressive are the thousands of zinc-containing proteins that require zinc for conferring a three dimensional structure that allows them to regulate replication of DNA and transcription of RNA. These proteins form the class called 'zinc fingers' and regulate the fundamental biologic process of translating genetic information to functional proteins. At least 3% of all proteins encoded for by the human genome have zinc fingers, and this has led Berg to coin the term 'galvanization of biology' to acknowledge the importance of this metal in human physiology.

While it is beyond the scope of this chapter to review many of the zinc containing biomolecules (see Table 13.2 for an overview of important examples), a few will be highlighted that have specific relevance to cutaneous biology and supporting the clinical observations reviewed above. Matrix metalloproteinases (MMPs) are zinc dependent proteases capable of degrading many molecules important in wound healing, including signaling factors as well as the structural proteins of the extracellular matrix (including collagen and elastin). Wound healing is inherently an intensive protein synthesis process, thus the zinc finger proteins DNA and RNA polymerases, which control protein synthesis, are critical throughout this process. The anti-inflammatory role observed clinically for zinc, relevant both in wound healing as well as in other dermatitis conditions, may lie partially in the importance of alkaline phosphatase (AP). AP requires multiple zinc ions and is involved

Summary of major zinc biomolecules			
Enzyme	**Chemical function of zinc**	**Physiological function of biomolecule**	**Relevant to skin?**
Alcohol dehydrogenase	Catalyzes oxidation of alcohols (esp. ethanol) to aldehydes	Liver metabolism	—
Carboxypeptidase	Catalyzes hydrolysis of C-terminal peptide residues	Protein digestion for nutrition	—
Thermolysin	Catalyzes hydrolysis of peptides	—	—

Matrix metalloproteinases
  Collagenase (MMP-1)
  Elastase (MMP-12)
  Gelatinase (MMP-2)
	Catalyzes hydrolysis of matrix proteins	Formation of extracellular matrix
		  Hydrolysis of collagen
		  Hydrolysis of elastin
		  Hydrolysis of gelatin
			
			Yes
			Yes
			—

β-Lactamase	Catalyzes hydrolysis of β-lactam rings (e.g., penicillin)	—	
Carbonic anhydrase	Catalyzes hydration of CO_2	Physiology of CO_2 transport and physiological buffering	—
Nuclease P1	Catalyzes formation of 5' single-stranded nucleotides from RNA and DNA	—	—
Superoxide dismutase	Catalyzes dismutation of superoxide anion into O_2 and H_2O_2	Scavenges damaging superoxide	Yes
Phosphotriesterases	—	—	—
Alkaline phosphatase	Catalyzes hydrolysis of phosphate mono-esters	—	Yes
Leucine aminopeptidase	Catalyzes hydrolysis of leucine N-terminal peptide residues	—	—
Phospholipase C	Cleaves bond between head group and lipid moiety of phospholipids	—	—
Metallothionein	Binding of zinc	Storage of zinc	Yes

Zinc finger class
  DNA Polymerases
  RNA Polymerase
	Confers conformation to facilitate nucleotide binding	Nucleic acid metabolism
		  Replication of DNA
		  Transcription of RNA
			
			Yes
			—

α-Amylase	—	—	—
Aspartate transcarbamoylase	—	—	—

Table 13.2 Summary of major zinc biomolecules

in adenosine monophosphate metabolism, which has a role in restraining an inflammatory response. The breadth of the impacts of these zinc biomolecules on the wound healing process is represented schematically in Figure 13.1.

The observed antioxidant activity of zinc may have its roots in multiple effects: zinc is a component of both superoxide dismutase and metallothionein, both of which have strong antioxidant activity; zinc may also displace more harmful metal ions (such as copper and iron) which cause oxygen based free radical formation due to their oxidation-reduction activity; zinc does not have this capacity to generate radicals since it dose not undergo redox activity.

While this survey barely skims the surface of relevant zinc biochemistry, it should provide sub-

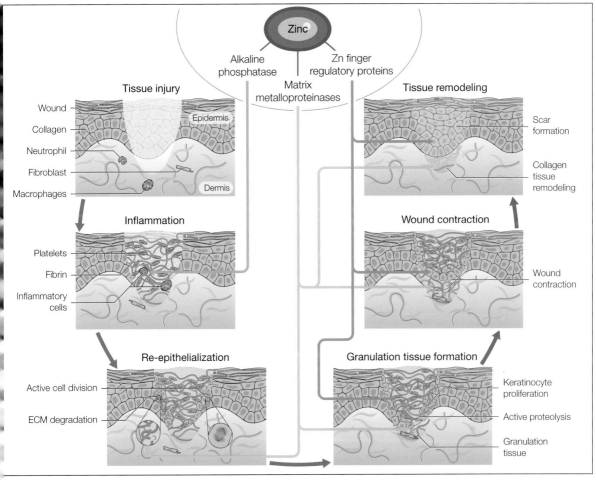

Fig. 13.1 An overview of the key functional steps in the wound healing process of skin with an indication of the places and functions of zinc in this process

stantial confidence that the empirical and clinical observations on the importance of zinc to skin health are indeed real and based on a firm scientific foundation.

Copper in Cosmeceutical Products

Materials

The number of copper compounds commonly used in personal care products is far less than for zinc. There are 19 copper materials listed within the INCI, none of which are accepted by the FDA as safe and effective for OTC topical drugs. As with zinc, the normal form is ionic Cu^{2+}, with various counterions that can impact solubility. The nature of the counterion and the resultant impact on bioavailability is not well known and requires substantial

expertise in product pharmacology to achieve the desired benefit. Copper also has a very strong affinity for other product matrix ingredients that must be carefully monitored to minimize negative effects either to the matrix or the copper itself. As mentioned above, copper also has the potential for oxidation-reduction activity, which can enhance reactive oxygen species formation.

Basis for use of copper materials
Clinical perspective

Animals fed copper-deficient diets suffer at least two abnormal skin conditions: melanin pigment level is decreased and collagen synthesis is impaired with a resultant loss in physical properties. As with zinc, copper appears to play a role in healing damaged skin. Recent data demonstrated that a copper–peptide complex (glycyl-L-histidyl-L-lysine, GHK) enhances the expression of extracellular matrix macromolecules in an animal wound repair model. For this reason, copper peptides are found in a number of dermatologic preparations to enhance wound healing. This wound healing technology was adapted to the cosmeceutical moisturizer marketplace in the form of daily wear products with claims of minimizing wrinkles presumably by enhancing collagen synthesis. It is important to note that copper is a difficult metal to penetrate the skin. In the cosmeceutical formulations, the copper is bound to a protein peptide to enhance skin penetration and presumably confer biologic activity.

Scientific foundation

Copper is also ubiquitous in all cells, but the overall amount in the body, 0.1 g, is far lower than that of zinc. As with other metals, copper is primarily bound to enzymes, over 100 have been structurally characterized; major ones are summarized in Table 13.3. Melanins are responsible for skin pigmentation, providing a natural photoprotective effect. Synthesis of melanin requires the copper based enzyme tyrosinase. The role that copper plays in damage repair is probably based on several copper containing enzymes: lysyl oxidase cross-links molecules of tropocollagen to form collagen and an as-yet unidentified enzyme is involved in cross-linking proteins by disulfide bond formation (this one is probably specifically important in the kinky hair formed as a symptom of Menke's syndrome). Antioxidant activity is most likely also beneficial for damage repair and can be traced to the copper enzymes superoxide dismutase (which has both copper and zinc ions) and ceruloplasmin.

Selenium in Cosmeceutical Products

While selenium is recognized as an essential trace element, it is quite rare both in the body and in personal care products. There are only four selenium compounds listed in the INCI compilation. One of the compounds, selenium sulfide, is accepted by the FDA for dandruff treatment.

Selenium has been reported to reduce the risk of nonmelanoma skin cancer in humans. Most of the skin effects reported for selenium involve antioxidant activity. This is based on dietary deficiency studies in which the signs of oxidative stress increase with decreasing selenium intake. The largest topical use of selenium exploits the antifungal activity of selenium sulfide for use in antidandruff shampoos.

There are 11 characterized selenium proteins and enzymes. The largest class is of glutathione peroxidases which catalyze the reduction of potentially damaging reactive oxygen species such as hydrogen peroxide and lipid peroxides by coupling to the oxidation of

Summary of major copper biomolecules			
Enzyme	Chemical function of copper	Physiologic function of biomolecule	Relevant to skin?
Cytochrome c oxidase	Electron transfer (redox)	Generation of energy in mitochondria	—
Superoxide dismutase	Catalyzes dismutation of superoxide anion into O_2 and H_2O_2	Scavenges damaging superoxide	Yes
Tyrosinase	Oxidizes tyrosine to dihydroxyphenylalanine (DOPA)	Melanin production	Yes
Dopamine β-hydroxylase	Hydroxylation of dopamine to form norepinephrine	Catecholamine production	—
Lysyl oxidase	Catalyzes oxidation of lysine to reactive aldehyde	Cross-linking of collagen and elastin	Yes
Ceruloplasmin	Binding of Cu	Copper transport	—
Unidentified	—	Cross-linking of keratin (disulfide bonds)	Yes
Factor V	Stimulates formation of thrombin	Blood clotting	—

Table 13.3 Summary of major copper biomolecules

glutathione. This supports the clinical observations regarding antioxidant activity; it is not known whether this function also plays a role in reduced tumor incidence. Selenium is added to a variety of cosmeceutical moisturizers presumably for its ability to reduce collagen damage from reactive oxygen species thus decreasing cutaneous aging.

Strontium in Cosmeceutical Products

There is even less known about strontium and skin, as there are no known strontium-containing proteins. There are eight strontium-containing salts listed in the INCI Dictionary.

The primary use for strontium in personal care products appears to be as an anti-irritant. While the proposed mechanism involves direct interaction between strontium ion and Type C nociceptors, the published data does not allow the differentiation of the possibility of chemical interaction between strontium and the potentially irritating species (α-hydroxy acids). More study is needed to firmly establish strontium scientifically.

Currently, strontium is used in a variety of cosmeceutical moisturizers and physician administered alpha hydroxy acid peel formulations. The strontium is said to function as an anti-inflammatory, thus minimizing skin redness and the resultant stinging following exposure of the facial to high concentration alpha hydroxy acids. It is unclear whether the effect of strontium in these applications is due to topical effects on the skin barrier or due to alterations in the inflammatory cascade.

Summary

The wide use of metal ions in skin care products was initially based primarily on empiricism. From this brief review of the potential scientific data supporting use of the metals, it appears in many cases there is real basis for understanding why topically applied metals can be beneficial to skin. Of the metals reviewed here, zinc, copper, selenium, and strontium, varying degrees of scientific pedigree were found in support of their utility. Established and well based benefits of zinc include both healing damaged skin as well damage prevention. Copper appears to have similar damage repair benefits, though these are less well established scientifically. Selenium's antioxidant activity is based on specific enzymatic activity; strontium's anti-irritancy activity requires additional scientific support.

Further Reading

Ågren MS 1992 Influence of two vehicles for zinc oxide on zinc absorption through intact skin and wounds. Acta Dermato-Venereologica 71:153–156

Albergoni V 1998 Physiological properties of copper and zinc. In: Rainsford KD, Milanino R et al (eds) Copper and zinc in inflammatory and degenerative diseases. Kluwer, pp 7–17

Berg JM, Shi Y 1996 The galvanization of biology: a growing appreciation for the roles of zinc Science 271:1081–1085

Danks DM 1991 Copper deficiency and the skin. Oxford University Press, New York, pp 1351–1361

Goldsmith LA (ed) 1991 Physiology, biochemistry, and molecular biology of the skin, 2nd edn. Oxford University Press, New York

Hostÿnek JJ 1998 Toxic potential from metals absorbed through the skin. Cosmetics and Toiletries 113:33–42

Hostÿnek JJ 1999 Metals in personal care products. Cosmetics and Toiletries 114:47–56

Hostÿnek JJ 2000 Chromium, cobalt, copper and iron: metals in personal care products. Cosmetics and Toiletries 115:52–65

Hostÿnek JJ, Maibach HI 2001 Lead, manganese and mercury: metals in personal care products. Cosmetics and Toiletries 116:26–36

Hostÿnek JJ, Maibach HI 2002 Nickel compounds in cosmetics. Cosmetics and Toiletries 117:24–30

Hostÿnek JJ, Maibach HI 2002 Silver, titanium and zirconium: metals in cosmetics and personal care products. Cosmetics and Toiletries 117:26–36

Hostÿnek JJ, Maibach HI 2002 Tin, zinc and selenium: metals in cosmetics and personal care products. Cosmetics and Toiletries 117:32–42

Mullin CH, Frings G, Abel J, Kind PP, Goerz G 1987 Specific induction of metallothionein in hairless mouse skin by zinc and dexamethasone. Journal of Investigative Dermatology 89:164–166

Neldner KH 1991 The biochemistry and physiology of zinc metabolism. Oxford University Press, New York, pp 1329–1350

Parat MO, Richard MJ, Meplan C, Favier A, Beani JC 1999 Impairment of cultured cell proliferation and metallothionein expression by metal chelator NNN'N'-tetrakis-(2-pyridylmethyl)ethylene diamine. Biological Trace Element Research 70:51–68

Pence BC, Delver E, Dunn DM 1994 Effects of dietary selenium on UVB-induced skin carcinogenesis and epidermal antioxidant status. Journal of Investigative Dermatology 102:759–761

Pirot F, Millet J, Kalia YN, Humbert P 1996 In vitro study of percutaneous absorption, cutaneous bioavailability and bioequivalence of zinc and copper from five topical formulations Skin Pharmacology 9:259–269

Rittenhouse T 1996 The management of lower extremity ulcers with zinc-saline wet dressings versus normal saline wet dressings. Advances in Therapeutics 13:88–94

Rostan EF, DeBuys HV, Madey DL, Pinnell, SR 2002 Evidence supporting zinc as an important antioxidant for skin. International Journal of Dermatology 41:606–611

Sheretz EF, Goldsmith LA 1991 Nutritional influences on the skin. Oxford University Press, New York, pp 1315–1328

Siméon A, Wegrowski Y, Bontemps Y, Marquart F 2000 Expression of glycosaminoglycans and small proteoglycans in wounds: modulation by the tripeptide-copper complex glycyl-L-histidyl-L-lysine-Cu^{2+}. Journal of Investigative Dermatology 115:962–968

Skaare AB, Rolla G, Barkvoll P 1996 The influence of triclosan, zinc or propylene glycol on oral mucosa exposed to sodium lauryl sulfate. European Journal of Oral Science 105:527–533

Tasaki M, Hanada K, Hashimoto I 1993 Analyses of serum copper and zinc levels and copper/zinc ratios in skin diseases. Journal of Dermatology 20: 21–24

Warren R, Schwartz JR, Sanders LM, Juneja PS 2002 Attenuation of surfactant-induced interleukin 1α expression by zinc pyrithione. Exogenous Dermatology 2:23–27

Zhai H, Hannon W, Hahn GS, Pelosi A, Harper RA, Maibach HI 2000 Strontium nitrate suppresses chemically induced sensory irritation in humans. Contact Dermatitis 42:98–100

Cosmeceutical Moisturizers

14

James Q. Del Rosso

Introduction

Dermatologists are frequently asked questions by patients about skin care products, such as 'Is there a specific moisturizer that you recommend?'. It is common for practitioners to select from an array of samples, or to become familiar with a few brand name products through personal familiarity or the random experiences of individual patients. A thorough understanding of the features of moisturizer formulations, and their differences, provides the clinician with a greater ability to recommend products appropriately and confidently. Various factors related to formulation science impact on the type and extent of clinical benefit achieved and the potential for unwanted effects (i.e. skin irritation, lack of aesthetic appeal).

Two basic processes that function in concert to maintain the overall health of skin are cleansing and moisturizing. Cleansing allows for removal of external debris, natural cutaneous secretions, and microorganisms. Moisturizers are an important component of basic skin care, especially in conditions where clinical or subclinical alteration of the epidermal barrier and/or reduced epidermal water content are present. Such conditions include low ambient humidity, and clinically evident xerosis due to genetic tendency (e.g. ichthyosis) or underlying disease states (e.g. atopic dermatitis, hypothyroidism, diabetes), or use of products or medications associated with epidermal barrier disruption such as harsh cleansers, astringents, and some topical medications. The myriad of moisturizer products available confounds rational product selection. The bottom line is to maintain a 'simplest is best approach', especially as many product claims, special additives, and carefully marketed 'prestige products' are backed by little to no scientific evidence supporting their benefit or extraordinary expense.

This chapter reviews the fundamental principles related to formulating various types of moisturizer formulations and the current understanding of skin barrier physiology and function. Specific components of moisturizers, their functions, and resultant clinical effects are discussed.

Maintenance of Normal Skin Integrity and Water Content

Cutaneous water balance, homeostasis, and normal skin appearance require the presence of an intact epidermal barrier. The epidermal barrier is composed of two functioning components: (i) a *cellular protein matrix* composed of an intertwined and layered lattice of keratinocytes ('bricks') with an uppermost layer of thin stratum corneum cells (corneocytes) and (ii) an *intercellular lipid bilayer matrix* ('mortar'). Proper function and maintenance of both components assures skin integrity, water balance, hydration, and orderly corneocyte desquamation. Disturbance of either of the epidermal components produces increased transepidermal water loss (TEWL), resulting in xerotic skin changes, characterized by dryness, scaling, roughness, fine fissuring, and associated pruritus. The ideal range of stratum corneum water content is 20–35%; reduction to below 10% water content results in visibly evident xerotic skin changes.

Role of corneocytes and natural moisturizing factor

The epidermis is in constant flux, as corneocytes traverse from below and ultimately desquamate. In the presence of adequate water content, desquamation occurs upon enzymatic degradation of desmosomes, allowing for separation and shedding

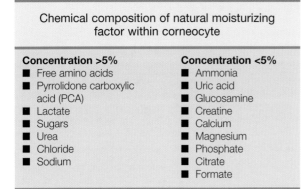

Box 14.1 Chemical composition of natural moisturizing factor within corneocyte

of superficial corneocytes. Unlike normal skin, xerotic skin is characterized by retained corneodesmosomes within desquamating stratum corneum, resulting in shedding of 'clumps' of corneocytes visibly apparent as flakes or scales, as opposed to imperceptible desquamation of single corneocyte cells. Stratum corneum chymotryptic enzyme activity, integral to the hydrolysis of corneodesmosomes and the physiologic process of desquamation, is reduced in soap-induced dry skin as compared to normal skin.

The moisture content of corneocytes is maintained by small hygroscopic compounds which have been collectively categorized under the term 'natural moisturizing factor' (NMF). The components of NMF include filaggrin derived amino acids, pyrrolidone carboxylic acid (PCA), lactate, sugars, and several electrolytes (Box 14.1). If stratum corneum water content falls below a critical level, enzymatic function required for normal desquamation is impaired, leading to corneocyte adhesion and accumulation of corneocytes on the cutaneous surface. These aberrant changes correspond with the visible appearance of dryness, roughness, scaling, flaking, chafing, and fissuring.

Role of intercellular lipids

An important component of epidermal proliferation and differentiation is the formation of a permeability barrier composed of a programmed combination and ratio of lipids. Stratum corneum lipids are synthesized predominantly within the nucleated cells of the epidermis and are largely autonomous from circulating lipids. Lipid synthesis is regulated primarily by changes in epidermal barrier status. Epidermal barrier lipids are mostly composed of equimolar concentrations of free fatty acids, cholesterol, and ceramides. Lower quantities of cholesterol sulfate and nonpolar lipids are also present. The bipolar nature of lipids comprising the intercellular matrix allows for the formation of alternating lipid layers with hydrophilic 'heads' and hydrophobic 'tails'. This orderly arrangement forms a barrier which controls water permeability and movement between epidermal cells (regulation of TEWL) and seals water soluble hygroscopic compounds (NMF) within corneocytes, thus maintaining intracellular water content. Epidermal lipids are also collected within lamellar bodies (Odland bodies) which are located within keratinocytes of the upper epidermis and function to biochemically convert newly synthesized lipids to an organized membrane structure (lamellar unit membrane structure). Lamellar bodies deliver proteolytic enzymes required for desquamation of corneocytes to the interstitium and convert 'precursor lipids' into vital barrier function lipids such as ceramides. As cornification occurs in the upper epidermis, a phospholipid enriched plasma membrane is converted to a ceramide-rich bilayered membrane. At least seven subfractions of ceramides have been identified, accounting for up to 50% of stratum corneum lipid content by weight. Loss of epidermal lipids that are critical components of the lamellar epidermal barrier results in increased TEWL, a reduction in skin plasticity and the adverse sequelae related to decreased stratum corneum water content as described above. Interestingly, significant reduction in multiple subfractions of ceramides has been noted in both lesional and nonlesional skin of patients with atopic dermatitis.

Physiologic Epidermal Barrier Repair

The homeostatic signal which correlates with maintenance and repair of epidermal barrier function is TEWL. When TEWL increases by as little as 1%, a physiologic signal initiates barrier repair by upregulating lipid synthesis. Disturbances in epidermal barrier permeability induce a physiologic response to restore barrier function with normalization occurring within hours to days; the time course of restoration of barrier function is dependent on the extent of the insult, the age of the patient, and the patient's overall health status. Recovery of the epidermal barrier occurs as extracellular lipids are secreted into the stratum corneum interstitium by

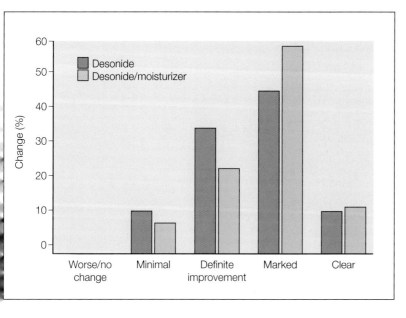

Fig. 14.1 Physicians' global assessment of improvement with a topical corticosteroid alone versus a moisturizer in combination with a topical corticosteroid

keratinocytes underlying the site of insult and are organized into lamellar membrane unit structures. Within 30 minutes, lamellar bodies are deposited from the outer granular layer, followed within the next 4 hours by synthesis of fatty acids and cholesterol and over the next 6–9 hours by increased ceramide production.

Clinical Impact of Moisturizers

In the presence of intrinsic or extrinsic factors that promote barrier disruption and reduced epidermal water content, moisturizers, especially those with optimized components, simulate the role of epidermal lipids in promoting and restoring epidermal barrier function. Externally applied lipids have been shown to intercalate between corneocytes and can mitigate surfactant induced skin irritation. Application of nonphysiologic lipids such as petrolatum allows for restoration of barrier function by permeating within the interstium of the stratum corneum and creating a diffuse hydrophobic phase. Studies evaluating the application of physiologic lipids as moisturizers suggest that these lipids can be incorporated into the formation of barrier lipids and lamellar units and do not appear to downregulate physiologic lipid production in skin. However, based on in vitro murine models, the use of physiologic lipids in moisturizers appears to require the inclusion of all three lipid components (ceramide, cholesterol, free

fatty acids) in optimized concentrations, otherwise barrier recovery may be impaired (Fig. 14.1).

Significance of Moisturizer Application Frequency

Due to the loss of applied product imposed by the continuous natural process of epidermal desquamation and limitations of product substantivity, persistent efficacy provided by moisturizer use requires repeated application on a daily basis.

Evaluation of moisturizing properties after discontinuation of treatment with moisturizers (regression phase analysis) has demonstrated longlasting effects for several days after use of both lanolin based and cetyl alcohol/petrolatum/polyglycerylmethacrylate based moisturizer preparations (Fig. 14.2).

Significant Components of Moisturizer Formulations

The 'real world' usage of a moisturizer formulation requires noticeable efficacy and cosmetic acceptability. With regard to efficacy, it is important to recognize that the term *moisturizer* does not imply that moisture (water) is being added to the skin. Rather, a properly designed moisturizer formulation contains *occlusive*, *humectant*, and *emollient* ingredients. The occlusive component retards evaporation and water loss by forming a hydrophobic film on the skin

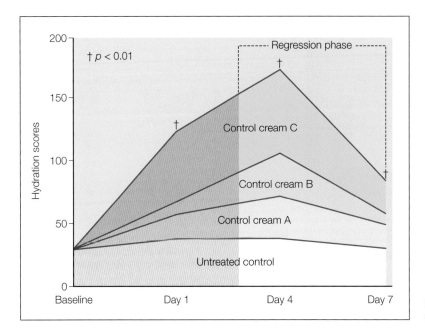

Fig. 14.2 Regression analysis of selected moisturizing creams

surface and within the superficial interstitium between corneocytes. Humectant compounds attract water from the dermis and harbor water into the outer epidermal layer ('from the inside out'). In climate conditions characterized by ambient humidity exceeding 70%, humectant compounds can also attract and trap water from the environment ('from the outside in'). The combination of occlusive and humectant ingredients provide complementary actions in achieving and maintaining epidermal hydration and barrier function (Fig. 14.3). Emollient ingredients, described as being capable of 'filling the crevices' between fragmented collections of desquamating corneocytes, are the third major component of moisturizer formulations. Emollients contribute to clinical efficacy and cosmetic elegance by imparting a smooth, soft texture to the skin surface.

Occlusive ingredients

Occlusive agents are often greasy and are most effective when applied onto slightly dampened skin. Examples of occlusive ingredients include petrolatum, lanolin, mineral oil, and silicone derivatives (dimethicone, cyclomethicone) (Box 14.2). The use of lanolin is limited by odor, expense, and potential allergenicity. Mineral oil is frequently used due to its favorable texture ('feel'), but is limited in its ability to reduce TEWL. The term 'oil free' implies that

the formulation does not contain mineral or vegetable oils. Silicone derivatives are not greasy and when used alone impart a protective effect with limited moisturizing quality. They are often used in combination with petrolatum to impart a more cosmetically favorable texture as petrolatum alone is perceived by many consumers as 'too greasy'.

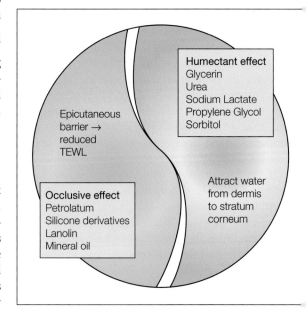

Fig. 14.3 Basic moisturizer components

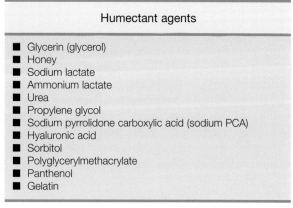

Box 14.2 Occlusive agents

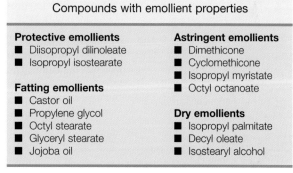

Box 14.3 Humectant agents

Humectant ingredients

Several compounds are added to moisturizers due to their humectant quality, attracting water from the dermis into the epidermis. Many humectant compounds also exhibit emollient properties when applied to skin. Examples of compounds that are commonly used in moisturizer formulations due to their humectant properties are listed in Box 14.3. It is important that a humectant agent when used as a moisturizer component be combined with an occlusive ingredient as application of a humectant alone can increase TEWL. For example, topical glycerin (glycerol) when applied alone to skin increases TEWL by 29%.

Emollient ingredients

Emollients are frequently 'oily' substances that include a vast array of compounds ranging from esters to long chain alcohols. Although emolliency does not necessarily correlate with reduction in TEWL, emollient characteristics do correlate with consumer satisfaction and product preference as a smooth skin texture is expected after moisturizer application. Examples of compounds with emollient properties are listed in Box 14.4. Some compounds may be used due to their emollient qualities and compatibility with other components used in specific formulations. Unlike astringent alcohols (e.g. isopropyl alcohol, ethyl alcohol), emollient alcohols (e.g. cetyl alcohol, stearyl alcohol) are not drying and impart a

Box 14.4 Compounds with emollient properties

smooth texture to skin upon application. Ester type emollients include octyl stearate, isopropyl myristate, oleyl oleate, cetearyl isononanoate, and PEG-7 glyceryl cocoate. Depending on inherent properties, emollients may be classified as protective, fatting, dry, or astringent (Box 14.4).

Esthetic Characteristics and Special Moisturizer Additives

Formulation characteristics

The majority of moisturizers are formulated as lotions (oil-in-water emulsion) or creams (water-in-oil emulsion). Lotion formulations are thinner and are compatible with daytime facial use; characteristic basic components include mineral oil, propylene glycol, and water. Night creams and replenishing or 'therapeutic' formulations are composed of heavier lipids such as petrolatum or lanolin derivatives, mineral oil, and water. Correlation of specific formulations with 'skin type' is significant, as specified ingredient combinations are made more compatible with dry, normal, or oily complexions by adjusting oil–water ratios and the heaviness of occlusive ingredients and emollients. For example, dimethicone and cyclomethicone are nongreasy, noncomedogenic emollients that are commonly used in 'oil free' facial moisturizers targeted for patients with 'oily skin'. Oil-absorbent compounds such as talc or kaolin may be added to absorb excess sebum and reduce 'facial shine'.

Conclusion

As the primary goals of moisturizer use are to maintain skin integrity and appearance by retaining skin water content, preventing TEWL, and initiating barrier repair when cutaneous insult arises, the most important formulation ingredients are humectant, occlusive, and emollient components. Proper balancing of these components results in the development of clinically effective and cosmetically appealing formulations.

Further Reading

Del Rosso JQ 2003 Understanding skin cleansers and moisturizers: the correlation of formulation science with the art of clinical use. Cosmet Dermatol 16:19–31

Draelos ZD 1995 Moisturizers. In: Draelos ZD (ed) Cosmetics in dermatology, 2nd edn. Churchill Livingstone, New York, pp 83–95

Draelos ZD 1995 Skin cleansers. In: Draelos ZD, ed. Cosmetics in dermatology, 2nd edn. Churchill Livingstone, New York, pp 207–214

Draelos ZD 2000 Therapeutic moisturizers. Dermatology Clinics 18:597–607

Fluhr J, Holleran WM, Berardesca E 2002 Clinical effects of emollients on skin. In: Leyden JJ, Rawlings AV (eds) Skin moisturization. Marcel Dekker, New York, pp 223–243

Flynn TC, Petros J, Clark RE, et al 2001 Dry skin and moisturizers. Clinics in Dermatology 19:387–392

Gensler HL 1997 Prevention of photoimmunosuppression and photocarcinogenesis by topical niacinamide. Nutrition and Cancer 29:157–162

Grubauer G, Feingold KR, Elias PM 1987 The relationship of epidermal lipogenesis to cutaneous barrier function. Journal of Lipid Research 28:746–752

Hanifin JM, Hebert AA, Mays SR, et al 1998 Effects of a low-potency corticosteroid lotion plus a moisturizing regimen in the treatment of atopic dermatitis. Current Therapeutic Research 59:227–233

Imokawa G, Abe A, Jin Y, et al 1991 Decreased level of ceramides in stratum corneum of atopic dermatitis: an etiologic factor in atopic dry skin? Journal of Investigative Dermatology 96:523–526

Jackson EM 1996 Moisturizers: adjunct therapy and advising patients. American Journal of Contacta Dermatitis 7:247–251

Johnson AW 2002 The skin moisturizer marketplace. In: Leyden JJ, Rawlings AV (eds) Skin moisturization. Marcel Dekker, New York, pp 1–30

Kirsner RS, Froehlich CW 1998 Soaps and detergents: understanding their composition and effect. Ostomy/Wound Management 44(3A):62S–69S

Kligman A 1978 Regression method for assessing the efficacy of moisturizers. Cosmetics and Toiletries 93:27–32

Lazar AP, Lazar P 1991 Dry skin, water, and lubrication. Dermatologic Clinics 9:45–51

Loden M, Andersson A-C, Lindberg M 1999 Improvement in skin barrier function in patients with atopic dermatitis after treatment with a moisturizer cream. British Journal of Dermatology 140:264–267

Loden M 1997 Barrier recovery and influence of irritant stimuli in skin treated with a moisturizing cream. Contact Dermatitis 36:256–260

Ludwig A, Dietel M, Schafer G, et al 1990 Nicotinamide and nicotinamide analogues as antitumor promoters in mouse skin. Cancer Research 50:2470–2475

Mao-Qiang M, Brown BE, Wu-Pong S, et al 1995 Exogenous nonphysiologic vs physiologic lipids. Divergent mechanisms for correction of permeability barrier dysfunction. Archives of Dermatology 131:809–816

Menon GK, Feingold KR, Elias PM 1992 Lamellar body secretory response to barrier disruption. Journal of Investigative Dermatology 98:279–289

Presland RB, Jurevic RJ 2002 Making sense of the epithelial barrier: what molecular biology and genetics tell us about the functions of oral mucosal and epidermal tissues. Journal of Dental Education 66:564–574

Proksch E, Elias PM 2002 Epidermal barrier in atopic dermatitis. In: Bieber T, Leung DYM (eds) Atopic dermatitis. Marcel Dekker, New York, pp 123–143

Rawlings AV, Canestrari DA, Dobkowski B 2004 Moisturizer technology versus clinical performance. Dermatologic Therapy 17:49–56

Rawlings AV, Harding CR, Watkinson A, Scott IR 2002 Dry and xerotic skin conditions. In: Leyden JJ, Rawlings AV (eds) Skin moisturization. Marcel Dekker, New York, pp 119–144

Rawlings AV, Harding CR 2004 Moisturization and skin barrier function. Dermatologic Therapeutics 17:43–48

Salka BA 1997 Emollients. Cosmetics and Toiletries 112:101–106

Shurer NY, Plewig G, Elias PM 1991 Stratum corneum lipid function. Dermatologica 183:77–94

Tabata N, O'Goshi K, Zhen XY, et al 2000 Biophysical assessment of persistent effects of moisturizers after daily applications: evaluation of corneotherapy. Dermatology 200:308–313

Wehr RF, Krochmal L 1987 Considerations in selecting a moisturizer. Cutis 39:512–515

Yamamoto A, Serizawa S, Ito M, et al 1991 Stratum corneum lipid abnormalities in atopic dermatitis. Archives of Dermatological Research 283:219–223

Zettersten EM, Ghadially R, Feingold KR, et al 1997 Optimal ratios of topical stratum corneum lipids improve barrier recovery in chronically aged skin. Journal of the American Academy of Dermatology 37:403–408

Skin Lightening Agents

15

Marta I. Rendon, Jorge I. Gaviria

Introduction

Hyperpigmentation is a common skin problem that is particularly prevalent in middle aged and elderly individuals. It is cosmetically important and can greatly detract from both appearance and quality of life, particularly in cultures where smooth skin is valued as a sign of health or in cultures that are beauty conscious. Hyperpigmented skin lesions may be postinflammatory as a sequel to acne, trauma, chemical peels, or laser therapy. Exogenous causes, particularly ultraviolet (UV) light exposure, are a common factor in pigmentary abnormalities such as melasma, solar lentigines, and ephelides (Fig. 15.1) Exposure to certain drugs and chemicals as well as the existence of certain disease states can result in hyperpigmentation (Box 15.1).

The treatment of acquired hyperpigmentation has traditionally been challenging and frequently

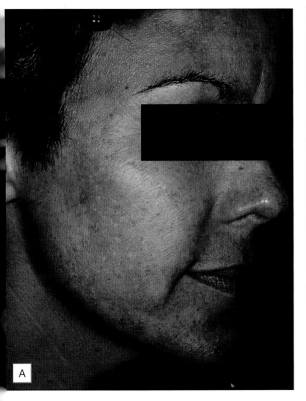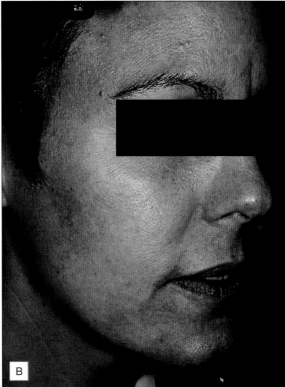

Fig. 15.1 The typical appearance of melasma with reticulated hyperpigmented plaques. (**A**) Before cosmeceutical treatment. (**B**) Eight weeks after cosmeceutical treatment

Acquired hyperpigmentation

Skin diseases and conditions
- Melasma
- Riehl's melanosis
- Poikiloderma of Civatte
- Erythromelanosis follicularis
- Linea fusca
- Post inflammatory hyperpigmentation

Exogenous causes
Ultraviolet exposure (e.g. melasma, solar lentigines, ephelides)
Photosensitizing agents (e.g. berloque dermatitis due to bergamot oil, furocoumarines)
Drugs (e.g. estrogens, tetracyclines, amiodarone, phenytoin, phenothiazines, sulfonamides)
Cosmetics

Other causes
Pregnancy
Liver disease
Addison's disease
Hemochromatosis
Pituitary tumors

Box 15.1 Acquired hyperpigmentation

Depigmenting agents and reported effect on the melanin synthetic pathway

Before melanin synthesis
- Tyrosinase transcription:
  Tretinoin

During melanin synthesis
- Tyrosynase inhibition:
  Hydroquinone
  4-Hydroxyanisole
  4-S-CAP and derivatives
  Arbutin
  Aloesin
  Azelaic acid
  Kojic acid
  Emblica
  Tyrostat
- Peroxidase inhibition:
  Phenols
- Product reduction and ROS scavengers:
  Ascorbic acid
  Ascorbic acid palmitate

After melanin synthesis
- Tyrosinase degradation:
  Linoleic acid
  α-Linolenic acid
- Inhibition of melanosome transfer:
  Serine protease inhibitors
  Lecthins and neoglycoproteins
  Soybean/milk extracts
  Niacinamide
- Skin turnover acceleration:
  Glycolic acid
  Lactic acid
  Linoleic acid
  Liquiritin
  Retinoic acid
  Helix aspersa Müller

4-S-CAP = 4-S-cystaminylphenol

Box 15.2 Depigmenting agents and reported effect on the melanin synthetic pathway. (Modified from Briganti S, Camera E, Picardo M 2003 Chemical and instrumental approaches to treat hyperpigmentation. Pigment Cell Research 16:1–11)

discouraging. Many of the agents that have been used cause skin irritation, require many months of regular use before results are apparent, or are only partly effective. Patient compliance with therapy must be strict. Sun avoidance and the religious use of a high sun protection factor (SPF) sunblock are mandatory for successful treatment.

Skin Lightening Cosmeceuticals

Multiple depigmenting cosmeceuticals are currently available, although published clinical evidence to support their effectiveness is lacking. These skin lightening compounds work by removing undesired pigment by acting at one or more steps in the pigmentation process (Box 15.2). Since tyrosinase is the rate limiting enzyme for melanin biosynthesis, many of the cosmeceuticals for skin lightening exert their effect on this enzyme.

Hydroquinone

For many years, the phenolic compound hydroquinone has been the most widely and successfully used skin lightening agent for the treatment of melasma, postinflammatory hyperpigmentation, and other disorders of hyperpigmentation (Fig. 15.2).

Hydroquinone occurs naturally in many plants as well as in coffee, tea, beer, and wine. Hydroquinone depigments skin by inhibiting the conversion of tyrosine to melanin. It has been shown to decrease tyrosinase activity by 90%. It may also inhibit DNA and RNA synthesis, as well as degrade melanosomes.

In the USA, hydroquinone is available over the counter (OTC) in strengths up to 2%. Most prescription strength hydroquinone formulations contain 3–4%, but concentrations as high as 10% may be available through compounding pharmacies.

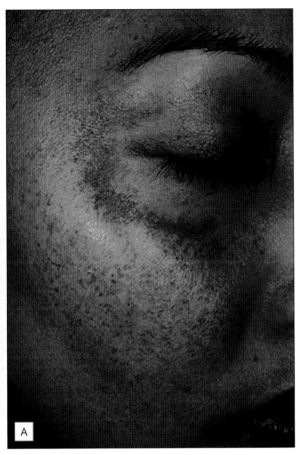 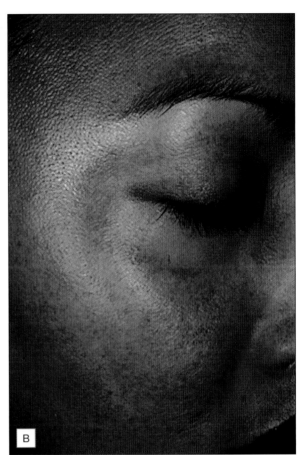

Fig. 15.2 **(A)** The appearance of facial melasma before treatment. **(B)** Improvement in hyperpigmentation following hydroquinone therapy (8 weeks after treatment)

Also, several new combination agents are now available in the USA. A prescription drug containing 4% hydroquinone, tretinoin, and a low potency fluorinated steroid, fluocinolone acetonide, is effective and safe in the treatment of melasma. Other combination products contain glycolic acid, vitamin C, and/or retinol to function as penetration enhancers for the hydroquinone active.

Hydroquinone is generally considered safe. Common side effects are skin irritation or contact dermatitis, which can be treated with topical steroids. A rare but serious side effect of hydroquinone is the development of exogenous ochronosis, a sooty hyperpigmentation in the treatment area, which may be difficult to reverse. Exogenous ochronosis appears to be prevalent among darker complected individuals when hydroquinone is used at high concentrations or for prolonged periods even at low concentrations.

For this reason, hydroquinone is restricted in several African countries and highly regulated in many Asian countries. Because of potential mutagenic properties, hydroquinone is also banned as an OTC depigmenting agent in the European Union and Japan. As a result of the restrictions, alternative depigmenting agents are increasingly being used either as monotherapy or in combination with hydroquinone or other skin lightening agents. Alternating the use of hydroquinone with one of these alternative agents in 4 month cycles will help prevent side effects such as irritation as well as decreasing the risk of exogenous ochronosis.

Natural cosmeceuticals for dyspigmentation

Increasing interest in the use of natural actives, as well as the need to find an alternative to hydroquinone, has led to research on a variety of dyspigmentation

Natural depigmenting agents

- Aloesin
- Arbutin
- Azelaic acid
- Glycolic acid
- Kojic acid
- Licorice extract
- Melatonin
- Niacinamide
- Paper mulberry
- Retinol
- Soy extracts
- Vitamin C

Box 15.3 Natural depigmenting agents

Active ingredients found in skin lightening kojic acid combination products

- Arbutin
- Asefitida extract
- Cranberry extract
- GABA
- Glycolic acid
- Hydroxy acid
- Laurel berry derivates
- Licorice extract
- Moisturizers
- Mulberry extract
- Vitamin C

Box 15.4 Active ingredients found in skin lightening kojic acid combination products

treatment cosmeceuticals derived from natural ingredients (Box 15.3).

Kojic acid

Kojic acid is a tyrosinase inhibitor derived from various fungal species such as *Aspergillus* and *Penicillium*. It is used in food processing to prevent browning and to promote the reddening of unripe strawberries. It is used in Asia both topically as a skin lightening agent, and also in the diet.

Kojic acid is used in concentrations between 1 and 4% and is often more effective in combination with other ingredients (Box 15.4). Kojic acid has been reported to have a high sensitizing potential and may cause irritant contact dermatitis. However, it is useful in patients who cannot tolerate hydroquinone and studies show it may be combined with a topical corticosteroid to reduce irritation. Skin lightening products that contain kojic acid are typically used twice per day for 1 or 2 months or until the desired effect is achieved.

Licorice extract—glabridin

Licorice extract is obtained from the root of *Glycyrrhiza glabra linneva*. Its main active ingredient is 10–40% glabridin. Glabridin offers 50% inhibition of tyrosinase activity with no attendant cytotoxicity and has been shown to be 16 times more efficacious than hydroquinone.

The combination of licorice extract with other ingredients yields good skin lightening responses (Box 15.5). New formulations containing licorice

Active ingredients found in skin lightening licorice extract combination products

- Arbutin
- Hyaluronic acid
- Hydrating agents
- Kojic acid
- Moisturizing complex
- Mulberry extract
- Tyrosine peptides
- Vitamin C-phosphate
- Vitamin E

Box 15.5 Active ingredients found in skin lightening licorice extract combination products

extract are under development for the treatment of dermal melasma.

Bearberry and arbutin

Bearberry (*Arctostaphylos uva ursi*), 'the bear's grape', has been named from the notion that bears eat the fruit even though it has an unpleasant flavor. The main constituents of bearberry are a crystallizable glucoside known as arbutin (hydroquinone-beta-D-glucopyranoside) and methyl arbutin, both with skin lightening properties. The skin lightening effect occurs via inhibition of melanosomal tyrosinase activity rather than suppression of tyrosinase synthesis.

While the effective concentration for arbutin in skin lightening has not been determined, it has been noted that its efficacy is less than that of kojic acid. Several products that contain arbutin alone or in combination in concentrations of 1% with other depigmenting agents are available.

Paper mulberry

Paper mulberry extract is a tyrosinase inhibitor, which is isolated from the roots of an ornamental tree, *Broussonetia papyrifera*. In a Korean study, the tyrosinase inhibition activity of paper mulberry was compared to that of hydroquinone and kojic acid. The 50% inhibitory concentration of paper mulberry extract was reported to be 0.396% versus 5.5% for hydroquinone and 10% for kojic acid. A patch test using 1% paper mulberry extract showed a lack of significant skin irritation at 24 and 48 hours. Although paper mulberry has shown effects on tyrosinase inhibition, there are currently no studies evaluating its use as a cosmeceutical in pigmentary disorders.

Soy

Soy has become a recently popular cosmeceutical in facial moisturizers to even skin discoloration. Natural soybeans contain the small proteins Bowman–Birk inhibitor (BBI) and soybean trypsin inhibitor (STI). The mechanism of action of soy is different from that of hydroquinone, kojic acid, or glabridin. Interference with the PAR-2 pathway by STI has been shown to reduce dyspigmentation by reducing the phagocytes of melanosomes by keratinocytes, thus reducing melanin transfer. It is important to note that this cosmeceutical effect is present only with fresh soy milk and not with pasteurized soy milk, since the STI is rapidly degraded.

Vitamin C

Topical vitamin C products can be derived from such natural sources as fruits and vegetables, as discusssed in Chapter 8, which is solely devoted to vitamin C. Vitamin C interferes with pigment production at various oxidative steps of melanin synthesis by interacting with copper ions at the tyrosinase active site and reducing dopaquinone. A stable derivative, magnesium L-ascorbic acid-2-phosphate (MAP), has been shown to lighten dyspigmentation.

Melatonin

Melatonin is a hormone that is secreted by the pineal gland in response to sunlight. In addition to its effects on diurnal rhythms in mammals, it has been shown in vitro to inhibit melanogenesis in a dose related manner. It does affect tyrosinase activity, suggesting that its effect occurs more proximally in the melanogenesis pathway. It has been shown to inhibit cyclic AMP driven processes in pigment cells. The concentration needed for effective cosmeceutical skin lightening in human skin has not yet been established. It has been shown to have anti-inflammatory activity at a dosage of $0.6 \, \text{mg/cm}^2$.

Glycolic acid

Glycolic acid, an alpha-hydroxy acid derived from sugarcane, is an important cosmeceutical (discussed in detail in Chapter 16) that has skin lightening effects. At low concentrations, glycolic acid has an epidermal discohesive effect, which results in more rapid desquamation of pigmented keratinocytes. Like retinoids, glycolic acid shortens the cell cycle so that pigment is lost more rapidly. At higher concentrations, glycolic acid results in epidermolysis. Several studies have shown that the removal of superficial layers of epidermis with glycolic acid peels at concentrations of 30–70% can enhance the penetration of other topical skin lighteners such as hydroquinone.

When glycolic acid is used in the treatment of postinflammatory hyperpigmentation or melasma, it has been suggested that it should be initiated at low concentrations to avoid skin irritation or induce post-inflammatory hyperpigmentation, especially in dark skinned individuals. The use of hydroquinone both prior to and after the peel can lessen the risk of such pigmentary changes. Also, the addition of glycolic acid to hydroquinone formulations seems to increase efficacy due to enhanced penetration.

Aloesin

Aloesin is a natural hydroxychromone derivative isolated from aloe vera which inhibits tyrosinase at noncytotoxic concentrations, probably acting as a competitor inhibitor on DOPA oxidation and as a non-competitor on tyrosine. In vivo, the combination of aloesin and arbutin synergistically inhibit ultraviolet induced melanogenesis.

Niacinamide

Niacinamide is the amide form of vitamin B_3. Niacinamide affects pigmentation by inhibiting the transfer of melanosomes from the melanocyte to the epidermal keratinocytes. Studies have shown the effectiveness of 3.5% niacinamide combined with retinyl palmitate for the improvement of hyperpigmentation.

Azelaic acid

Azelaic acid is a naturally occurring dicarboxylic acid derived from *Pityrosporum ovale*. Its lightening effect appears to be selective and most apparent in highly active melanocytes, with minimal effects in normally pigmented skin.

Azelaic acid at a concentration of 20% was found to be a more effective treatment than 2% hydroquinone and produces both a greater lightening of pigmented lesions and reduction in lesion size. Azelaic acid at concentrations of 15% or 20% applied twice daily for 3–12 months produced clinical and histologic resolution in facial lentigo maligna. It has also been used successfully to treat rosacea, solar keratosis, and hyperpigmentation associated with burns and herpes labialis.

Azelaic acid is generally well tolerated and can be used for extended periods. Its most frequent side effects include transient erythema and cutaneous irritation characterized by scaling, itching, and burning, which generally resolve after 2–4 weeks of application.

Other skin lightening products

For other compounds, the in vitro data are promising, however no sufficient in vivo studies are available to judge their clinical efficacy. Emblica, a compound isolated from *Phyllanthus emblica* fruits, is native to tropical southeastern Asia. The compound, a chelator for iron and copper, reduces ultraviolet induced skin pigmentation at a 1% concentration and has a presumed effect on tyrosinase inhibition and expression. Unsaturated fatty acids, such as oleic and linoleic acid, suppress pigmentation in vitro. Linoleic acid in vivo shows a skin lightening effect on UVB induced pigmentation without toxic melanocyte effects. An extract from the Chilean snail of the species *Helix aspersa* Müller has been used with success in the treatment of melasma and hyperpigmentation. Tyrostat, an extract of a plant native to Canada's northern Prairie region, acts by inhibiting melanin

synthesis. These are but a few of the many botanical and naturally derived agents in the literature that are touted for their ability to lighten skin. They are briefly presented here to give the reader an idea of the tremendous variety of cosmeceutical actives available to the cosmetic chemist.

Retinoids and retinoid combination therapy

Naturally occurring retinoids and retinol are derived from vitamin A. Retinol and retinoids have been used to treat pigmentary disorders including melasma and the postinflammatory hyperpigmentation that is a frequent sequel to acne.

While the actual mechanism of action of retinoid as depigmenting agents is not clear, in animal studies it has been shown to inhibit tyrosinase induction. In an early paper from Kligman and Willis in 1975, it was suggested that tretinoin may exert its depigmenting action by means of dispersion of pigment granules in keratinocytes with a loss of supranuclear caps in the basal layer. Retinoids may also interfere with pigment transfer to keratinocytes. Additionally, retinoids accelerate epidermal turnover causing keratinocytes to be shed more quickly, also leading to pigment loss.

Tretinoin is included in a triple combination dyspigmentation formulation currently approved for the treatment of melasma, as well as in several prescription acne and antiaging products in concentrations of 0.04–0.1%. Retinol is sold in OTC formulations and is less effective for the treatment of dyspigmentation and less irritating than tretinoin. Retinol 0.15% is an ingredient with 4% hydroquinone and ultraviolet A (UVA) and UVB sunscreens in a cream that is used to treat disorders of hyperpigmentation. Other products include ultraviolet A(UVA) and UVB sunscreens in their formulations.

Summary

As the population ages, dyspigmentation due to photoaging will be more common. Hyperpigmentation from other causes, such as melasma and postinflammatory conditions, are also of increasing concern as patients realize that the unsightly brown discoloration can be improved with dermatologic treatment (Fig. 15.3).

While there are numerous cosmeceutical skin lightening agents, more extensive controlled clinical trials are needed to assess their safety and efficacy.

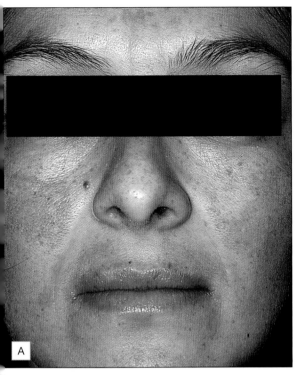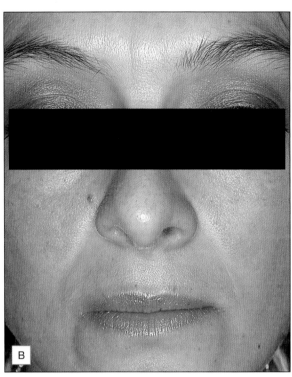

Fig. 15.3 The increasing US population of women with darker skin makes hyperpigmentation treatment an important cosmetic concern. (**A**) Before cosmeceutical treatment. (**B**) Eight weeks after cosmeceutical treatment

Further Reading

Adebajo SB 2002 An epidemiological survey of the use of cosmetic skin lightening cosmetics among traders in Lagos, Nigeria. West African Journal of Medicine 21:51–55

Baumann L 2004 Depigmenting agents. In: Day DJ (ed) Understanding hyperpigmentation. What you need to know. Continuing Medical Education monograph. Intellyst Medical Communications. Aurora, CO

Briganti S, Camera E, Picardo M 2003 Chemical and instrumental approaches to treat hyperpigmentation. Pigment Cell Research 16:1–11

Cameli N, Marmo W, Gaeta A, Calderini G, Picardo M 2001 Evaluation of clinical efficacy of a mixture of depigmenting agents. Pigment Cell Research 14:406

Draelos ZD 2004 Several active naturals aid in the prevention of photoaging. Highlights of a symposium: the role of natural ingredients in dermatology. Skin and Allergy News Supplement January: 4

Guevara IL, Pandya AG 2003 Safety and efficacy of a 4% hydroquinone combined with 10% glycolic acid, antioxidants, and sunscreen in the treatment of melasma. International Journal of Dermatology 42:966–972

Hakozaki T, Minwalla L, Zhuang J, et al 2002 The effect of niacinamide on reducing cutaneous pigmentation and suppression of melanosome transfer. British Journal of Dermatology 147:20–31

Holloway VL 2003 Ethnic cosmetic products. Dermatologic Clinics 21:743–749

Jones K, Hughes J, Hong M, Jia Q, Orndorff S 2002 Modulation of melanogenesis by aloesin: a competitive inhibitor of tyrosinase. Pigment Cell Research 15:335–340

Kollias N, Wallo W, Pote J, et al 2003 Documentation of changes in cutaneous pigmentation incorporating advances in imaging technology. Scientific Poster Presented at American Academy of Dermatology 61st Annual Meeting, San Francisco, California, March 21–26

Lim JT 1999 Treatment of melasma using kojic acid in a gel containing hydroquinone and glycolic acid. Dermatologic Surgery 25:282–284

Pérez-Bernal E, Muñoz-Pérez MA, Camacho F 2000 Management of facial hyperpigmentation. American Journal of Clinical Dermatology 1:261–268

Piamphongsat T 1998 Treatment of melasma: a review with personal experience. International Journal of Dermatology 37:897–903

Rendon MI 2003 Melasma and post-inflammatory hyperpigmentation. Cosmetic Dermatology 16:9–17

Sarkar R, Bhalla M, Kanwar AJ 2002 A comparative study of 20% azelaic acid cream monotherapy versus sequential therapy in the treatment of melasma in dark skinned patients. Dermatology 205:249–254

Seiberg M, Paine C, Sharlow E, et al 2000 Inhibition of melanosome transfer results in skin lightening. Journal of Investigative Dermatology 115:162–167

Exfoliants: AHAs and BHAs

16   *Cherie M. Ditre*

Introduction

Exfoliation is defined from the Latin *exfoliatio* meaning falling off in scales or layers. Since many dermatologic conditions are either due to or associated with an inability to exfoliate due to excessive corneocyte cohesion, it appears that chemical exfoliation of some epidermal elements would provide a therapeutic benefit. In addition, this accelerated cell loss and sloughing which is the basis of chemexfoliation has been found to beneficially impact the skin's appearance. These cosmetic benefits attributed to skin exfoliation has been long known since the time of the ancient Egyptians, their observation that simply bathing in sour milk, now known to contain the bioactive ingredient lactic acid, yielded softer and smoother skin thereby improving the skin's luster and appearance. Dermatologists have been interested in chemical exfoliants since 1882 when Unna, a German dermatologist, first described the properties of salicylic acid, resorcinol, phenol and trichloroacetic acid as a chemical peeling agent.

Nowadays, we have many means of inducing skin exfoliation. These agents are chemical, mechanical, and thermal from lasers or light based sources. This section will concentrate on those chemical agents known as AHAs (alpha hydroxy acids), BHAs (beta hydroxy acids), and PHAs (poly hydroxy acids) that have found a resurgence in their popularity for both the therapeutic as well as the cosmetic benefit that they impart to the skin. It has been long touted that their benefits are due to exfoliation alone. Currently then, the FDA classifies AHAs as a cosmeceutical for this and other superficial reactions on the skin.

Depending on their formulation, vehicle, acid type, pH, concentration, and body area treated, these acids can provide a wide range of skin benefits. There is still controversy surrounding these agents as well as others, and this chapter will discuss this, along with the exfoliation process risk and benefit ratios to the skin.

Alpha Hydroxy Acids (AHAs)

Definition

AHAs are a group of organic carboxylic acids that have been popularized since they are felt to be natural substances. The name is derived from their chemistry, an hydroxyl group attached to the alpha carbon adjacent to the acid moiety. Indeed many AHAs are found naturally occurring in the body, but when used in skin products or procedures these agents are synthetically derived. Nonetheless, synthetic AHAs function as those derived from organic sources.

The simplest molecule of AHAs and indeed the prototype is glycolic acid (derived from sugarcane) with the lowest molecular weight and a pK_a of 3.83. It is water soluble and has been used in its partially neutralized form for topical home care products and in a free acid form in peeling products. Lactic acid (derived from sour milk) with a molecular weight of 91 is felt to work best in its L form. It has been found in topical home care products and in Jessner's peeling solution. Tartaric acid (derived from grapes) is the antioxidant and is used in some home care products. Citric acid (derived from citrus fruits) is a larger charge AHA but with similar skin benefits.

Histologic effects

It has been long held that lower concentrations of AHAs, when applied topically, reduce the thickness of the hyperkeratotic stratum corneum by reducing corneocyte cohesion in the lower levels of the stratum corneum. When applied in higher concentrations and at low pH values, these same AHAs can cause epidermolysis as they have been found to work at the desmosomal attachment sites of the basalar layer. This effect can then produce varying degrees of exfoliation of the skin and therefore AHAs are useful in the management of various cosmetic and dermatologic conditions such as dry skin, seborrheic dermatitis, callosities, acne (Fig. 16.1), scarring (Fig. 16.2), actinic and seborrheic keratoses, and warts as well as photodamaged skin.

Mechanism of action

The mechanism of action of AHAs has not been fully determined. It is postulated that AHAs act as a chelating agent and thereby decrease local

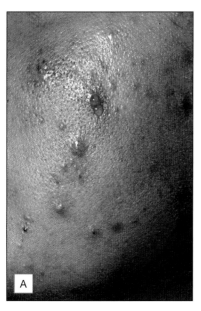
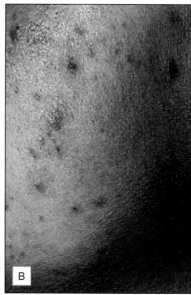

Fig. 16.1 Acne treatment can be enhanced through the use of glycolic acid peels. (**A**) Before. (**B**) After

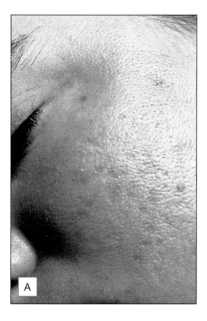
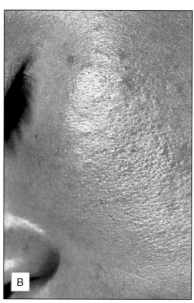

Fig. 16.2 The appearance of acne scarred skin can be minimized with repeated alpha hydroxy acid peels. (**A**) Before. (**B**) After

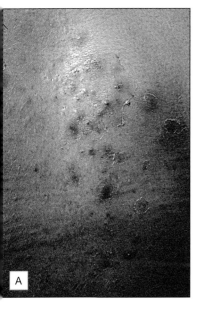 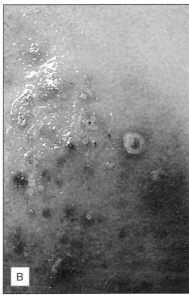

Fig. 16.3 Whitening of the skin following application of an alpha hydroxy acid peeling solution indicates cellular adhesion disruption and the initiation of exfoliation. (**A**) Before. (**B**) After

calcium ion concentrations from cation dependent cell adhesion molecules. This calcium loss from cadherins of desmosomes, adherens junctions, and tight junctions causes a decrease in desmosomal attachments. This makes the usually protected endogenous stratum corneum chymotryptic enzymes on cadherins vulnerable to proteolysis. When calcium is decreased then cellular adhesions are disrupted and exfoliation takes place (Fig. 16.3).

Another proposed mechanism for AHA induced exfoliation is an increase in apoptosis. In one study, lactic acid was shown to cause a concentration dependent increase in apoptotic cells. In this same study, vascular endothelial growth factor (VEGF) was increased at least 2.5 fold over vehicle control with either a 1.5 or 3% concentration of lactic acid (LA). Angiogenin secretion was decreased by LA in a concentration dependent manner. It was concluded that topical AHAs modulate secretion of cytokines by keratinocytes and that this regulation may account in part for their effects in skin disorders as well as photoaging. Another study in 2003 confirms that glycolic acid (GA) directly accelerates collagen synthesis by fibroblasts, and modulates matrix degradation and collagen synthesis through keratinocyte released cytokines (Fig. 16.4). The primary mediator for this matrix degradation is interleukin 1α (IL-1α).

In our study of AHAs (GA, LA, and CA) at a 25% concentration, it was shown that there was an increase in dermal dendrocytes and mast cell activation. It was postulated then that AHAs may cause upregulation of epidermal and dermal markers by stimulating transforming growth factor beta (TGF-β) which in turn causes activation of dermal dendrocytes and mast cell release.

Role in moisturization

Unlike salicylic acid, AHAs have the ability not only to cause exfoliation but also moisturization. This dual nature of AHAs has been noted but not completely understood. It is postulated that the AHAs induced increased mucopolysaccharide content, in particular dermal glycosaminoglycans (GAGs), in the skin, which may account for the increased moisturization. It was shown in one study that 20% GA treatment of forearm skin as compared to vehicle demonstrated an increase in hyaluronic acid content in the epidermis and dermis and an increase in collagen mRNA gene expression in the AHA treated sites only.

There is relatively little data on the effects of AHA on stratum corneum lipids. In their unpublished data, Motta and Berardesca indicate that an increase production of ceramides occurs with AHAs use. This would provide one explanation for the moisturization and barrier fortification that these products deliver (Fig. 16.5).

Role in skin barrier function

The major concern with long term use of AHAs is the possibility of disruption of skin barrier function.

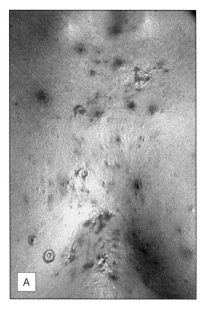
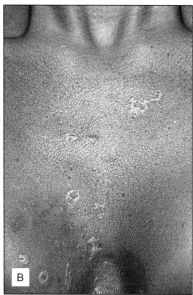

Fig. 16.4 Alpha hydroxy acid peels can be used on the chest to improve acne and skin texture. (**A**) Before. (**B**) After

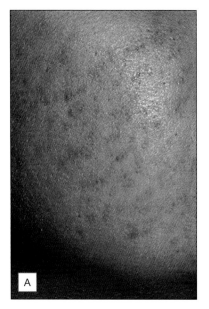
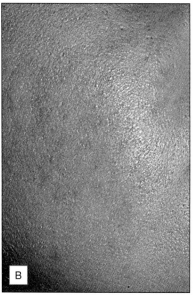

Fig. 16.5 Improvement in skin texture following an alpha hydroxy acid peel is demonstrated. (**A**) Before. (**B**) After

Several studies have addressed this. In 1997, Berardesca et al applied to six test sites the following: three different AHAs (glycolic acid (GA) pH 4.4, lactic acid (LA) pH 4.4, tartaric acid (TA) pH 3.4), a PHA (gluconolactone (GLU) pH 4.3) all in 8% concentration, a vehicle (VE) and an untreated skin control (UNT) over 4 weeks. Each of these sites were then subjected to a 5% sodium lauryl sulfate (SLS) challenge patch test under occlusion for 6 hours. Barrier function and skin irritation were then evaluated immediately after the removal of the SLS patches and at 24 and 48 hours later. There were no significant differences in the transepidermal water loss (TEWL) after AHA and PHA at week 4. The vehicle treated site actually showed an increase in water loss compared with the untreated control. This was felt to be due to the vehicle being slightly alkaline at pH 8.2. After SLS challenge, GLU and TA treated sites resulted in a significantly lower water loss compared to vehicle, untreated control, and GA at 24 and 48 hours. They concluded that all AHAs/PHAs can both improve barrier reactivity and increase resistance to surfactant induced skin irritation. This effect was more marked, however, with gluconolactone and tartaric acid treated sites. This unique effect of GLU and TA was postulated to be due to their antioxidant properties.

In this study, the authors tried to explain the observation that AHAs and PHAs impart a brightening effect or glow to the appearance of the skin. This effect was postulated to be due to the thinner more compact stratum corneum after AHA/PHA treatment which better reflects light. Surprisingly, this effect was found to be still present even after SLS challenge, a known inducer of lackluster, dry, scaly skin. It was concluded from the study that AHAs/PHAs impart a measurable skin brightening effect at about week 4 of treatment and, more importantly, they protect the skin from the aggressive challenge of surfactants.

In 2001, Kim et al applied a 5% GA and a 5% LA to hairless mice daily over a 2 week period. They found no significant difference in TEWL and skin capacitance when comparing the mice skin treated with the AHAs versus vehicle alone. They did find on electron microscopy that the AHA treated skin showed an increase in the number and secretion of lamellar bodies and a decrease in stratum corneum layers compared to the epidermis of vehicle treated alone. They concluded that AHAs in low concentrations may improve skin barrier function in mice by inducing an enhanced desquamation and an increase in the number and secretion of the lamellar bodies without increasing TEWL. This may be a unique function of the AHAs, again explaining their exfoliating and moisturizing capabilities.

In 2004, Song et al found that skin barrier function is damaged after a GA peel and also after aluminum oxide microdermabrasion but recovers within 1–4 days after treatment. Therefore, these authors felt that repeat peeling at 2 weeks intervals would allow sufficient time for the skin to recover.

Effects on UVB induced skin tumors

GA may exert inhibitory effects on UVB induced skin tumor development by blocking UVB induced apoptosis through inhibition of c-fos expression and activation of AP-1. This effect may also be due to inhibition of p53–p21 response pathways. GA was applied bid after UV irradiation given 5 d/wk to hairless mice. Transcription factors AP-1 and nuclear factor kappa B (NF-κB) activation was significantly lower in UV and GA treated skin compared with activation in UV irradiated skin alone. There was also decreased expression of UV induced cell cycle regulatory proteins, proliferative cell nuclear antigen (Ag) (PCNA), cyclin D1, cyclin E, and the associated subunits cyclin dependent kinase 2 (cdk2) and cdk4. The expression of signal mediators p38 kinase, jun N-terminal kinase (jnk), and mitogen activated protein kinase (MEK) was lower in GA treated skin compared with expression in UV treated skin alone. Therefore GA reduced tumor development. This protective effect of GA was quantitated to be a 20% reduction in skin tumor incidence, a 55% reduction in tumor multiplicity (number of tumors/mouse), and a 47% decrease in number of large tumors (>2 mm). GA was tested for maternal and developmental toxicity in pregnant rats and their pups when the pregnant rat was given GA in water over gestational days 7 through 21. At doses of 150 mg/kg there was no observed effect level (NOEL) in maternal or developmental toxicity. However, there were reported levels at doses that were four times higher than this.

Photosensitivity

In 2003, the backs of 29 Caucasians were treated daily with 10% GA (pH 3.5) and compared to placebo in a randomized double blind study over 4 weeks and then subjected to treatment with UV light at 1.5 MED. GA caused enhanced sensitivity to UV light as measured by sunburn cell induction and lowered MED's. This effect abated after 1 week off the GA treatment. The conclusion of the authors was that short term (1 month) application causes photosensitivity. In other unpublished data, AHAs may increase the need for sunscreen to a level equivalent to surfactant use, i.e. washing the skin with soap and water, namely spf 2, to adequately protect from photosensitivity. There is no published data about the long term use of GA and photosensitivity. However since 2000 the FDA has been undertaking an AHA photocarcinogenicity study and is working with the National Toxicology Program to continue to study AHA safety.

Effects on pigmentation

Interestingly, in that same year an in vitro study showed that GA and LA in doses of 300 or 500 μg/mL suppressed melanin formation by

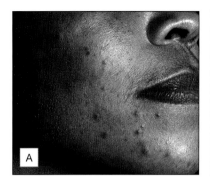
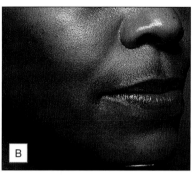

Fig. 16.6 Alpha hydroxy acids can be used to improve the skin texture and color of persons with deeply pigmented skin. (**A**) Before. (**B**) After

directly inhibiting tyrosinase activity. Adjusting the pH up to 5.6 did not affect tyrosinase activity and this effect was then deemed independent of these AHAs acidic nature. The authors postulate that GA and/or LA might work on pigmented lesions by accelerating epidermal turnover and by directly inhibiting melanin formation in melanocytes. There have been conflicting clinical studies showing no benefit to a positive benefit in patients with hyperpigmented skin conditions. It is this author's belief that the AHAs may actually work clinically by enhancing penetration of other bleaching agents such as hydroquinones or retinoids and/or by directly inducing skin turnover which improves the appearance of hyperpigmentation due to hyperkeratinization (Fig. 16.6).

Cosmeceutical effects

In 1996, topical 8% GA and LA creams were compared in a double blind, vehicle controlled randomized clinical trial of the effects on photodamaged skin of 74 women aged 40–70 years over 22 weeks. The study showed that AHA creams were well tolerated and found to be modestly beneficial in ameliorating the clinical signs of photodamage. After 10 weeks of treatment, both GA and LA significantly reduced mottled hyperpigmentation of the forearms compared with the vehicle. This effect was maximized by 14 weeks of treatment. At the end of this study, only LA showed a continued significant advantage over the vehicle. AHA induced significant reductions in skin sallowness as observed at 10 weeks, maximized at 14 weeks, and maintained throughout the 22 weeks of the study over vehicle. There was a 16% greater dimunution of tactile roughness with AHAs as compared to vehicle alone.

Only the subjects using AHAs noted improvement from baseline in the number of fine wrinkles, firmness, age spots, or eveness of color.

In our study in that same year, it was shown that AHAs (GA, LA, and CA) all produced an improvement in photoaging markers. Histologically, it was shown that AHAs in a 25% concentration could cause epidermal and papillary dermal thickening, yield a more undulating rete ridge pattern, increase acid mucopolysaccharides, improve the quality of the elastic fibers, and increase the collagen density.

Combination with other antiaging agents

Another study described the use of 15% GA versus 0.1% estradiol versus the combination of GA/estradiol on postmenopausal women. Sixty-five patients were treated with one agent alone or in combination to one side of the face, and with the vehicle to the opposite side, for 6 months. This study showed that epidermal thickness increased by 23% with estradiol, 27% with glycolic acid, and 38% with the combination.

Kligman et al looked at the compatibility of AHAs with retinoids. They reported that in 20 adolescents with moderate acne vulgaris the use of AHAs with either 0.025% or 0.05% tretinoin was tolerated and that there were only mild adverse subjective reactions which occurred in both placebo versus AHA treated skin sites. In the photoaged group, 20 women aged 39–60 years were given tretinoin 0.05% for the first 2 months which was then increased to 0.1% for the remaining 4 months. GA 8% was applied to the entire face. The manifestations of stinging, dryness, itching, and occasional mild peeling and erythema were noted in the first 6 weeks and then lessened. There were no more complaints than usually encountered with tretinoin alone. At the end of the study, 50% of the patients had moderate effacement of wrinkles. Two thirds of the patients felt that their skin had less dry scaling and that the skin's surface was definitely smoother. It was felt that the combination of AHA and retinoids caused no more difficulty than the use of tretinoin alone. It is postulated that there is a synergistic effect with the two agents.

Salicylic Acid

Salicylic acid is a phenolic aromatic acid, 2-hydroxy-benzoic acid or o-hydroxy benzoic acid. It has been popularized as a beta hydroxy acid but this description has been refuted chemically since the hydroxyl and carboxyl groups are directly attached to an aromatic benzene ring. These groups can then exhibit an acidic property like its analog, phenol. In AHAs, BHAs like tropic acid, and PHAs, the hydroxyl and carboxyl groups are attached to an aliphatic or alicyclic carbon chain and the hydroxyl group is neutral in chemical property.

Salicylic acid is used in cosmetic formulations as a denaturant, hair conditioning agent, and skin conditioning agent, and is available in a wide range of cosmetic products at concentrations ranging from 0.0008% to 3%. SA is fat soluble and this property makes it useful in patients with oily skin.

Mechanism of action

It has also been contested that the mechanism of action of salicylic acid at concentrations from 2% to 12% is simply due to keratolysis of the stratum corneum without effect on deeper skin components. This draws the contrast between the AHAs, which have been touted to modulate keratinization at the lower levels of the stratum corneum adjacent to the stratum granulosum (see above). However, there is some data to suggest that SA works on the intercellular spaces between corneocytes in the stratum corneum.

One recent study indicates that SA acts at the level of transcription to downregulate the production of fibrinogen, fibronectin, and alpha hemolysin virulence factors necessary for bacterial replication in host tissues. Whether SA affects bacterial production in acne has not been reported here.

Toxicity

Salicylates are absorbed percutaneously and approximately 10% of applied salicylates can remain in the skin. This has created a controversy over the risk of salicylism due to SA application over a large surface or compromised skin over a sustained period of time. Salicylism has been shown to occur with methyl salicylate ointments and high concentrations of SA on widespread areas of hyperkeratoic skin but there are no known cases resulting from SA acne products. Therefore, it is best to be cautious when using SA in childhood, pregnancy, lactation, and concomitant drug therapy, simply because relevant drug studies are lacking. Nonetheless, an exposure assessment of a representative cosmetic salicylate product used on a daily basis estimated that the exposure would be only 20% of the level seen with ingestion of a 'baby' aspirin (81 mg) on a daily basis. Little acute toxicity (LD_{50} in rats $>2\,g/kg$) via a dermal exposure route is seen for SA. Subchronic dermal exposures to undiluted methyl salicylate were associated with kidney damage. Methyl salicylate is used as a denaturant and flavoring agent (0.0001–0.6%).

Hairless SKH/hr1 mice were irradiated with ultraviolet B (UVB) light for 14 weeks and then were subjected with or without treatment every 2 weeks to 30% salicylic acid in PEG (polyethylene glycol) for a total of 18 weeks. In this study it was interesting to note that the total number of skin tumors were greatly reduced in the treated versus the control mice and skin tumor development was also slower in the treated versus the control mice. Fractions of T and B lymphocytes and natural killer cells from spleens of both groups of mice were comparable, and interferon gamma production did not differ. It was then suggested by the authors that chemical peeling with salicylic acid in PEG may help to prevent as well as to reduce the number of UVB induced skin tumors.

Safety

Because of the possible use of these ingredients as well as the AHAs as exfoliating agents, a concern exists that repeated use may effectively increase exposure of the dermis and epidermis to UV radiation. It was concluded by the Cosmetic Ingredient Review Expert Panel that the risk of increased UV radiation damage with the use of any exfoliant, including salicylic acid and salicylates, necessitated the cosmetic industry to take steps to formulate ingredients that are nonirritating with these exfoliating agents so as not to increase sun sensitivity, or to include directions for the daily use of sun protection. Available data were not sufficient to establish a limit on concentration of these ingredients, or to identify the minimum pH of formulations containing these ingredients, such that no skin irritation would occur. With the information that is presently available, the Cosmetic Ingredient Review Expert Panel reached the conclusion that when formulated in this way these ingredients are safe. It is interesting to note that ethylhexyl salicylate (formerly known as octyl salicylate) is used as a fragrance ingredient, sunscreen agent, and UV light absorber (0.001–8%).

Combining with other agents

Salicylic acid is reported to enhance percutaneous penetration of some agents (e.g. vitamin A), but not others (e.g. hydrocortisone). Its use as an antiaging agent has also been debated. It is anecdotally reported to be superiorly tolerated in rosacea skin types compared with GA. Clearly it is useful because of its effect on oily skin types with acne vulgaris.

Conclusion

Larger cohort studies need to be done to fully evaluate the efficacy as well as the mechanism of action of PHAs a well as the AHAs and BHAs (SA). The safety and toxicity of these agents are thought to be well controlled when formulated in a non-irritating vehicle and when combined with sunscreen. It is this author's belief that these agents do indeed increase the efficacy of other combined agents and that with further studies this will be more clearly understood.

Further Reading

Akhavan A, Bershad S 2003 Topical acne drugs: review of clinical properties, systemic exposure and safety. American Journal of Clinical Dermatology 4:473–492

Alpha-hydroxy acids: unapproved uses or indications 2004 SKINmed 3(3):141–144

Berardesca E, Distante F, Vignoli GP, Oresajo C, Green B 1997 Alpha hydroxyacids modulate stratum corneum barrier function. British Journal of Dermatology 137:934–938

Bernstein EF, Brown DBM, Schwartz MD, Kaidbey K, Ksenzenko SM 2004 The polyhydroxyl acid gluonolactone protects against UV radiation in an in vitro model of cutaneous photoaging. Dermatologic Surgery 30:189–195, discussion 196

Bernstein EF, Lee J, Brown DP, Yu R, Van Scott EJ 2001 Glycolic acid increases type I collagen mRNA and hyaluronic acid content of human skin. Dermatologic Surgery 27:429–433

Brody HJ 1997 Chemical peeling and resurfacing, 2nd edn. Mosby, St Louis, MO, p 1

Corcuff P, Fiat F, Gracia AM, Leveque JL 1996 Hydroxy acid induced desquamation of the human stratum corneum: A comparative ultrastructural sudy. 19th International Federation Society of Cosmetic Chemists Congress, Sydney, Australia (3):85–94

Cosmetic Ingredient Review Expert Panel 2003 Safety assessment of salicylic acid. International Journal of Toxicology 22(suppl 3):1–108

Ditre CM, Griffin TD, Murphy GF, et al 1996 Effects of alpha hydroxy acids on photoaged skin: a pilot clinical, histologic, and ultrastructural study. Journal of the American Academy of Dermatology 34:187–195

Ditre CM, Nini KT, Vagley RT 1996 Introduction: practical use of glycolic acid as a chemical peeling agent. Journal of Geriatric Dermatology 4(suppl B):2B–7B

Dorland's Illustrated Medical Dictionary, 30th edn 2003 WB Saunders, Philadelphia

Edison BL, Green BA, Wildnauer RH, Sigler ML 2002 A polyhydroxy acid skin care regimen provides antiaging effects comparable to an alpha-hydroxyacid regimen. Cutis 73:14–17

Grimes PE 1999 The safety and efficacy of SA chemical peels in darker racial ethnic groups. Dermatologic Surgery 25:18–22

Grimes PE, Green BA, Wildnauer, RH, Edison BL 2004 The use of polyhydroxy acids (PHAs) in photoaged skin. Cutis 73(suppl 2):3–13

Kim TH, Choi EH, Kang YC, Lee SH, Ahn SK 2001 British Journal of Dermatology 144:267–273

Kligman AM 1995 The compatibility of combinations of GA and tretinoin in acne and in photoaged facial skin. Journal of Geriatric Dermatology 3(suppl A):25A–28A

Leyden JJ, Lavker RM, Grove G, Kaidbey K 1994 Alpha hydroxy acids are more than moisturizers. Issues and perspectives of AHAs. Cosmetic Dermatology October(suppl):33A–37A

Okana Y, Abe Y, Masaki H, et al 2003 Biological effects of glycolic acid on dermal matrix metabolism mediated by dermal fibroblasts and epidermal keratinocytes. Experimental Dermatology 12(suppl 2):57–63

Rendl M, Mayer C, Weninger W, Tschachler E 2001 Topcially applied lactic acid increases spontaneous secretion of vascular endothelial growth factor by human reconstructed epidermis. British Journal of Dermatology 145:3–9

Song JY, Kang HA, Kim MY, Park YM, Kim HO 2004 Damage and recovery of skin barrier function after glycolic acid chemical peeling and crystal microdermabrasion. Dermatologic Surgery 30:390–394

Usuki A, Ohashi A, Sato H, et al 2003 The inhibitory effect of GA and LA on melanin synthesis in melanoma cells. Experimental Dermatology 12(suppl 2):43–50

Van Scott EJ, Ditre CM, Yu RJ 1996 Alpha-hydroxyacids in the treatment of signs of photoaging. Clinics in Dermatology 14:217–226

Van Scott EJ, Yu RJ 1995 Actions of alpha hydroxy acids on skin compartments. Journal of Geriatric Dermatology 3(suppl A):19A–24A

Van Scott EJ, Yu RJ 1989 Alpha hydroxy acids: therapeutic potentials. Canadian Journal of Dermatology 1(5):108–112

Van Scott EJ, Yu RJ 1989 Alpha hydroxy acids: procedures for use in clinical practice. Cutis 43:222–228

Veda S, Mitsugi K, Ichige K, et al 2002 New formulation of chemical peeling agent: 30% SA in polyethylene glycol. Journal of Dermatologic Sciences 28:211–218

Wang X 1999 A theory for the mechanism of action of the AHAs applied to the skin. Medical Hypotheses 53:380–382

Yu RJ, Van Scott EJ 1994 Alpha-hydroxy acids: science and therapeutic use. issues and perspectives of AHAs. Cosmetic Dermatology October(suppl):1–6

Yu RJ, Van Scott EJ 1996 Bioavailability of alpha-hydroxy acids in topical formulations. Cosmetic Dermatology 9:54–62

Yu RJ, Van Scott EJ 1997 Salicylic acid: not a beta-hydroxy acid. Cosmetic Dermatology 10:27 [letter to the editor]

17 Peptides and Proteins

Mary P. Lupo

Introduction

The main purpose of cosmeceuticals is to improve the appearance of aging skin. In dermatology, there are often many ways to accomplish any particular goal. One method to reverse cutaneous signs of aging is through the use of prescription retinoids, such as tretinoin and tazarotene. However, these substances are irritating to the skin resulting in the peeling and stinging characteristic of barrier damage. In recent years, the trend in cosmeceuticals has been for products that improve the appearance of aging skin without the irritation of topical retinoids. This has resulted in the popularity of peptides, which have demonstrated cosmeceutical effects both in vitro and in vivo that could result in clinical aging skin improvement. This chapter discusses the current use of cosmeceutical peptides to aid the practicing dermatologist in understanding the science behind these new ingredients and how to utilize them for cutaneous antiaging treatment.

Terminology and Definitions

Peptides are short chains of amino acid sequences that make up larger proteins. There are three categories of peptides currently being used in cosmeceutical products (Box 17.1). This increase in peptide technology has arisen because of the technology to synthesize fragments that mimic peptide sequences in collagen and elastin with the ability to stimulate

---

Cosmeceutical peptides

- Signal peptides
- Carrier peptides
- Neurotransmitter blocking peptides

Box 17.1 Cosmeceutical peptides

---

production of new collagen and elastin. Other peptides are currently available that function primarily as carriers of cofactors for important enzymatic steps in collagen production. Peptide fragments also exist that are able to block neurotransmitter release. Since some wrinkling of the skin is caused by collagen breakdown, while other wrinkles are caused by hyperkinetic facial muscle movement, peptides that have actions to inhibit or reverse these actions could have clinical antiaging cosmeceutical benefits.

Indications and Biologic Activity

Clinically, photoaged skin has wrinkles that are coarse, while the wrinkles of naturally aged skin are much finer. Both of these wrinkles are due, in part, to the loss of collagen in the skin. Chronologically aged skin shows decreased production of new collagen, as well as increased proteolytic activity resulting in increased collagen degradation. Aging fibroblasts show decreased synthesis of mRNA for type I collagen, which is the major collagen in the skin. Also, in skin cell cultures, aging fibroblasts proliferate at a slower rate than fetal fibroblasts. Therefore, natural aging is at least partly the result of the limited replicative capacity of dermal fibroblasts, as well as the overexpression of proteolytic activity of matrix metalloproteinase 1 (MMP-1, interstitial collagenase).

Additionally, both photoaged and naturally aged human skin have lower procollagen type I mRNA and protein compared to younger skin. The balance between collagen synthesis and collagen breakdown appears to be different in the same individual from photoaged to naturally aged skin. While both show greater MMP activity, it is even higher in the skin aged from UV radiation exposure. The precocious elastosis seen in actinically damaged skin is also at least partially responsible for the difference in the appearance of sun induced versus age induced wrinkling. The elastotic degeneration of sun damaged skin may be due to chronic injury to the fibroblasts that results in thicker elastotic fibers with accentuated microfibral dense masses. In the photoaged skin, both mRNA and protein production are reduced when compared to sun protected skin of the same individual. UV radiation is well known to stimulate MMP-1, which in turn damages and degrades collagen. It is likely that the degraded and damaged collagen has a further deleterious effect on dermal fibroblast function after repeated injury. Thus, there is a need for cosmeceuticals capable of either increasing collagen regeneration or preventing its further demise. Peptides and proteins for antiaging purposes were developed with this end in mind.

Signal peptides

It is well recognized that the ability to stimulate proteins of the extracellular matrix, including collagen and elastin, or diminishment of the activity of collagenase, or both could result in clinical improvement of the wrinkles and lines that are seen in both photoaged and naturally aged skin. Thus, direct stimulation of the collagen producing human dermal fibroblasts or downregulation of fibroblast collagenase production are the mechanisms by which a cosmeceutical may clinically improve lines and wrinkles. Bioactive peptides were originally developed as part of wound healing research on the growth and stimulation of human skin fibroblasts. These same peptides are now being studied for their ability to act as growth factors via activation of protein kinase C, a key enzyme for cell growth and migration. Wound studies of human keratinocyte cultures show a stimulatory effect from topical application of neuropeptides, such as gastrin releasing peptide. Certain amino acid chains in specific lengths and sequences have been found to stimulate human skin dermal fibroblast growth in vitro. One study of elastin derived peptides showed that valine-glycine-valine-alanine-proline-glycine (VGVAPG) significantly stimulated human skin fibroblast production, probably mediated through a binding of the peptide to a plasmalemmal receptor of human skin fibroblasts. This same hexapeptide sequence has been found to stimulate human dermal skin fibroblasts, downregulate elastin expression, and to be chemotactic for fibroblasts. Other studies have shown the peptide sequence tyrosine-tyrosine-arginine-alanine-

aspartame-aspartame alanine to inhibit procollagen C-protenase, which cleaves C propeptide from type I procollagen. This could result in decreased collagen breakdown. A specific amino acid sequence, lysine-theronine-theronine-lysine-serine, found on type I procollagen, has been found to stimulate feedback regulation of new collagen synthesis resulting in an increased production of extracellular matrix proteins. This particular pentapeptide has made the transition from research to practical application. The five amino acid chain has been linked to a lipophilic fatty acid, palmitic acid, in order to enhance skin stability and improve skin delivery. Penetration enhancers are very important in cosmeceutical peptide technology, since penetration of these large molecular weight molecules is difficult and efficacy cannot be achieved without entry into the skin.

Carrier peptides

Another function of peptides in cosmeceuticals is to stabilize and deliver metals such as copper, an important trace element necessary for wound healing and enzymatic processes. There are several ways in which copper, if delivered into the skin, may have anti-skin-aging benefits. Free radicals have frequently been implicated in both chronologic and actinic aging because they cause damage to collagen. Superoxide dismutase acts as an important antioxidant and requires copper as a cofactor. In addition, lysyl oxidase, an important enzyme in collagen and elastin production, is also dependent on copper. It has been postulated that the tripeptide glycyl-L-histidyl-L-lysine (GHK) facilitates copper uptake by cells. Copper spontaneously complexes with this tripeptide, which is found on the alpha II chain of human collagen. Its release from the collagen helix during wounding or inflammation may result in a feedback stimulation of new collagen. The GHK sequence has been found to stimulate collagen synthesis by fibroblasts as well as increasing levels of both MMP-2 and MMP-2 mRNA. It also increases the level of tissue inhibitors of metalloproteases TIMP-1 and TIMP-2. As such, it is believed to aid in dermal tissue remodeling. Therefore, the tripeptide alone may be beneficial as a signal peptide. The major effect of this peptide, however, is felt to be the delivery of copper into the skin as an active rather that the GHK peptide as an active. Laboratory studies on both experimental rat and cultured human fibroblasts have demonstrated stimulation of both type I collagen and glycosaminoglycan synthesis by the copper–peptide complex. In addition, chondroitin sulfate and dermatin sulfate were also enhanced. This type of data has resulted in incorporation of the copper tripeptide complex in facial cosmeceutical creams.

Neurotransmitter inhibiting peptides

Recently a new hexapeptide called argireline has been synthesized and alleged to have antiwrinkle activity. This peptide, acetyl-glutamyl-glutamyl-methyoxyl-glutaminyl-arginyl-arginylamide, inhibits neurotransmitter release by interference with the formation or stabilization of the protein complex required to drive calcium dependent exocytosis when studied with in vitro models. These in vitro studies have resulted in incorporation of this peptide into certain cosmeceutical products. The clinical results of this peptide's inhibitory effect on neurotransmitter release may raise the threshold for minimal muscle activity, requiring more signal to achieve movement and thus reducing subconscious muscle movement over time. If delivered to targeted facial muscles, there could be a decrease in dynamic facial lines and wrinkles.

Peptide mechanisms of action

The recurring theme in peptide studies is that protein subfragments of collagen and elastin, which are liberated during cellular processes, can act as feedback stimulators of their own neosynthesis. They can, in essence, signal or at least mimic the signals that result in synthesis of new proteins of the extracellular matrix. Carrier proteins, by contrast, have the primary function in cosmeceuticals of delivering ionized elements such as copper into the skin where the copper then may have benefits for enhanced collagen production. Lastly, the mechanism of action of neurotransmitter inhibiting peptides is to act as a blocking agent at the docking vesicle for the release of neurotransmitters. However, for any type of peptide to be biologically active in vivo, it must be first stabilized in the product and adequately delivered into the viable dermis or musculature where these processes occur.

Cosmeceutical Peptide Use

Small chain peptides in specific sequences may be able to imitate some biological processes to stimulate repair, while other oligopeptides may inhibit processes that accelerate the signs of aging in the skin (Fig. 17.1). The major benefit of signal peptides and carrier peptides is to enhance collagen production without the irritation that is seen with prescription retinoids (Figs 17.2 and 17.3). Cosmeceutical peptides have the advantage of not increasing transepidermal water loss thus preserving the barrier function that is often compromised with the use of retinoids. The optimal way to incorporate peptides into a skin care protocol is to use them after applying topical retinoids to reduce dehydration and irritation (Fig. 17.4). The peptides, such as signal and carrier peptide products, may be used with retinoids daily to improve tolerance of the retinoid and result in better patient compliance.

Adverse Effects of Peptide

As with most cosmeceutical preparations, the major concern is one of allergic contact dermatitis. The daily casual use of these products will determine whether or not an allergy is present. Manifestations of allergic contact dermatitis would be an erythematous papular rash with itching. Thus proteins and peptides are some of the most common allergens. With copper delivery into the skin, there are theoretical concerns of free ions triggering reactions like the Fenton reaction, which results in free radical generation.

In general, however, these peptide cosmeceuticals are safe in the currently marketed formulations.

Summary

Cosmeceutical peptides are currently in the marketplace and their success is reflected in commercial sales. Limited studies both in vitro and in vivo are often used to determine the benefit of ingredients in cosmeceutical products. Peptides have a body of knowledge regarding their utility as cell regulators, but further research is required to determine their long term effects as cosmeceuticals in the anti-aging arena.

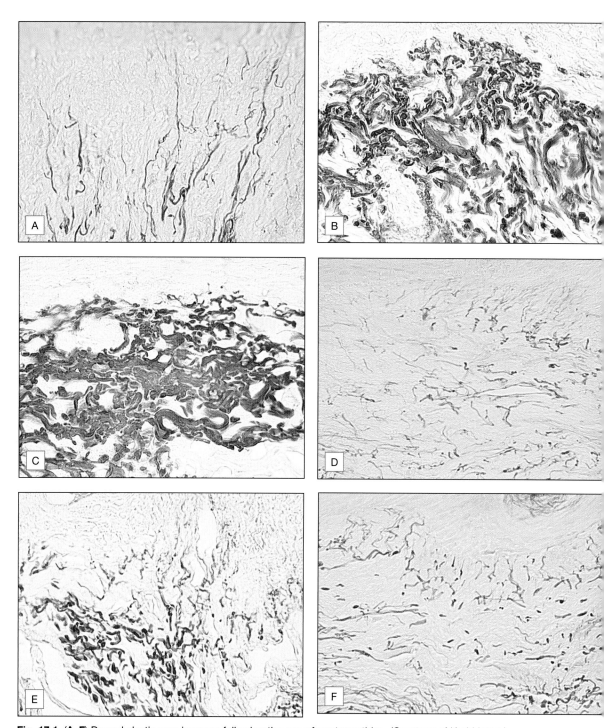

Fig. 17.1 (**A–F**) Dermal elastin may increase following the use of pentapeptides. (Courtesy of Karl Lintner)

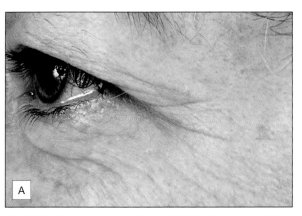
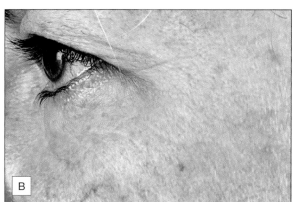

Fig. 17.2 The appearance of periorbital fine lines and wrinkles following 4 months' use of a pentapeptide: example 1. (**A**) Before. (**B**) After. (Courtesy of Karl Lintner)

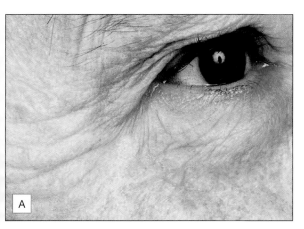
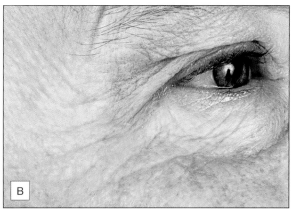

Fig. 17.3 The appearance of periorbital fine lines and wrinkles following 4 months' use of a pentapeptide: example 2. (**A**) Before. (**B**) After. (Courtesy of Karl Lintner)

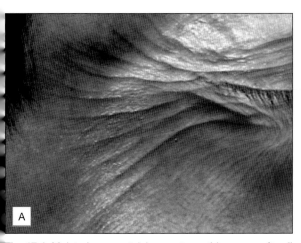
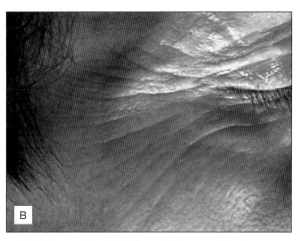

Fig. 17.4 Moisturizers containing pentapeptides may soften lines of facial expression. (**A**) Before. (**B**) Four months after. (Courtesy of Karl Lintner)

Further Reading

Blanes-Mira C, Clemente J, Jodas G, et al 2002 A synthetic hexapeptide (argireline) with anti-wrinkle activity. International Journal of Cosmeceutical Science 24:303–310

Chung JH, Seo JY, Choi HR, et al 2001 Modulation of skin collagen metabolism in aged and photoaged human skin in vivo. Journal of Investigative Dermatology 117:1218–1224

Katayama K, Armendariz-Borunda J, Raghow R, et al 1993 A pentapeptide from type I collagen promotes extracellular matrix production. Journal of Biological Chemistry 268:9941–9944

Khorramizadeh MR, Tredget EE, Telasky C, et al 1999 Aging differentially modulates the expression of collagen and collagenase in dermal fibroblasts. Molecular and Cellular Biochemistry 194:99–108

Lintner K 2002 Promoting production in the extracellular matrix without compromising barrier. Cutis 70(6S):13–16

Simeon A, Emonard H, Hornebeck W, Maquart FX 2000 The tripeptide–copper complex glycyl-L-histidyl-L-lysine-Cu^{2+} stimulates matrix metalloprotinase-II expression by fibroblast cultures. Life Sciences 67:2257–2265

Simeon A, Wegrowski Y, Bontemps J, Maquart FX 2000 Expression of glycosaminoglycan and small proteoglycans in wounds: modulation by the tripeptide–copper complex glycyl-L-histidyl-L-lysine-Cu^{2+}. Journal of Investigative Dermatology 115:962–968

Varoni J, Spearman D, Perone P, et al 2001 Inhibition of type I procollagen synthesis by damaged collagen in photoaged skin and by collagenase-degraded collagen in vitro. Journal of American Pathology 158:931–942

Nutritional Antioxidants

18

Karen E. Burke

Dermatologists today have the capability of preventing damage to normal skin and even retarding the skin's natural aging through the use of cosmeceuticals. Especially during the past decade, research has demonstrated the efficacy of many topical nutrients, particularly antioxidants—some not synthesized by humans and therefore essential (vitamins C and E), some self-synthesized (α-lipoic acid, ubiquinone), and some exogenous (genistein). The challenge is to make topical formulations which attain percutaneous absorption of active forms and which maintain antioxidant activity. Such cosmeceuticals could protect as well as reduce and reverse manifestations of aging skin.

α-Lipoic Acid

R-Alpha lipoic acid (αLA) is synthesized in the mitochondria of plants and animals, including humans. Natural αLA is covalently bound to protons via lysine; thus only minimal free αLA enters the circulation after biosynthesis or eating αLA-rich food. The lipoamide is a required co-factor for two enzymes in the citric acid cycle. It is also essential for the formation of a co-factor required in nucleic acid synthesis and for the metabolism of branched chain amino acids.

With oral supplements of free αLA, unbound αLA is transported to tissues. Free αLA is rapidly metabolized by the liver, so that the half-life in blood after absorption is only about 30 minutes, limiting the amount delivered. High tissue levels are short-lived since most free αLA is rapidly reduced to dihydrolipoic acid (DHLA), as shown in Figure 18.1.

Notwithstanding this transient availability, free αLA has been shown to be therapeutic for autoimmune liver disease by binding autoantibodies, heavy metal intoxication by trapping circulating metals, diabetic polyneuropathy by preventing oxidative damage and mushroom poisoning. Although not normally found in significant amounts in the skin, αLA is a good candidate for topical application:

- As a small, stable molecule, it could successfully be percutaneously absorbed.
- As a potent antioxidant it might protect from UV and other free radical environmental changes.
- Because it is soluble in both aqueous and lipid environments, it can interact with oxidants and antioxidants in many cellular compartments.

Indeed, αLA has been found to penetrate rapidly into murine and human skin to dermal and subcutaneous layers. Two hours after application of 5% αLA in propylene glycol, maximum levels of αLA were attained in the epidermis, dermis, and subcutaneous tissue. The stratum corneum concentration of αLA predicted the penetration and levels in

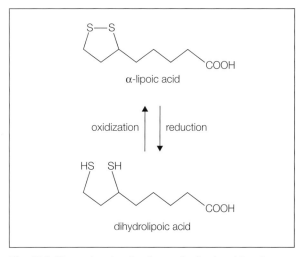

Fig. 18.1 The molecular structures of α-lipoic acid and dihydrolipoic acid

Antioxidant Activity of α-Lipoic Acid and DHLA		
	α-**Lipoic Acid**	**DHLA**
Antioxidant	+	++
Scavenges reactive oxygen species (ROS)	+	+
Chelates metals:		
Fe^{2+}, Cu^{2+}	+	−
Cd^{2+}	−	+
Regenerates endogenous antioxidants (vitamin E, vitamin C, glutathione, ubiquinol)	−	+
Repairs oxidatively damaged proteins	−	+
Pro-oxidant	+	+
+ activity; ++ greater activity; − no activity		

Table 18.1 Antioxidant Activity of α-Lipoic Acid and DHLA (Biewenga et al 1997)

the underlying skin. 5% of the αLA was converted to DHLA in both the epidermis and dermis, leading the researchers to conclude that both keratinocytes and fibroblasts reduce αLA.

Topical αLA with its metabolite DHLA could protect the skin from oxidative stress in several ways. Both αLA and DHLA are highly effective antioxidants as summarized in Table 18.1. DHLA is actually the more potent form. Both successfully scavenge reactive oxygen species (ROS) in vitro and in vivo. However, pro-oxidant activity has been observed. This occurs when an antioxidant reacts with a ROS scavenger, forming a product that is more harmful than the scavenged ROS. Fortunately αLA can act as an antioxidant against the pro-oxidant activity of DHLA (Biewenga GP et al). Both αLA and DHLA further provide antioxidant activity by chelating Fe^{2+} and Cu^{2+} (αLA) and Cd^{2+} (DHLA).

DHLA, unlike αLA, has the capacity to regenerate the endogenous antioxidants vitamin E, vitamin C, glutathione, and ubiquinol, as illustrated in Figure 18.2. This is clearly of great importance for skin, since UV exposure directly depletes especially ubiquinone and vitamin E as well as vitamin C, thereby stressing the other linked antioxidants. Regeneration of these major membrane and cytosol antioxidants gives cascading protection. Increases in the other important antioxidants (intracellular glutathione and extracellular cysteine) are noted when αLA is added to cell cultures. Vitamin E deficient animals do not show symptoms (weight loss, neuromuscular abnormalities) when supplemented with αLA.

Although αLA is a potent antioxidant, it provides **no** effective protection against UV-induced erythema or cell damage measured as sunburn cells. However, αLA (but not DHLA) acts as an anti-inflammatory agent by reducing the production and inhibiting the binding of transcription factors such as nuclear factor-$\kappa\beta$ (NF-$\kappa\beta$), thereby indirectly affecting the gene expression of inflammatory cytokines such as tumor necrosis factor alpha (TNF-α) and interleukins. DHLA (but not αLA) can repair oxidatively damaged proteins, which in turn regulate the activity of proteinase inhibitors such as α_1-AP, an inflammatory modulator. As antioxidants, both αLA and DHLA are directly anti-inflammatory by virtue of their quenching oxidants secreted by leukocytes and macrophages at sites of inflammation.

αLA may prove to retard and correct both intrinsic and extrinsic aging of the skin as well as other organs. By damaging DNA, the ROS continuously formed in normal metabolism may be largely responsible for the functional deterioration of organs with aging. A decrease in cellular protein and DNA as well as in αLA levels has been measured in aged rat liver, kidney, and spleen. Supplementation with αLA increases nucleic acid and protein levels in the elderly organs. Similarly, the age-related decrease of mitochondrial function in cardiac and brain cells can be improved with αLA supplementation. Clearly, aging skin might similarly benefit.

To evaluate possible improvement to photodamage, a split face study was done on 33 women. Topical application twice daily of 5% lipoic acid cream for 12 weeks decreased skin roughness by 50.8% (as measured by laser profilometry) when compared with the placebo. Clinical and photographic evaluation showed reduction in lentigenes and fine wrinkles. Clearly, topical αLA should be further studied by quantitative techniques to

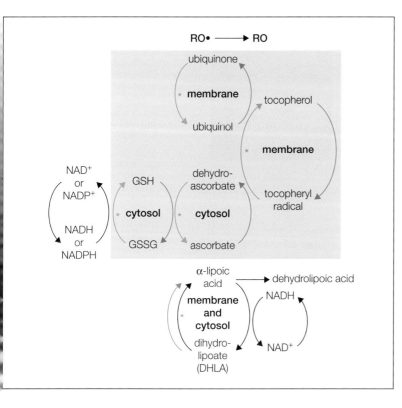

Fig. 18.2 Interactions of low molecular weight antioxidants. The reactions which directly quench oxygen free radicals(RO·) are indicated by the red arrows(RO·→RO); the reactions regenerating these antioxidants are indicated by the green arrows. Reactions with arrows touching are directly linked. RO· generated in a cell membrane is reduced by tocopherol, forming a tocopheryoxyl free radical which can in turn be quenched within the membrane by ubiquinol or at the membrane–cytosol junction by ascorbate (vitamin C). RO· generated in cytosol is directly reduced by ascorbate. The oxidized dehydroascorbate is reconverted to ascorbate by glutathione (GSH). Both α-lipoic acid and DHLA directly reduce oxygen free radicals. Also DHLA is itself a potent reducing agent which regenerates the oxidized forms of vitamin C, vitamin E, and oxidized glutathione (GSSH); this linkage is indicated by an asterix. (Adapted from diagram in Podda & Grundmann-Kollmann 2001, incorporating information from Biewenga et al 1997)

Fig. 18.3 The molecular structure of ubiquinone. The 'head' of the ubiquinone molecule is a fully substituted quinone ring which does not allow addition reactions with thiol groups in the cell (such as GSH). Ubiquinones vary by the length of the 'tail': Q_{10} has 10 isoprene units. Humans can synthesize Q_{10} out of the other coenzymes Q_1 to Q_9, though this ability decreases with age

confirm these results and to elucidate mechanisms of action.

Ubiquinone (Coenzyme Q_{10})

Ubiquinone (coenzyme Q_{10}, Fig. 18.3) is so named because it is ubiquitous in virtually all living cells, excluding some bacteria and fungi, although the level is quite variable. Since most human tissues synthesize ubiquinone, it is not considered to be a vitamin.

Ubiquinone is primarily located in the inner mitochondrial membrane where it is essential for the production of the ATP required for all vital cellular functions. Until recently, ubiquinone was thought to function only in energy transduction; however, with the discovery that ubiquinone is also an antioxidant within subcellular membranes, new roles are now being recognized. Ubiquinone can regenerate reduced tocopherol, as depicted in Figure 18.2. In fact, within membranes the amount of ubiquinone is from three to thirty times that of tocopherol. Without ubiquinone, the regeneration of tocopherol would be very slow.

The concentration of ubiquinone is highest in organs with high rates of metabolism such as heart, kidney, and liver, where it functions as an energy transfer molecule. In skin, the level of ubiquinone is relatively low, with 10-fold higher levels in the epidermis than in the dermis. Thus, the epidermis might potentially benefit from topical ubiquinone. Indeed, it has been demonstrated that ubiquinone can be topically absorbed. Application of ubiquinone in ethanol to porcine skin achieved 20% penetration into the epidermis and 27% into the dermis.

The fact that ubiquinone can serve not only as an energy generator but also as an antioxidant in the

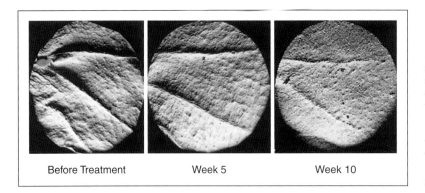

Fig. 18.4 Reduction of wrinkles with ubiquinone. Silicone replicas of the skin, analyzed by laser profilometry, show a significant reduction in the depth of periorbital fine lines and wrinkles in a 46 year old female after 10 weeks of twice daily application of ubiquinone cream (Eucerin Q10 Anti-Wrinkle Sensitive Skin Crème). (From Wrinkle Reduction Study 2003 In: Eucerin Q10 Product Compenium 2003, Beiersdorf Inc., Wilton, CT, p 11)

Before Treatment   Week 5   Week 10

skin has been investigated. In cultured human keratinocytes exposed to hydrogen peroxide, the detrimental increase in the activity of phospho-tyrosine kinase was suppressed and the loss of glutathione was prevented. Ubiquinone (0.3%) also suppressed the UVA-induced reduction of mito-chondrial membrane potential in fibroblasts from both young and old donors. Finally, the UV-induced oxidative damage to DNA in keratinocytes in vitro was reduced significantly with ubiquinone.

Ubiquinone can retard loss of hyaluronic acid and slowdown of cell division—both manifestations of intrinsic aging. Aged human fibroblasts in vitro produce less glycosaminoglycan and proliferate more slowly than young cells. The addition of ubiquinone increased levels of glycosaminoglycan as well as rates of cell division.

Ubiquinone further protects from the UVA-induced degradation of collagen. Both ubiquinone and vitamin E were shown in vitro to suppress fibroblast production of UVA-induced collagenase, thereby markedly retarding collagen breakdown. Ubiquinone suppressed collagenase expression over a longer period of time than did vitamin E.

Ubiquinone's antioxidant action in skin was confirmed in vitro by sophisticated ultra-weak photon emission (UPE). Increased antioxidants result in decreased UPE. Elderly volar skin demonstrated 33% reduction in antioxidant activity when compared with young skin. This was corrected after 1 week of twice daily topical application of 0.3% ubiquinone. After UVA irradiation, a decrease in anti-oxidant activity was noted; this loss was significantly corrected with topical 0.3% ubiquinone.

The efficacy of ubiquinol in reversing photoaging was further studied clinically. Ubiquinol cream (0.3%) was applied to one-half of the face and placebo to the other once daily for 6 months. Casts were made of the periorbital rhytides. The improvement can be appreciated in the photographs shown in Figure 18.4. Quantitative microtopography demonstrated a 27% reduction in the mean wrinkle depth.

Another clinical measure of photoaging is stratum corneum cell size. With deceased cell turnover time in aged skin, comeocytes become larger. Treatment once daily for 6 months with ubiquinone cream decreased comeocyte size equivalent to rejuvenation of 20 years. Thus, ubiquinone is an effective anti-oxidant protecting the dermal matrix from both intrinsic and extrinsic aging, making it a potentially important cosmeceutical.

Genistein

Genistein is an isoflavone cosmeceutical isolated from soy. Recent interest in genistein has been stimulated by epidemiological studies which correlate diets high in soy with reduced incidence of cardiovascular disease, osteoporosis, and certain cancers in humans.

The direct anticarcinogenic action of genistein is documented. Animal studies demonstrate protection against bladder, breast, colon, liver, lung, prostate and skin cancer with oral genistein, and dietary soy inhibits chemically induced skin cancer in mice. Growth of many in vitro cancer cell lines is inhibited by genistein. Genistein also arrests the growth and induces the differentiation of malignant melanoma cells in vitro and inhibits pulmonary metastases of malignant melanoma cells in vivo.

The mechanism by which genistein inhibits carcinogenesis may be through inhibition of tyrosine protein kinases (TPKs), the enzymes which phosphorylate proteins necessary for the regulation of cell division and transformation. Of particular importance is phosphorylation of TPK-dependent epidermal growth factor receptors (EGF-R), which are related to tumor promotion, including initiation of

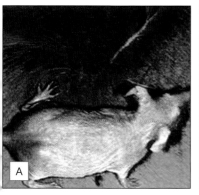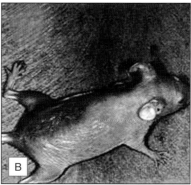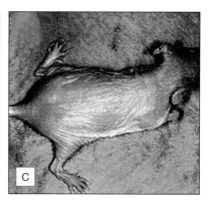

Fig. 18.5 Effect of genistein on UVB-induced acute skin burns in mice. Skh-1 hairless mice were treated topically with 5 µmol genistein 60 minutes before UVB at a dose of 1.8 kJ/cm² for 10 days. Photographs were taken 24 hours after last UVB irradiation. (**A**) Negative control (sham irradiation). (**B**) Vehicle before UVB. (**C**) 5 µmol genistein before UVB. (Wei et al 2003)

transcription factors, release of inflammatory mediators (as prostaglandins), and stimulation of cell proliferation. Genistein was found to downregulate both UVA- and UVB-induced EGF-R phosphorylation in human epidermoid carcinoma cells in vitro. In mouse skin, genistein also blocks the UVB-induced expression of the photo-oncogenes c-*fos* and c-*jun* which promote cell proliferation in oncogenesis. Similarly, genistein retards UV-induced apoptotic changes—including caspace-3 and p21-activated kinase 2 activation of human epidermal carcinoma cells and phosphokinase Cδ in human keratinocytes.

Genistein is also a potent antioxidant. Genistein scavenges peroxyl free radicals, thereby protecting against lipid peroxidation in vitro and in vivo. The decreased incidence of cardiovascular disease with high soy diets may be due to genistein's inhibiting the oxidation of low density lipoprotein (LDL) cholesterol in both aqueous and lipophilic environments. Of direct importance in protection from UV-induced skin damage, genistein has been shown to inhibit in vitro chemical and UV-induced DNA oxidation as well as psoralen plus UVA (PUVA) DNA damage. The fact that genistein also reduces erythema and histologic inflammation caused by PUVA may have implications for PUVA therapy by reducing possible short and long term adverse reactions.

Topical genistein (10 µmol/cm²) protects against acute and chronic UV damage to the skin. After exposure of Skh:1 hairless mice to UVB, topical genistein blocked acute skin burns and inhibited UVB-induced cutaneous wrinkling, as demonstrated clinically in Figures 18.5 and 18.6. Histologic analy-sis confirmed that topical genistein blocks the signs of chronic photodamage—epidermal hyperplasia and reactive acanthosis with nuclear atypia (Fig. 18.7). At a molecular level, UV-induced damage to DNA (as measured by the biomarker 8-hydroxy-2'-deoxyguanosine) was reduced. Inhibition of acute UV-induced erythema with topical genistein (5 µmol/cm²) was also demonstrated in humans: topical genistein (applied 30 minutes before UVB) inhibited by one minimal erythema dose (MED) the UVB-induced erythema as shown in Figure 18.8. Thus, topical genistein may protect human skin against photodamage.

Equally impressive is the fact that topical genistein also inhibits skin cancer, a consequence of chronic UVB damage. Both the incidence and the multiplicity of UVB-induced skin tumors in Skh:2 hairless mice were reduced by about 90% after 25 weeks of UVB exposure. Figure 18.9 shows protection from carcinogenesis of representative mice treated with genistein before UVB exposure. Also, after chemical induction and promotion of skin tumors, topical genistein inhibited tumor cell number by 60–75%.

Another possible dermatologic benefit of genistein is as a phytoestrogen. The skin has both α and β nuclear estrogen receptors through which estrogen binding can regulate linked genes of proliferation and differentiation. Genistein has a 30-fold higher affinity for ERβ than ERα, but a greater ERα agonist activity than ERβ. Though estradiol has 700-fold more ERα and 45-fold more ERβ activity than genistein, the possible biologic effect of genistein through dietary soy isoflavones may be important. Oral and topical estrogen increase the collagen

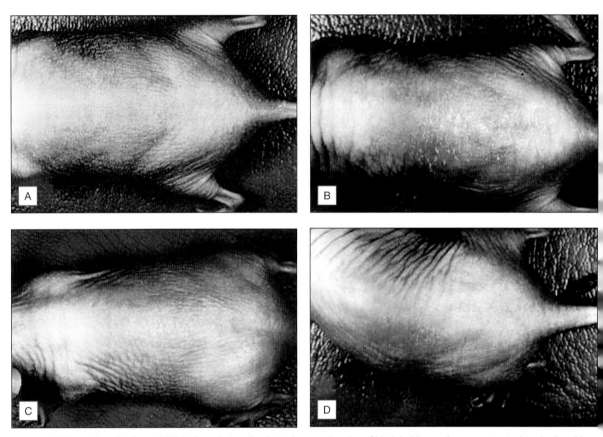

Fig. 18.6 Effect of genistein on UVB-induced chronic photodamage in mice. Skh-1 hairless mice were treated topically with 5 μmol genistein 60 minutes before or 5 minutes after twice weekly UVB at a dose of 0.3 kJ/cm^2 for 4 weeks. Photographs were taken 24 hours after last UVB irradiation. (**A**) Negative control (sham irradiation). (**B**) Vehicle plus UVB. (C) 5 μmol genistein before UVB. (**D**) 5 μmol genistein after UVB. (Wei et al 2003)

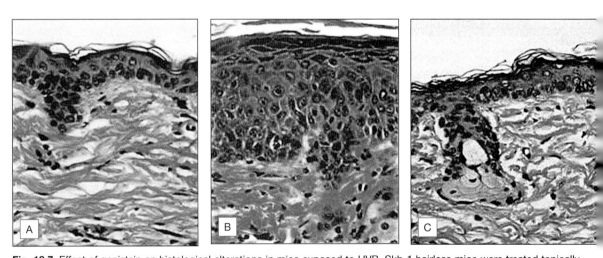

Fig. 18.7 Effect of genistein on histological alterations in mice exposed to UVB. Skh-1 hairless mice were treated topically with 5 μmol genistein 60 minutes before UVB at a dose of 0.3 kJ/cm^2 twice weekly for 4 weeks. Mice were killed 24 hours after the last UVB irradiation and skin specimens were taken for histology. (**A**) Negative control (sham irradiation). (**B**) Vehicle plus UVB. (C) 5 μmol genistein before UVB. (Wei et al 2003)

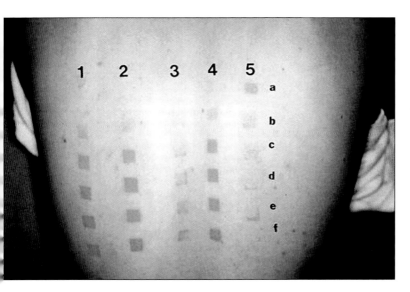

Fig. 18.8 Effect of genistein on UVB-induced erythema in human skin. The study was performed in the phototherapy unit in the Department of Dermatology, Mount Sinai Hospital. UVB fluences used a range from 0 to 100 mJ/cm². Genistein was applied to dorsal skin either 60 minutes before or 5 minutes after UVB exposure. Photographs were taken 24 hours after UVB irradiation. A minimal erythema dose (MED) for this individual was 40 mJ/cm². Lane 1: Vehicle before UVB; lane 2: no treatment before or after UVB; lane 3: 1 µmol genistein/cm² of skin before UVB; lane 4: 1 µmol genistein/cm² of skin after UVB; and lane 5: dose response of topical genistein applied before UVB (1 MED) at a dose ranging from 0.05 to 5 µmol/cm². (Wei et al 2003)

content of skin which diminishes with aging. This effect is especially dramatic in women during and after menopause. Genistein may reduce the atrophic appearance of aging skin both by preventing photodamage through inhibition of metalloproteinases in human skin (independent of sunscreen effect) and by stimulating collagen synthesis. Thus, topical genistein shows promise not only in protecting the skin against acute and chronic photodamage but also in enhancing the diminished collagen synthesis of normal intrinsic aging.

Summary

Nutritional antioxidants represent a novel category of cosmeceuticals. There is no doubt that higher levels are achieved in the skin through topical application than with oral supplementation, thus providing a protective antioxidant reservoir in the skin. Current research indicates that topical ubiquinone and genistein may provide UV photoprotection. In addition, they, as well as topical α-lipoic acid, may retard both intrinsic aging and photoaging. Topical antioxidants continue to be an important area of cosmeceutical research.

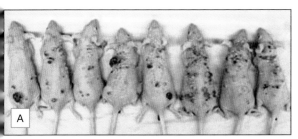
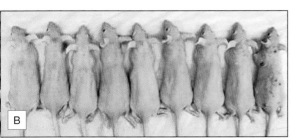
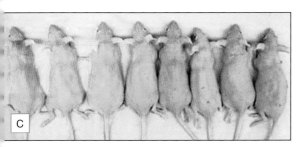

Fig. 18.9 Representative photograph of inhibition of photocarcinogenesis in mice treated with genistein. (**A**) Hairless mice irradiated with 0.3 kJ/m² thrice weekly for 25 weeks. (**B**) Mice treated with 1 µmol genistein before UVB exposure. (**C**) Mice treated with 5 µmol genistein before UVB irradiation. (Wei et al 2003)

Further Reading

Aklyama T, Ishida J, Nakagawa S, et al 1987 Genistein, a specific inhibitor of tyrosine-specific protein kinases. Journal of Biological Chemistry 262:5592–5595

Beitner H 2003 Randomized, placebo-controlled, double blind study on the clinical efficacy of a cream containing 5% alpha-lipoic acid related to photoaging of facial skin. British Journal of Dermatology 149:841–849

Biewenga GP, Haenen GRMM, Bast A 1997 The pharmacology of the antioxidant lipoic acid. General Pharmacology 29:315–331

Crane, FL 2001 Biochemical functions of coenzyme Q_{10}. Journal of the American College of Nutrition 20:591–598

Hoppe U, Bergemann J, Diembeck W, et al 1999 Coenzyme Q_{10}, a cutaneous antioxidant and energizer. BioFactors 9:371–378

Pinnell SR, Lin J-Y, Lin F-H, et al 2004 Alpha lipoic acid is ineffective as a topical photoprotectant of skin. Poster presentation, 62nd Annual Meeting of the American Academy of Dermatology, Washington, DC

Podda M, Grundmann-Kollmann M 2001 Low molecular weight antioxidants and their role in skin ageing. Clinical and Experimental Dermatology 26:578–582

Podda M, Traber MG, Packer L 1997 Chapter 10: Alpha-lipoate: antioxidant properties and effects on skin. In: Fuchs J, Packer L, Zimmer G (eds) Lipoic acid in health and disease. Dekker, New York, pp 163–180

Podda M, Zollner TM, Grundmann-Kollmann M, et al 2001 Activity of alpha-lipoic acid in the protection against oxidative stress in skin. Current Problems in Dermatology 29:43–51

Shyong EQ, Lu YH, Lazinsky A, et al 2002 Effects of the isoflavone (genistein) on psoralen plus ultraviolet A radiation (PUVA)-induced photodamage. Carcinogenesis 23:317–321

Stocker R 2003 Coenzyme Q_{10}. The Linus Pauling Institute Micronutrient Information Center Online. Available: http://lpi.oregonstate.edu/infocenter/othernuts/coq10/

Varila E, Rantalia I, Oikarinen A, et al 1995 The effect of topical oestradiol on skin collagen of post-menopausal women. British Journal of Obstetrics and Gynaecology 102:985–989

Wei H, Saladi R, Lu Y, et al 2003 Isoflavone genistein: photoprotection and clinical implications in dermatology. Journal of Nutrition 133:3811S–3819S

19 Endogenous Growth Factors as Cosmeceuticals

Richard E. Fitzpatrick

Introduction

Exposure to ultraviolet radiation causes cumulative damage that accelerates normal chronologic aging and exacerbates injury to skin tissue, resulting in photodamage. Consumer interest in correcting signs of photodamage, such as wrinkles, dyspigmentation, sagging, and surface roughness, is increasing as the population ages, particularly as the 'Baby Boomer' segment reaches middle age. Treatments include topical retinoids and antioxidants, chemical peels, dermabrasion, laser, and various lifting surgeries, depending on the severity of skin damage.

Within the last decade researchers have focused on the pathophysiology of photodamage and have found correlations with certain aspects of acute and chronic wound healing. Of specific interest to cosmeceutical manufacturers are the effects of growth factors in the process of wound healing. Growth factors are regulatory proteins that mediate signaling pathways between and within cells. After a wound has been inflicted, a variety of growth factors flood the wound site and interact synergistically to initiate and coordinate each phase of wound healing. This process is complex and not completely understood. Most studies have evaluated the role of single growth factors in controlled wound-healing environments. These studies demonstrate the importance of growth factors in the repair of damaged tissue, but research into the phases of wound healing has demonstrated that it is the interaction of multiple growth factors that is vital to tissue regeneration. Cosmeceutical manufacturers have taken notice of the positive results of clinical studies showing accelerated wound healing and have begun to include growth factors in products designed to mitigate damage from chronologic aging and sun exposure.

Photodamage Effects on Skin Tissue

Photodamage occurs predominantly within the epidermis and the upper papillary dermis. Histologic studies demonstrate that ultraviolet exposure disrupts the normal architecture of connective tissue within the dermis. The dermal extracellular matrix is composed primarily of type I collagen, although type III collagen, elastin, proteoglycans, and fibronectin are also included in smaller amounts. Ultraviolet exposure decreases collagen and elastin and alters the crosslinked structure of collagen and elastin fibers within the dermal extracellular matrix. Abnormal elastic material containing elastin and fibrillin accumulates and appears to occupy areas of lost collagen. This deposition of abnormal elastic material is called solar elastosis. Glycosaminoglycans (GAGs), a type of proteoglycan that is a component of the extracellular matrix, are polysaccharide molecules that bind to water, forming a hydrated, space filling polymer between collagen and elastin fibers that helps support skin tissue. In photodamaged skin GAGs are abnormally deposited in the elastotic tissue rather than between collagen and elastin fibers. The clinical result of decreased collagen and elastin and disruption of the normal support architecture is the appearance of wrinkles, sagging skin, uneven pigmentation, hyperpigmentation, and thickened or leathery skin texture. Although in chronologic aging skin also develops wrinkles, photodamaged skin is differentiated histologically by the presence of solar elastosis.

Growth Factors in Wound Healing

Hundreds of growth factors have been identified. Those that are important in wound healing include cytokines involved in immune response and phagocytosis, and growth factors that induce the synthesis of new collagen, elastin, and GAGs, the components of the dermal extracellular matrix that are abnormally affected by ultraviolet radiation. Table 19.1 lists the functions of the most important growth factors in wound healing.

Wound healing is dependent on the *synergistic interaction* of many growth factors. After injury, cytokines and other growth factors flood the wound site to mediate the inflammatory response, promote new cell growth, and decrease wound contraction and scarring. The process of wound healing is commonly divided into four overlapping phases that describe physiologic responses to injury. These phases include hemostasis, inflammation, proliferation, and remodeling. Table 19.2 summarizes each phase of wound healing. During hemostasis, platelets release various cytokines and other growth factors at the wound site to promote chemotaxis and mitogenesis. In the inflammatory stage, neutrophils and monocytes migrate to the wound site in response to specific cytokines and growth factors to initiate phagocytosis and to release additional growth factors that will attract fibroblasts. The proliferation phase is marked by epithelialization, angiogenesis, granular tissue formation, and collagen deposition. During proliferation, keratinocytes restore barrier function to the skin and secrete additional growth factors that stimulate the expression of new keratin proteins. Fibroblasts produce collagen that is deposited in the wound bed. This cycle of collagen production and growth factor secretion continues in a type of autocrine feedback loop of continuous wound repair.

The remodeling phase is the final step in the wound repair process and typically lasts several months. It is during remodeling that the extracellular matrix is reorganized, scar tissue is formed, and the wound is strengthened. Type III collagen deposited during the proliferation phase is gradually replaced by type I collagen, which is more tightly crosslinked and provides more tensile strength to the matrix than type III collagen. Cells at the wound

Growth factors in wound healing	
Growth factors and cytokines	**Properties/actions**
Vascular endothelial growth factor (VEGF)	Mediates angiogenesis Chemotactic for endothelial cells Mitogenic for endothelial cells and keratinocytes
Hepatocyte growth factor (HGF)	Mediates tissue organization and regeneration
Platelet-derived growth factor (PDGF)	Chemotactic for fibroblasts and macrophages Mitogenic for fibroblasts, smooth muscle cells, and endothelial cells
Epidermal growth factor (EGF)	Mediates angiogenesis Chemotactic for endothelial cells Mitogenic for fibroblasts, endothelial cells, and keratinocytes
Granulocyte colony stimulating factor (G-CSF)	Mediates angiogenesis Mitogenic for hematopoietic cells
Transforming growth factor beta (TGF-β)	Mediates angiogenesis Chemotactic for fibroblasts, keratinocytes, and macrophages Mitogenic for fibroblasts and smooth muscle cells Inhibits endothelial cells, keratinocytes, and lymphocytes Regulates matrix proteins including collagen, proteoglycans, fibronectin, and matrix degrading proteins
Keratinocyte growth factor	Mediates tissue organization and regeneration
Interleukins (IL-6 and IL-8)	Chemotactic for inflammatory cells and keratinocytes Mitogenic for lymphocytes and keratinocytes

Table 19.1 Growth factors in wound healing. (Sources: Fitzpatrick RE, Rostan EF. Reversal of photodamage with topical growth factors: a pilot study. *J Cosmet Laser Ther* 2003;5:25–34; Moulin V. Growth factors in skin wound healing. *Eur J Cell Biol*. 1995 Sep;68(1):1-7)

site secrete several growth factors with specific functions related to remodeling and matrix formation. For example, collagen and fibronectin synthesis are initiated by TGF-β, while PDGF and TGF-β stimulate fibroblasts to produce GAGs and modulate the proliferation of smooth muscle cells. Other growth factors modify the vasculature. Over time, cell density increases, and skin tissue is strengthened.

Specific growth factors directly initiate activity that promotes wound healing as well as modifying the activities of matrix cells and other growth factors. Growth factors are capable of both stimulating and inhibiting specific actions. The activity of growth factors is modulated through other growth factors and through various intrinsic factors that interact to achieve homeostasis and balance during wound healing. Research continues to uncover more information about the functions of individual growth factors during wound healing and, importantly, the synergistic interaction of growth factors with each other and with other components of wound healing. Whether the presence or absence of a single growth factor is significant in wound healing is not yet known. Current understanding suggests that it is the interaction of many growth factors that is significant, with no single growth factor being solely determinant in the outcome of wound healing.

Treating Photodamaged Skin

The most aggressive approach in the treatment of photodamage has been to remove damaged skin and foster the growth of healthy new epidermal and papillary dermal layers. Acid peels and dermabrasion are effective in destroying damaged skin, but it is difficult to precisely control the amount of surface tissue removed. Adverse effects from these procedures may include erythema, scarring, hyperpigmentation, or hypopigmentation. Ablative skin resurfacing with the CO_2 laser also has been widely used to remove photodamaged skin by vaporizing outer skin layers. Lasers can be precisely controlled so the amount of tissue removed is predictable. However, the removal of the epidermis results in a partial thickness open wound that may take weeks to heal and presents the same risks for erythema, scarring, and dyspigmentation as acid peels and dermabrasion. Nonablative laser resurfacing appears to stimulate dermal healing and new collagen formation without removing the epidermis. Studies of nonablative laser treatment of photodamaged skin have demonstrated statistically significant improvement in clinical grading of skin damage with only transient erythema and minimal side effects, and biopsies have quantified post-treatment formation of new dermal collagen. Histologic evaluation of traditional ablative laser wounds reveals the expression of EGF, TGF-β, PDGF, and fibroblast growth factors, as well as wound healing activity that is identical to the phases of wound healing initiated from surgically inflicted wounds. Similarly, nonablative laser techniques appear to result in subclinical thermal wounds that initiate the wound healing process and presumably the release of growth factors.

Phases of cutaneous wound healing	
Phase	**Activities**
Hemostasis	Neutrophils, platelets, and plasma proteins infiltrate the wound and initiate vasoconstriction Platelets release clotting factors to initiate coagulation Platelets then release cytokines and other growth factors that attract neutrophils, macrophages, monocytes, and other cells necessary for cutaneous healing
Inflammation	Neutrophils initiate phagocytosis and attract macrophages Macrophages continue phagocytosis and release additional growth factors and cytokines, which attract fibroblasts to the wound, promote angiogenesis, and stimulate keratinocyte growth
Proliferation (also known as granulation)	Fibroblasts synthesize collagen New collagen fibers begin to form a matrix, or scaffold, for additional fibroblast attachment
Remodeling (also known as maturation)	Collagen fibers are remodeled, or crosslinked, into an organized matrix Additional collagen fibers attach to the matrix and are assembled into new tissue Wound contraction and tissue strengthening occurs

Table 19.2 Phases of cutaneous wound healing

Topical Application of Growth Factors

Individual growth factors (e.g. TGF-β, EGF, PDGF, etc.) have been shown to accelerate wound healing in both acute and chronic wounds. Photodamaged skin is similar to a chronic wound that may not progress to complete tissue remodeling. Total healing of photodamaged skin is unlikely because the surface area of the injury is too large to be completely repaired, and ongoing cumulative damage continues to occur daily. It is estimated that only 15 minutes of sun exposure can induce enough damage to collagen and elastic fibers to require remodeling activity. A mixture of multiple growth factors derived from a three dimensional tissue culture of human fibroblasts was used in a pilot study designed to evaluate the effects of growth factors applied topically to treat photodamaged skin. The objective in using multiple growth factors was to stimulate the remodeling phase of wound healing in which many growth factors work synergistically. The selection of growth factors used in the pilot study was based on preliminary data that demonstrated the efficacy of this combination in stimulating the proliferation of fibroblasts and keratinocytes and increasing collagen secretion. The study included 14 patients with photodamaged skin (Fitzpatrick class II). Each patient applied the mixture of growth factors twice daily for 60 days. Baseline and 60 day results were evaluated using 3 mm punch biopsies and optical profilometry. A total of 11 of 14 patients (78.6%) showed clinical improvement at 60 days. New collagen formation in the Grenz zone increased by 37%, and epidermal thickening increased by 27%. Additional evaluation of this combination of growth factors in a larger study of 250 patients with photodamaged skin who were treated for 3 months demonstrated improvements in skin hydration, roughness, dyspigmentation, blotchiness, and wrinkles.

Combination Approaches: Laser Plus Topical Growth Factors

Laser resurfacing and topical application of growth factors have each been shown to improve clinical signs of photodamage and to stimulate the formation of dermal collagen. Depending on whether CO_2 or nonablative resurfacing is used, some degree of erythema will occur, and the process of wound healing will take time. A human fibroblast derived temporary skin substitute was approved in 1997 for use as a temporary wound covering for mid-dermal to indeterminate depth wounds. This skin substitute has been used extensively in patients with partial thickness burns. In addition to providing a protective barrier, this temporary skin substitute contains growth factors secreted by the tissue culture and allows fibroblasts to proliferate and secrete dermal collagen, matrix proteins, and growth factors. Study of the use of fibroblast derived temporary skin after CO_2 laser resurfacing produced faster healing and less pain and inflammation than traditional postoperative measures.

The degree of clinical improvement and histologic improvement seen with nonablative resurfacing is very similar to that seen with the use of topical growth factors. This is logical, since they both appear to involve the same mechanisms for improvement. The simultaneous use of both would be expected to result in an enhanced response and this approach is taken by many physicians.

For noninvasive, nonablative laser resurfacing, the post-treatment application of growth factors in a topical formulation may provide benefit in accelerated or improved wound healing.

Risks Associated with Growth Factors

There are no proven risks associated with the topical application of growth factors, other than the potential for allergic reactions in patients with hypersensitivities to these substances. The protein molecules are too large to be absorbed, and there is even some controversy about whether they can penetrate the epidermis. However, theoretical concerns have been raised about the potential for growth factors to stimulate the development of melanomas. This theory is based on the presence of receptors for some growth factors, such as VEGF, in various types of melanomas. In addition, certain growth factors are expressed by cancerous cells, while others are thought to alter the environment around cancerous cells to promote tumor growth. For example, VEGF, which is a key factor in tumor neoangiogenesis, is expressed by some types of skin tumors. Whether increased VEGF expression contributes to tumor growth is uncertain, however. Exogenous VEGF added to melanoma cells was shown in one study to increase cell proliferation, but increased expression of VEGF in another study did not result in melanoma cell proliferation. By contrast, VEGF expression in squamous cell carcinomas of the head and neck was shown to produce a significant inhibitory effect on cell proliferation and tumor cell migration. Whether VEGF contributes to tumor cell proliferation or is produced in response to the growth of a tumor is unknown. To date, studies of growth factors and their association with tumors have focused on their expression by the tumor. It is unlikely that topically applied VEGF would affect tumor proliferation. Similarly, TGF-β has been alternately reported to decrease or promote cancer progression. Generally, this growth factor has been found to have inhibitory effects on tumor growth, but the activity of TGF-β in cancerous tissue is complex and has not been fully explained. As with VEGF, studies have focused on TGF-β expressed by tumor and other types of cells. Topical application is unlikely to either inhibit or promote cancer growth.

Another concern about the application of growth factors is whether they could contribute to hypertrophic scarring. Specifically, it has been postulated that TGF-β may increase the potential for scarring during wound healing due to its function in activating fibroblasts, which synthesize collagen, and because elevated levels of TGF-β have been noted at the site of dermal injury. But these findings cannot be extrapolated to suggest a causative role for TGF-β in the development of hypertrophic scarring. It has been suggested that an abnormal response of proliferative scar fibroblasts to TGF-β stimulation may contribute to the development of keloid and burn scars, but evaluation of patients with a genetic proclivity for the development of keloid scars failed to demonstrate a relationship between TGF-β plasma levels and keloid formation. Increased levels of TGF-β have been noted at the site of dermal wounds, but whether this growth factor contributes to scarring or is produced in response to scar development is unclear. With regard to the topical application of growth factors, there is no clinical evidence that they induce abnormal scarring, and anecdotal observations have failed to reveal any activity of growth factors that would produce an abnormal wound healing response. In fact, the current understanding of growth factor activity in the wound healing environment reveals a balance of both stimulatory and inhibitory actions that are carefully modulated to achieve homeostasis.

Conclusions

Studying the role of growth factors in cutaneous wound healing has led to research demonstrating positive cosmetic and clinical outcomes in photodamaged skin (Fig. 19.1). Although the topical use of growth factors is an emerging treatment approach, initial studies suggest that dermal collagen production and clinical improvement in photodamage appearance are substantial. Further, the increase in dermal collagen produced by topical growth factors can be measured quantitatively by biopsy. Although the functions of growth factors in the natural wound healing process are complex and incompletely understood,

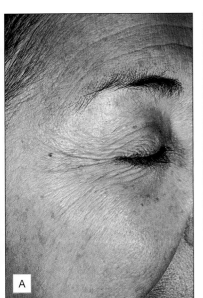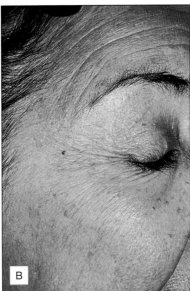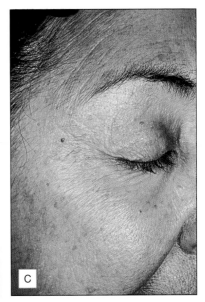

Fig. 19.1 An example of the clinical effects observed while using a growth factor containing moisturizer. (**A**) Baseline. (**B**) Month 3. (**C**) Month 6

it appears that wound healing is dependent on the synergistic interaction of many growth factors. Currently, most studies of single growth factors provide limited understanding within a narrow scope. The most promising research suggests that multiple growth factors used in combination may stimulate the growth of collagen, elastin, and GAGs. The use of a multiple growth factor topical formulation appears to provide a promising first line treatment for mild to moderate photodamaged skin. Combination with laser therapy for more severe damage has not been studied but may provide additional benefit.

Further Reading

Alam M, Hsu TS, Dover JS, et al 2003 Nonablative laser and light treatments: histology and tissue effects—a review. Lasers in Surgery and Medicine 33:30–39

Bayat A, Bock O, Mrowietz U, et al 2003 Genetic susceptibility to keloid disease and hypertrophic scarring: transforming growth factor beta$_1$ common polymorphisms and plasma levels. Plastic and Reconstructive Surgery 111:535–543

Bernstein EF, Andersen D, Zelickson BD 2000 Laser resurfacing for dermal photoaging. Clinics in Plastic Surgery 27:221–240

Bernstein EF, Brown DB, Urbach F, et al 1995 Ultraviolet radiation activates the human elastin promoter in transgenic mice: a novel in vivo and in vitro model of cutaneous photoaging. Journal of Investigative Dermatology 105:269–273

Bernstein EF, Ferreira M, Anderson D 2001 A pilot investigation to subjectively measure treatment effect and side-effect profile of non-ablative skin remodeling using a 532 nm, 2 ms pulse-duration laser. Journal of Cosmetic Laser Therapy 3:137–141

Bernstein EF, Fisher LW, Li K, et al 1995 Differential expression of the versican and decorin genes in photoaged and sun-protected skin. Comparison by immunohistochemical and northern analyses. Labortaory Investigations 72:662–669

Bernstein EF, Underhill CB, Hahn PJ, et al 1996 Chronic sun exposure alters both the content and distribution of dermal glycosaminoglycans. British Journal of Dermatology 135:255–262

Brown GL, Nanney LB, Griffen J, et al 1989 Enhancement of wound healing by topical treatment with epidermal growth factor. New England Journal of Medicine 321:76–79

El-Domyati M, Attia S, Saleh F, et al 2002 Intrinsic aging vs. photoaging: a comparative histopathological, immunohistochemical, and ultrastructural study of skin. Experimental Dermatology 11:398–405

Fisher GJ, Wang ZQ, Datta SC, et al 1997 Pathophysiology of premature skin aging induced by ultraviolet light. New England Journal of Medicine 337:1419–1428

Fitzpatrick RE 2000 TNS Recovery Complex aids in the healing of sun-damaged skin improving hydration, roughness, dispigmentation, and wrinkles. Soc Invest Dermatol 2000. May 11–14th, Chicago, IL Poster

Fitzpatrick RE, Rostan EF 2003 Reversal of photodamage with topical growth factors: a pilot study. Journal of Cosmetic Laser Therapy 5:25–34

Fournier N, Dahan S, Barneon G, Rouvrais C, Diridullou S, Lagarde JM, et al 2002 Nonablative remodeling: a 14 month clinical ultrasound imaging and profilometric evaluation of a 1540 nm Er : Glass laser. Dermatologic Surgery 28:926–931

Goldberg DJ 2000 New collagen formation after dermal remodeling with an intense pulsed light source. Journal of Cutaneous Laser Therapy 2:59–61

Goldman R 2004 Growth factors and chronic wound healing: past, present, and future. Advances in Skin and Wound Care 17:24–35

Graeven U, Fiedler W, Karpinski S, et al 1999 Melanoma-associated expression of vascular endothelial growth factor and its receptors FLT-1 and KDR. Journal of Cancer Research and Clinical Oncology 125:621–629

Hardaway CA, Ross EV, Paithankar DY 2002 Nonablative cutaneous remodeling with a 1.45 micron mid infrared diode laser; phase II. Journal of Cosmetic Laser Therapy 4:9–14

Herold-Mende C, Steiner HH, Andl T, et al 1999 Expression and functional significance of vascular endothelial growth factor receptors in human tumor cells. Labortaory Investigations 79:1573–1582

Kao B, Kelly KM, Majaron B, Nelsun JS, et al 2003 Novel model for evaluation of epidermal preservation and dermal collagen remodeling following photorejuvenation of human skin. Lasers in Surgery and Medicine 32:115–119

Lazar-Molnar E, Hegyesi H, Toth S, Falus A 2000 Autocrine and paracrine regulation by cytokines and growth factors in melanoma. Cytokine 12:547–554

Lewis MP, Lygoe KA, Nystrom ML, et al 2004 Tumour-derived TGF-beta$_1$ modulates myofibroblast differentiation and promotes HGF/SF-dependent invasion of squamous carcinoma cells. British Journal of Cancer 90:822–832

Liu B, Earl HM, Baban D, et al 1995 Melanoma cell lines express VEGF receptor KDR and respond to exogenously added VEGF. Biochemical and Biophysical Research Communications 217:721–727

Miyachi Y, Ishikawa O 1998 Dermal connective tissue metabolism in photoageing. Australasian Journal of Dermatology 39:19–23

Moulin V 1995 Growth factors in skin wound healing. European Journal of Cell Biology 68:1–7

Mustoe TA, Pierce GF, Morishima C, Deuel TF 1991 Growth factor-induced acceleration of tissue repair through direct and inductive activities in a rabbit dermal ulcer model. Journal of Clinical Investigation 87:694–703

Mustoe TA, Pierce GF, Thomason A, et al 1987 Accelerated healing of incisional wounds in rats induced by transforming growth factor-beta. Science 237:1333–1336

Naughton GK, Pinney E, Mansbridge J, Fitzpatrick RE 2001 Tissue-engineered derived growth factors as a topical treatment for rejuvenation of photodamaged skin. Soc Invest Dermatol 2001. Poster

Omi T, Kawana S, Sato S, Honda M, et al 2003 Ultrastructural changes elicited by a non-ablative wrinkle reduction laser. Lasers in Surgery and Medicine 32:46–49

Polo M, Smith PD, Kim YJ, Wang X, Ko F, Robson MC 1999 Effect of TGF-beta$_2$ on proliferative scar fibroblast cell kinetics. Annals of Plastic Surgery 43:185–190

Ramont L, Pasco S, Hornebeck W, Maquart FX, Monboisse JC 2003 Transforming growth factor-beta$_1$ inhibits tumor growth in a mouse melanoma model by down-regulating the plasminogen activation system. Experimental Cell Research 291:1–10

Roberts AB, Sporn MB, Assoian RK, et al 1986 Transforming growth factor type beta: rapid induction of fibrosis and angiogenesis in vivo and stimulation of collagen formation in vitro. Proceedings of the National Academy of Sciences USA 83:4167–4171

Rosenberg L, de la Torre J. Wound healing, growth factors. Online. Available: http://www.emedicine.com/plastic/topic457.htm. 18 Feb 2004

Ross EV, Sajben FP, Hsia J, et al 2000 Nonablative skin remodeling: selective dermal heating with a mid-infrared laser and contact cooling combination. Lasers in Surgery and Medicine 26:186–195

Rostan E, Bowes LE, Iyer S, Fitzpatrick RE 2001 A double-blind, side-by-side comparison study of low fluence long pulse dye laser to coolant treatment for wrinkling of the cheeks. Journal of Cosmetic Laser Therapy 3:129–136

Tanzi EL, Williams CM, Alster TS 2003 Treatment of facial rhytides with a nonablative 1450-nm diode laser: a controlled clinical and histologic study. Dermatologic Surgery 29:124–128

Uitto J 1993 Collagen. In: Fitzpatrick TB, Eisen AZ, Wolff K, Freedberg IM, Austen KF, eds. Dermatology in general medicine, vol 1, 4th edn. McGraw-Hill, New York, pp 299–314

Yu W, Naim JO, Lanzafame RJ 1994 Expression of growth factors in early wound healing in rat skin. Lasers in Surgery and Medicine 15:281–289

Sunscreens

20

Dee Anna Glaser, Heidi Ann Waldorf

Introduction

Increased outdoor leisure time, decreased clothing coverage, a diminishing stratospheric ozone layer, and the rise in popularity of indoor tanning have added up to a significant increase in ultraviolet (UV) radiation exposure in the last century. Skin cancer represents over 50% of all cancers in the USA annually; the incidence of melanoma alone has more than tripled in the past two decades. Although UV radiation's role as a cutaneous carcinogen was reported in the medical literature as early as the 1930s, and in the lay press in the 1940s and 1950s, general public recognition of the danger is a much more recent phenomenon. Additionally, increasing awareness of the causal relationship between UV exposure and the signs of aging, including wrinkling and dyspigmentation, has triggered widespread interest in sun protective products as cosmeceuticals.

In 1978, the US Food and Drugs Administration (FDA) reclassified sunscreens from 'cosmetics', intended to minimize sunburn and promote tanning, to over-the-counter 'drugs', intended to reduce the harmful effects of UV radiation on skin structure and function. However, it was not until May 1999 that the FDA published its final monograph addressing the testing and labeling of sunscreen products for the prevention of UVB damage, i.e. sunburn. Although implementation was scheduled for December 2002, the effective date of the sunscreen monograph was delayed pending the development of a proposed amendment to define requirements for broad spectrum UV coverage including UVA. The FDA anticipates that this new effective date will not occur before January 2005.

Chemical Sunscreens

The first commercial chemical sunscreen was introduced in 1928; it contained benzyl salicylate and benzyl cinnamate. In 1942, p-aminobenzoic acid (PABA) ointment was shown to be an effective sunburn protectant. This advance led to the development of many new sunscreen agents. The most recent FDA monograph includes 14 chemical sunscreen agents considered safe and effective for use in over-the-counter products.

The FDA-approved chemical sunscreens and the maximum allowed concentration for each are listed in Table 20.1. These 'sunscreen active ingredients' are defined as absorbing, reflecting, or scattering radiation in the ultraviolet range at wavelengths of 290–400 nm. The chemical (also called organic or soluble) sunscreen active ingredients prevent sunburn by absorbing UV radiation as photons of light energy that are transformed into harmless long wave radiation and then re-emitted as heat. The FDA defined maximum (instead of minimum) concentrations of each to avoid subjecting consumers to unnecessarily high levels of any active ingredient in

Sunscreen active ingredients: chemical	
Active ingredient	**Maximum concentration (%)**
Aminobenzoic acid (PABA)	15
Avobenzone	3
Cinoxate	3
Dioxybenzone	3
Homosalate	15
Methyl anthranilate	5
Octocrylene	10
Octyl methoxycinnamate	10
Octyl salicylate	5
Oxybenzone	6
Padimate O	8
Phenylbenzimidazole sulfonic acid	4
Sulisobenzone	10
Trolamine salicylate	12

Table 20.1 Sunscreen active ingredients: chemical

sunscreen combination products. This provision also recognizes that final product testing, not the concentration of each active ingredient, determines efficacy.

Physical Sunscreens

Opaque topical agents applied thickly on the skin surface have been used for decades to protect against sunburn. During the Second World War, red veterinary petrolatum was used by the military as a physical sunblock. In the 1950s, it became commonplace to see lifeguards and fair skinned children at the beach with solid white streaks of zinc oxide paste on their noses, lips, and cheeks. These products were messy and not conducive to widespread application. Over the last decade, cosmetic industry technology has been applied to the development of micronized versions of titanium dioxide and zinc oxide. With particle sizes of less than 0.2 μm, these formulations are nearly imperceptible on all but the darkest skin tones making them much more appealing.

Traditionally, physical agents used to prevent sunburn were called 'sunblocks' while chemical agents were 'sunscreens.' The terminology is misleading because it suggests that the former merely scatter or reflect UV radiation. In fact, the physical (also called inorganic or insoluble) agents, titanium dioxide and zinc oxide, also act as semiconductors that absorb UV radiation and release it as heat. The use of the term 'chemical-free' for sunscreens containing only physical, not chemical, sunscreen agents is also confusing for consumers, since all active and inactive ingredients have been obtained and/or combined through some chemical process. The US FDA-approved maximum concentration of these agents in sunscreen is listed in Table 20.2.

Rating Efficacy

With appropriate ultraviolet protection, exposed individuals do not suffer significant cutaneous DNA

Sunscreen active ingredients: physical	
Active ingredient	**Maximum concentration (%)**
Titanium dioxide	25
Zinc oxide	25

Table 20.2 Sunscreen active ingredients: physical

damage, sunburn cell formation, or immunosuppression. Clinically, suncreen use significantly reduces the occurrence of actinic keratoses, nonmelanoma skin cancer, and skin aging. Daily application of sunscreen decreases the number of acquired nevi in children. Although intermittently raised as an issue, sunscreen use does not cause secondary vitamin D deficiency.

The ultraviolet spectra relevant to cutaneous damage are UVB (290–320 nm) and UVA (320–400 nm). Ultraviolet A radiation is further classified as UVA II (320–340 nm) and UVA I (340–400 nm). Clinically, excessive acute UVB exposure results in the classic sunburn. Multiple acute UVB assaults early in life have been linked with basal cell carcinoma and melanoma. The development of actinic keratoses and squamous cell carcinoma are more closely causally linked to chronic UVB exposure. Absorption of UVB by DNA mutates the p53 tumor suppressor gene and initiates the formation of pyrimidine dimers, an elevated level of which are mutagenic and linked to cutaneous carcinogenesis.

UVA may be a more silent threat than the erythemogenic UVB. A significant amount of UVB is screened by the stratospheric ozone layer, so terrestrial surface sunlight contains 20 times more UVA than UVB. Unlike UVB, UVA can penetrate window glass, and is relatively unchanged by time of day, season, and altitude. UVA can produce tanning and dyspigmentation without preceding erythema. The longer wavelengths penetrate deep into the dermis causing many of the histologic and clinical changes associated with photoaging. UVA I causes immunosuppression through the depletion of Langerhans' cells and reduced activity of antigen presenting cells. UVA also indirectly damages DNA through the formation of oxygen free radicals, mechanisms thought to contribute to carcinogenesis. Indeed, studies in animal models suggest that UVA may play a significant role in the development of malignant melanoma.

Sunscreen ingredients differ in their absorption spectrum, as shown in Table 20.3. Ideally a sunscreen should provide protection against the full spectrum of ultraviolet radiation.

The sun protection factor (SPF) is the only internationally standardized measure of a sunscreen's ability to filter UV radiation. It is the ratio of the UV energy required to produce a minimal erythema dose (MED) on sunscreen protected skin to the UV energy required to produce an MED on unprotected skin (Box 20.1). The MED is the quantity of energy

Absorbance range of selected sunscreen active ingredients	
Sunscreen	**Absorbance range (nm)**
Aminobenzoic acid (PABA)	260–313
Homosalate	300–310
Cinoxate	270–328
Octyl methoxycinnamate	270–328
Octyl salicylate	300–310
Padimate O	290–315
Phenylbenzimidazole sulfonic acid	290–320
Trolamine salicylate	260–320
Methyl anthralinate	290–320
Oxybenzone	270–350
Sulisobenzone	270–360
Dioxybenzone	260–380
Avobenzone	310–400
Titanium dioxide	250–400
Zinc oxide	250–380

Table 20.3 Absorbance range of selected sunscreen active ingredients

Determination of sun protective factor (SPF) value

$$SPF = \frac{\text{Minimum erythema dose sunscreen protected skin (J/cm}^2\text{)}}{\text{Minimum erythema dose sunscreen unprotected skin (J/cm}^2\text{)}}$$

Box 20.1 Determination of sun protective factor (SPF) value

Sunscreen category designations	
Product category	**SPF**
Minimal sun protection product	$2 \leq SPF < 12$
Moderate sun protection product	$12 \leq SPF < 30$
High sun protection product	$SPF \geq 30$

Table 20.4 Sunscreen category designations

required to produce the first perceptible redness reaction of the skin with clearly defined borders. Energy is delivered utilizing a filtered light source simulating the solar emission spectrum with 94% of its output between 290 and 400 nm. (This mimics sunlight at sea level at a zenith angle of 10°.) For any given product, measurement must be done on between 20 and 25 test subjects of Fitzpatrick skin types I, II, and III. Test material is applied to an area of at least 50 cm^2 at a thickness of 2 mg/cm^2.

The SPF of a given over-the-counter topical sunscreen is determined by testing of that product as above. In accordance with FDA regulations, multiple sun protective active ingredients can be combined as long as each contributes a minimum SPF of at least 2 to the finished product. This requirement is meant to avoid the addition of unnecessary ingredients. It is important to note that certain ingredients are incompatible and, if combined, will reduce the final SPF of a product. For example, avobenzone is unstable when combined with cinnamates such as cinoxate, but is both stable and effective when combined with octocrylene. Conversely, combining other active ingredients can increase the level of sun protection by improving photostability. Both avobenzone and oxybenzone have been reported to undergo degradation after UV irradiance. The physical sunscreen ingredients, titanium dioxide and zinc oxide, have been shown to improve the survival of chemical sunscreens in vitro.

To help consumers chose a product best suited to the level of protection required, the FDA monograph divides sunscreens into three product category designations as listed in Table 20.4. Agents of SPF 30 or greater will be grouped together as 'high sun protection products', and labeled as '30 plus' or '30+', because SPFs over 30 offer only incremental benefits.

There are significant limitations to using SPF as a guideline for UV protection. The thickness of application used to measure SPF may be unrealistic under ordinary, nontest conditions, thereby giving the consumer false confidence while significantly lowering the functional SPF. Additionally, because it is based on MEDs, the SPF is an effective way to measure protection from UVB, but not UVA, radiation. As noted previously, UVA is far less erythemogenic than UVB, so a significant amount of UVA may be absorbed by skin protected from UVB before erythema is noted. Indeed, one concern is that the people who use high SPF value sunscreens (who might otherwise have limited their ultraviolet exposure due to a fear of sunburn) may remain outdoors longer and accumulate more UVA damage. These are two possible explanations for recent epidemiologic reports that seemingly link sunscreen use to the increased incidence of skin cancer.

There is currently no standardized agreed way to measure UVA protection. Table 20.5 outlines the in vivo and in vitro options available. Immediate

Methods of testing UVA protection		
Test	Skin types used	Time of reading
In vivo		
Immediate pigment darkening (IPD)	III–V	Immediate
Persistent pigment darkening (PPD)	II–IV	24 hours
Protection factor in the UVA (PFA or APF)	I–IV	24 hours
In vitro		
Critical wavelength (λ_c)		

Table 20.5 Methods of testing UVA protection

pigment darkening (IPD) measures the transient brown color that appears and fades within minutes of UVA exposure in vivo in darker skin types. The persistent pigment darkening (PPD) technique has an easier to assess endpoint: pigment due to melanin oxidation that can be measured 24 hours after exposure in vivo. The protection factor in the UVA (PFA) method is also read in vivo at 24 hours and assesses either erythema or tanning. The critical wavelength (λ_c) is that below which 90% of sunscreen's UV absorbance occurs in vitro between 290 and 400 nm. That means that a product with a λ_c of 340 nm would filter UVB and UVA II, but not UVA I.

In an effort to help the FDA develop more stringent guidelines, an American Academy of Dermatology (AAD) consensus conference was called in February 2000. It was recommended that only sunscreens satisfying protection against both UVB, represented by an SPF of at least 15, and UVA radiation, represented by a λ_c of at least 370 nm and a minimum fourfold increase in PPD or PFA value, be labeled 'broad spectrum'. The AAD also advised that any increase in SPF be accompanied by a proportional increase in the UVA protection.

The efficacy of a sunscreen is affected by environmental factors including humidity and activity. Since swimming and sweat inducing sports are most commonly warm weather, daytime, outdoor activities, the ability of a sunscreen to maintain its filtering abilities under wet conditions is critical. 'Water resistance' is defined as maintenance of the label SPF value after 40 minutes of water immersion in a fresh water pool, whirlpool, or jacuzzi, consisting of two 20-minute periods of moderate activity separated by a 20-minute rest period and concluded by air drying without toweling. To be 'very water resistant', the sunscreen must maintain its SPF over a test cycle including 80 minutes of moderate activity in water.

Dosage and Usage

Currently the emphasis on sunscreen use has shifted from monotherapy to being *one* step in limiting sun exposure. The fear that humans will increase their total UV exposure time when using sunscreens has prompted the medical community to incorporate a more global strategy of UV limits, along with the use of protective clothing, hats, and sunglasses. Sunscreens, however, play a very important role in the fight against skin damage induced by the sun, but the key is proper usage.

The current FDA standard for sunscreen application is 2 mg/cm^2 and yet studies suggest that actual usage is only 25–50% of the amount used to rate sunscreen SPF. The main problem with sunscreen effectiveness is the nonlinear relationship between the SPF rating and the amount applied to the skin (Fig. 20.1). Sunscreen application has been shown to be as little as 0.5 mg/cm^2 which would translate to an SPF of 8 or 15 when applying an SPF product of 30. To cover the average 1.73 m^2 adult, a total of 35 mL of sunscreen is required.

The question then centers on why there is such a large discrepancy between how much sunscreen is needed and the amount actually used. There are numerous possibilities, starting with the consumer. Some sunscreen users feel uncomfortable at the recommended doses. Products may feel thick and occlusive, and at the appropriate dose can look opaque. There is a lack of education and specific instructions. Directions on sunscreen labels can be

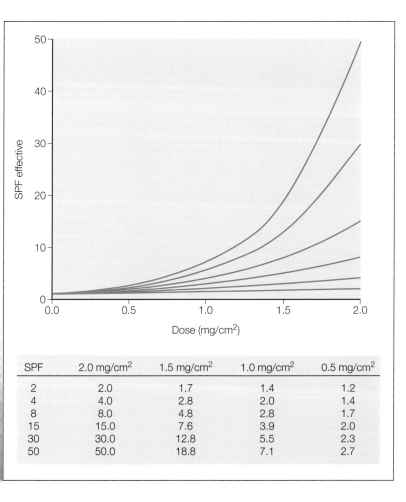

SPF	2.0 mg/cm^2	1.5 mg/cm^2	1.0 mg/cm^2	0.5 mg/cm^2
2	2.0	1.7	1.4	1.2
4	4.0	2.8	2.0	1.4
8	8.0	4.8	2.8	1.7
15	15.0	7.6	3.9	2.0
30	30.0	12.8	5.5	2.3
50	50.0	18.8	7.1	2.7

Fig. 20.1 Photoprotection from sunscreens. There is a nonlinear relationship between SPF and dose applied. To achieve the full SPF benefit, 2 mg/cm^2 of sunscreen needs to be applied to each body area

vague, with language such as 'apply liberally to all exposed areas prior to sun exposure'. The public may not understand how much is actually required, or may not have a good grasp on what 35 mL translates to clinically. This should be countered by relating the amount of product required with a common measurement that individuals can understand. Schneider (Fig. 20.2) suggests the 'teaspoon rule' based on the rule of nines used for calculating burn areas. With the teaspoon rule, an adult should apply approximately one-half teaspoon to each arm and to the face and neck. Six milliliters (just a little more than a teaspoon) should be applied to each leg, the chest, and to the back. This would amount to 33 mL being used. Another measurement most adults understand is the shot glass used to mix drinks. A shot glass is 30 mL and would approximate the requirement. Another method employed by some physicians is to recommend that patients apply twice or to put on two layers. This should

increase the amount applied and may help to reduce the numbers of 'missed' or 'skipped' areas. One of the biggest obstacles to proper dosing, however, is the desire by many Americans and Europeans to have tanned skin.

Besides the amount of sunscreen applied, there are a number of factors that also influence the protection equation and the best dosing regimen. These include resistance to water immersion and sand abrasion, reapplication, and the way products are applied. A mathematical study examined the relative importance of three sunscreen related factors: the amount of sunscreen applied, how the sunscreen was spread, and the UVA absorbing property of sunscreen. Diffey calculated that approximately 75% of the variance in UVA photoprotection achieved clinically depends upon how much product is applied. How well the product is applied and how well it absorbs UVA contributed almost equally to the remaining 25% of the variance.

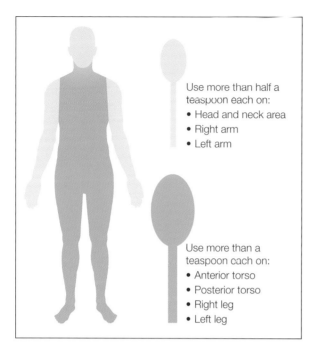

Use more than half a teaspoon each on:
- Head and neck area
- Right arm
- Left arm

Use more than a teaspoon each on:
- Anterior torso
- Posterior torso
- Right leg
- Left leg

Fig. 20.2 The 'teaspoon rule' can be used to guide patients on the appropriate amount of sunscreen required

Important in any discussion of sunscreen dosing is the proper timing for reapplication. Substantivity of a sunscreen is an indication of how well it maintains its degree of protection. Factors influencing the need for reapplication, include water activites, perspiration, rubbing of clothing or towels, and sand abrasion. It is generally recommended that the public reapply sunscreens every 2–3 hours and after swimming. This may not be sufficient, and reapplication of sunscreen at 20 minutes results in 60–85% of the UV exposure that would be obtained if the sunscreen were reapplied at 2 hours. Diffey advises that sunscreen be applied 15–30 minutes prior to sun exposure and reapplication of the product 15–30 minutes after sun exposure begins. Further reapplication will be necessary after activity that could remove sunscreen.

Adverse Events

Adverse events can be divided into direct reactions (Box 20.2) such as contact allergic reactions, and indirect sequelae such as increased UV exposure. The latter are more difficult to quantify and, to date, are less well defined.

Direct adverse effects of sun protective products

- Contact irritant dermatitis
- Contact allergic dermatitis
- Phototoxic reaction
- Photoallergic reaction
- Comedogenicity

Box 20.2 Direct adverse effects of sun protective products

Direct adverse events

Despite improvements in the formulations, there are still a number of reactions that occur, including idiosyncratic reactions to any of the components. With the higher SPF products, several active ingredients may be used in one formulation and at higher concentrations, increasing the potential for contact reactions. Companies, vying for consumers, are adding antioxidants, fragrances, preservatives, emulsifiers, and stabilizers, which can also cause adverse reactions.

Contact irritant reactions are by far the most common adverse event. Over 90% of cosmetic side effects are irritant reactions and half of these are subjective only. Also, some products may aggravate pre-existing conditions such as acne rosacea, atopic dermatitis, and seborrheic dermatitis. A true contact allergic reaction is typically seen 48 hours after exposure, and like other delayed hypersensitivity reactions presents with a spongiotic dermatitis. The offending agent acts as a hapten to bind with endogenous proteins and activates T lymphocytes. An immediate contact urticaria can be caused by sunscreens, with a wheal and flare reaction developing within 30–60 minutes after exposure. In one study using sunscreen or its vehicle, 19% (114 of 603 subjects) of the study population had adverse reactions. True allergic sensitization was seen in six, while 45 patients developed aggravation of their atopic dermatitis, 39 had a contact irritation, and 22 had nonspecific cosmetic intolerance.

Phototoxic and photoallergic reactions are possible with current sunprotectant products. A phototoxic reaction can occur when UV radiation is absorbed and can then be transferred to epidermal cells causing an exaggerated sunburn, or can promote photoexcitation of the agent. These reactive singlets or triplets can damage various portions of the cell including the cell membrane, DNA, and lysosomes. Padimate A, a PABA ester, was found to be quite phototoxic and was withdrawn from the market. A photoallergic reaction is a contact allergic reaction that requires UVR to transform the chemical into a sensitizer. Photoallergy most often involves the UVA portion of the UV spectrum. The use of effective UVA blockers should help to minimize UVA absorption and prevent photoallergic responses.

Indirect adverse events

The debate on vitamin D and sunscreens continues. Anywhere from 9% to 40% of Americans are deficient in vitamin D. Although vitamin D can be added to the diet in supplements, milk, cereal and other foods, 90% of requisite vitamin D is formed within the skin through the action of the sun. A number of studies point to a protective role of vitamin D in the pathogenesis of various malignancies, including colon, prostate, and breast cancer. Thus two separate but related adverse events are at least theoretically possible with the regular use of sunscreen: deficiency in vitamin D, and an increased risk of some internal cancers, especially, in those individuals who might already be at risk for vitamin D deficiency. This can be balanced with adequate dietary intake of vitamin D, supplemental use of vitamin D, or exposure to small amounts of sunlight. A study performed in Boston, Massachusetts, demonstrated that exposure of the body in a bathing suit to one minimal erythema dose of sunlight is equivalent to injecting about 10 000 IU of vitamin D. However more limited exposure, such as the hands, arms, and face, will require exposure two to three times a week at one-third to one-half a minimal erythema dose.

There has been additional concern that the use of sunscreen may actually increase the risk for developing melanoma, but an analysis of 14 studies published to date could not confirm an increased risk for melanoma developing after sunscreen use. There is concern that fair skinned individuals will increase their exposure to the sun with a false sense of security when using sunscreens. This is especially a problem if the sunscreen used has a high SPF rating but lacks adequate UVA coverage. Statistically US adolescents still have one or more summer sunburns and many adolescents reported having used sunscreen with a SPF of 15 or higher before receiving their most serious summer sunburn. These types of studies fail to demonstrate whether the teenagers would have sunburned without the use of a sunscreen, and would they indeed decrease risky sun behaviors if they did not have the aid of a sunscreen agent.

Thus the debate about indirect side effects is sure to continue for some time.

Ingredient-specific adverse events
Para-aminobenzoic acid

PABA is one of the oldest sunscreen agents employed in the USA. Side effects include contact irritation with stinging and burning, usually related to the alcohol base. In the 1980s, it was the most common cause of allergy to sunscreens, but the reactions to PABA have decreased due to its declining use.

Amyl dimethyl PABA and octyl dimethyl PABA

Padimate A and Padimate O were introduced as substitutes for PABA to reduce the numbers of reactions seen with PABA. A high proportion of patients using Padimate A did have burning, pruritus and erythema after sun exposure, and it was taken off the market. Padimate O is a viscous liquid that tends to remain on the surface of the stratum corneum with little penetration. It has a very low potential for sensitization.

Benzophenones

Benzophenones have a photoreactive carbonyl group. They respond to UVA radiation by electron resonance delocalization and can become potent allergic and UV-reactive photoallergic sensitizers. The incidence of allergic reactions to oxybenzone confirmed in photopatch series is 12%. Benzophenones are used extensively in cosmetics, and even in textiles, plastics, paints, varnishes, and other products. Thus benzophenone-sensitive patients may face many environmental exposures and challenges.

Cinnamates

Cinnimates are popular UVB sunscreens and uncommonly elicit photoallergic sensitization. They have been implicated in allergic reactions, however, and can cross-react with many related compounds including balsam of Peru, coca leaves, cinnamon oil, cinnaminic acid, and cinnamic aldehyde. The cinnamon derivatives are found in cosmetics, fragrances, flavorings, and products such as tobacco, toothpaste, vermouth, and colas.

Dibenzolymethanes

Avoenzone (Parsol 1789) is a butyl dibenzolymethane compound that, like other dibenzolymethanes, exhibits photolability. It is nonsensitizing in concentrations below 3%, but more potent formulations have elicited irritant and allergic reactions. Eusolex 8020 (available in Europe) is the more potent allergen and many reactions to avobenzone have been traced to an initial sensitization to Eusolex 8020. A camphor derivative, Eusolex 6300, also available in Europe, has caused several allergic reactions and can cross-react with Eusolex 8020.

Salicylates and anthranilates

Salicylates and anthranilates are weak UVB absorbers and so both are used in high concentrations. Despite this, they have been implicated in very few allergic reactions.

Physical sunblocks

The physical agents such as zinc oxide and titanium dioxide have unparalleled safety. They are inert compounds and have not been implicated in allergic sensitization.

New Research

Clearly there is a need for sunscreens that are efficacious at lower application densities to mimic what is frequently applied by the public in 'normal use' perhaps to $0.025–0.5 \, mg/cm^2$. Another area of improvement is in base or vehicle enhancement so that a better flow property would lessen uneven applications and allow for longer duration while still remaining cosmetically appealing. Sunscreens that are able to impart a 'tanned' appearance may have a role, especially for adolescents, such that it would encourage their usage.

As more is known about the contribution of UVA to photoaging and photocarcinogenesis, it is clear that there is a need for accurate quantification and standardized labeling of the UVA protection factor (Table 20.5).

The most promising research, however, lies in the use of additives that have a synergistic property with the sunscreen. Most notably, the addition of antioxidants could potentially limit the damage from UV photons and help to repair some of the genetic damage induced by UV photons that have penetrated the skin. Vitamin C has been demonstrated to modestly protect against UVB photodamage and UVA induced phototoxic responses. When combined with vitamin E there may be an even greater protection against cellular insult. Beta-carotene has been reported to be of value in the treatment of erythropoietic protoporphyria and may be able to inhibit UV promoted carcinogenesis. Selenium compounds, when topically applied in concentrations of less than 0.05%, reduce UV skin damage measured as less inflammation, less pigmentation, and retardation of skin cancer. Chelates such as ortho-phenanthroline, edetic acid, and dipyridylamine, bind metals such as iron, thus limiting their interactions with other materials and protecting against cellular damage from free radical oxygen. Topical chelate application prior to UV exposure is reported to reduce or delay visible skin wrinkling caused by UV exposure along with tumor formation.

It is important to remember that to date, innovations in sunscreens have had little direct effect on sun induced tumor incidence rates such as basal cell carcinoma and melanoma. This may be due to the additional use of tanning beds and other sun seeking behaviors, and current attitudes towards sun exposure and the continued appeal of 'tanned' skin. There are animal models and human studies that indicate that the use of high SPF sunscreen reduces the number of new actinic keratosis and leads to a reduction in recurrent squamous cell carcinomas.

When used appropriately and with other measures to help retard UV exposure such as behavior changes, and the use of clothing, sunscreens can be a very important tool.

Further Reading

Albert MR, Ostheimer KG 2003 The evolution of current medical and popular attitudes toward ultraviolet light exposure: Part 3. Journal of the American Academy of Dermatology 49: 1096–1106

Al Mahroos MA, Yaar M, Phillips TJ, et al 2002 Effect of sunscreen application on UV-induced thymine dimers. Archives of Dermatology 138:1480–1485

Bastuji-Garin S, Diepgen T 2002 Cutaneous malignant melanoma sun exposure, and sunscreen use: epidemiological evidence. British Journal of Dermatology 146(Suppl 1):24–30

Bissonnette R, Allas S, Moyal D, et al 2000 Comparison of UVA protection afforded by high sun protection factor sunscreens. Journal of the American Academy of Dermatology 43:1036–1038

Darlington S, Williams G, Neale R, et al 2003 A randomized controlled trial to assess sunscreen application and beta carotene supplementation in the prevention of solar keratoses. Archives of Dermatology 139:451–455

Diffey BL 1996 Sunscreens, suntans, and skin cancer: people do not apply enought sunscreen for protection. British Journal of Dermatology 313:942

Diffey BL 2001 Sunscreen isn't enough. Journal of Photochemistry and Photobiology B 64(2–3):105–108

Diffey BL 2001 Sunscreens and UVA protection: a major issue of minor importance. Photochemistry and Photobiology 74:61–63

Diffey BL 2001 When should sunscreen be reapplied? Journal of the American Academy of Dermatology 45:882–885

Foley P, Nixon R, Marks R, Frowen K, Thompson S 1993 The frequency of reactions to sunscreens: results of a longitudinal population-based study on the regular use of sunscreens in Australia. British Journal of Dermatology 128:512–518

Green A, Williams G, Neale R, et al 1999 Daily sunscreen application and betacarotene supplementation in prevention of basal-cell and squamous-cell carcinomas of the skin: a randomised controlled trial. Lancet 354:723–729

Hawk JL 2003 Cutaneous photoprotection. Archives of Dermatology 139:527–530

Lim HW, Naylor M, Honigsmann H, et al 2000 American Academy of Dermatology Consensus Conference on UVA protection of sunscreens: summary and recommendations. Journal of the American Academy of Dermatology 44:505–508

Meves A, Repacholi MH, Kehfuess EA 2003 Promoting safe and effective sun protection strategies. Journal of the American Academy of Dermatology 49:1203–1204

Mitchnick MA, Fairhurst D, Pinnell SR 1999 Microfine zinc oxide (Z-cote) as a photostable UVA/UVB sunblock agent. Journal of the American Academy of Dermatology 40: 85–90

Moloney F, Collins S, Murphy G 2002 Sunscreens safety, efficacy and appropriate use. American Journal of Clinical Dermatology 3:185–191

Naylor M, Boyd A, Smith D, Cameron GS, Hubbard D, Neldner K 1995 High sun protection factor sunscreens in the suppression of actinic neoplasia. Archives of Dermatology 131:170–175

Osborne J, Hutchinson P 2002 Vitamin D and systemic cancer: is this relevant to malignant melanoma? British Journal of Dermatology 147:197–213

Schneider J 2002 The teaspoon rule of applying sunscreen. Archives of Dermatology 138:838–839

Szczurko C, Dompmartin A, Michel M, Moreau A, Leroy D 1994 Photocontact allergy to oxybenzone: ten years of experience. Photodermatology, Photoimmunology and Photomedicine 10:144–147

US Food and Drug Administration 2003 Center for Food Safety and Applied Nutrition, Office of Cosmetics and Colors Fact Sheet. Sunscreens, tanning products, and sun safety

US Food and Drug Administration, HHS 1999 Sunscreen drug products for over-the-counter human use; final monograph. Federal Register 64(98)

21 Cosmeceuticals and Contact Dermatitis

Christen M. Mowad

Introduction

Cosmetics have been around for centuries. Cosmetics are defined by the Food, Drug and Cosmetic Act as 'articles intended to be rubbed, poured, sprinkled or sprayed or introduced into or otherwise applied to the human body or any part thereof for cleansing, beautifying, promoting attractiveness, or altering the appearance' and should not alter the structure or function of the skin. Drugs are defined as 'articles intended for use in the diagnosis, cure, mitigation, treatment or prevention of disease in man'. Cosmeceuticals are cosmetic products that contain bioactive ingredients with the intent to have a beneficial physiologic effect. There is no legal definition of cosmeceuticals. Cosmeceuticals fit somewhere between cosmetics and drugs. However, even water could be classified as a cosmeceutical given its effects on the hydration of the stratum corneum.

Unfortunately, sometimes the cosmeceutical products intended to enhance beauty can lead to a dermatitis that can be quite unsightly, uncomfortable, annoying and perplexing to the patient and the physician. Contact dermatitis is one of these adverse reactions and can be either irritant or allergic in nature, with the former being more common. Allergic contact dermatitis to cosmetics, personal care products, make-up, body washes, moisturizers, creams, nail, lip and hair care products, and the devices (i.e. sponges, applicators) used to apply them can result in a clinical dermatitis. These reports are well documented in the literature and clinically can appear as a well demarcated reaction at the location of product application. However, the dermatitis can be ectopic to the location the product is applied through transfer to a more sensitive area such as the face or eyelids. Reports of allergic contact dermatitis to cosmeceuticals are not as frequently reported in the literature as one would

expect given their widespread usage. This may be due in part to difficulty in testing these products and the lack of standardized allergens.

Vitamins

Contact dermatitis to cosmeceutical vitamins such as vitamin A (retinol), vitamin C (ascorbic acid), and vitamin E (tocopherol) has been reported in the literature. Vitamin A and its derivatives such as retinol, retinaldehyde, and retinyl palmitate typically produce an irritant contact dermatitis with dryness and skin irritation. This irritation is an unwanted side effect of retinization of the face, but cannot be avoided if the beneficial collagen regenerative effects are to be experienced. Irritant contact dermatitis can sometimes present identically to allergic contact dermatitis, but vesiculation and facial swelling are never an expected part of early retinization of the face. Allergic contact dermatitis to vitamin A is rare, but can be confirmed by positive patch testing. The vitamin A containing cream can be closed patch tested 'as is', but many times it is impossible to determine which of the many ingredients in the preparation is the culprit. Most large cosmeceutical manufacturers can provide a sample of the vitamin A raw material they use in their formulation for individual ingredient patch testing. The person to contact at the company and the address can be obtained from the Cosmetic Industry On Call brochure published as a joint effort between the American Contact Dermatitis Society (ACDS) and the Cosmetic, Toiletry, and Fragrance Association (CTFA). More information can be obtained at the CTFA web site at http://www.ctfa.org.

Vitamin C, also known as ascorbic acid, is another vitamin used topically to reverse signs of aging. It is difficult to formulate because it is easily oxidized to inactive products upon exposure to UV radiation or oxygen. Allergic contact dermatitis to topical vitamin C is rare, but irritation can occur due to the low pH effects of the asorbic acid on the skin. The same discussion regarding closed patch testing and ingredient procurement for vitamin A also applies to vitamin C.

Vitamin E, part of a family of compounds called tocopherols, is a common cause of both irritant and allergic contact dermatitis. Its role as a contact allergen is well documented, thus vitamin E represents the most common cosmeceutical vitamin to cause allergic contact dermatitis. Some of the reports have dealt with allergic reactions experienced to vitamin E found in a line of colored cosmetics manufactured in Europe. It appears that the manufacturer used food grade vitamin E instead of cosmetic grade vitamin E which accounted for the allergic contact dermatitis. Many of the casually reported cases of vitamin E allergy appear to be due to consumers breaking open vitamin E capsules intended for oral consumption and rubbing the oil onto wounds or scars to promote healing. While vitamin E formulated in this manner is safe for human oral consumption, it is not intended for topical application. Cosmetic grade vitamin E properly formulated in a moisturizing cream is rarely allergenic.

Hydroxy Acids

Hydroxy acids are a group of chemicals frequently found in cosmeceutical products. Irritant contact dermatitis to alpha hydroxy acids (AHAs), beta hydroxy acids (BHAs), and polyhydroxy acids (PHAs) are typically the form of irritant contact dermatitis. The larger size of PHAs reduces skin penetration, which also lessens the opportunity for irritant contact dermatitis to occur. More irritant reactions are seen with the AHAs, in the form of stinging and burning due to the low pH of these cosmeceuticals that rapidly penetrate the stratum corneum to reach the nerve endings in the dermis. AHAs that have been partially neutralized produce less contact dermatitis, but also do not produce dramatic antiaging effects. BHAs, such as salicylic acid, are oil soluble and do not penetrate the stratum corneum well. For this reason, irritant contact dermatitis is lessened, but can still occur in patients with compromised barrier function.

Botanicals

Botanicals form one of the largest categories o cosmeceutical ingredients in today's marketplace Given the push to nature in our increasingly healtl conscious society, botanicals are often seen by con sumers as natural safer alternatives to their syntheti counterparts. As a result of a strong driving force within the cosmetic industry toward natural products botanicals are a common cosmeceutical active ingre dient. Botanical additives are made from variou parts of the plant including the leaves, root, fruits stems, or flowers. The concentration, composition efficacy and antigenicity of a given plant extract ma) differ depending on the part of the plant from which it was obtained. Different antigens may also be present depending on the time of year the botanical was harvested and how the plant materia was processed prior to incorporation into a cosme ceutical. There are few systematic reviews on the subject of contact dermatitis and botanicals Although there are many cases of contact dermatiti to botanicals and essential oils in the literature, mos cases of allergic reactions that have been docu mented are single case reports. With the increasing use of botanicals in the cosmetic and cosmeceu tical arena, more reactions to these extracts are expected. This section will not review all of the individual case reports of allergic reactions to botanicals, rather it will serve to highlight some of the more common botanical culprits.

Aloe is a commonly used botanical extract for its soothing properties on wounds, burns, and irritated skin (Fig. 21.1). It is a mucilage containing thousands of individual chemical entities. This makes determination of the exact allergen impossible. Yet, case reports of allergic contact dermatitis are found in the literature. Patients who have experienced a suspected allergic contact dermatitis to aloe should simply learn to read ingredient labels and avoid products containing this botanical extract. It is not hard to avoid cosmeceuticals containing aloe.

Ginkgo biloba is another common botanical used primarily for its anti-inflammatory effects. There have been no reports of allergic contact dermatitis to this botanical documented in the literature.

Tea tree oil or melaleuca oil is derived from the Cheel shrub in Australia (Fig. 21.2). It has gained increasing popularity in a variety of shampoos and over-the-counter salon treatment products designed to minimize dandruff or seborrheic dermatitis. Tea tree oil can cause allergic contact dermatitis and

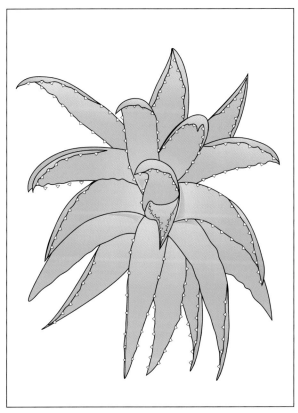

Fig. 21.1 Aloe vera mucilage is a possible cause of allergic contact dermatitis

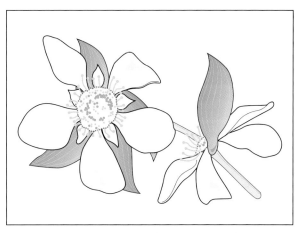

Fig. 21.2 Homeopathic dandruff shampoos may be a source of tea tree oil exposure

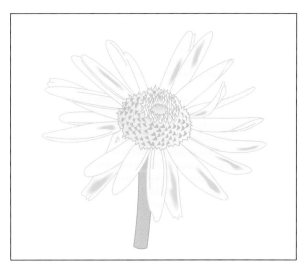

Fig. 21.3 Arnica montana is a medicinal plant capable of causing allergic contact dermatitis

in one study was found to be the most allergenic botanical extract. The constituent of the oil thought to cause the majority of allergic reactions is *d*-limonene; however, not all patients who react to tea tree oil react to *d*-limonene.

Curcumin is an antioxidant derived from turmeric root. Curcumin is a common additive to Middle Eastern and Indian food as a hot spice. Its use in these cultures dates back to the prerefrigeration era when curcumin was used as a food preservative. It is used in some cosmeceuticals to prevent the product from discoloring or oxidizing on the store shelf. Several currently marketed prestige cosmeceutical moisturizers contain curcumin to prevent the degradation of ceramides added to enhance the skin barrier. Curcumin is a cutaneous irritant and can cause stinging, burning, and itching in patients with atopic dermatitis or other barrier defects. There are also rare reports of allergic contact dermatitis resulting from topical contact with curcumin.

Witch hazel has been used as a cosmeceutical astringent, acne agent, and vasoconstrictor. It is a

cause of allergic contact dermatitis. Currently, witch hazel is a common additive to cosmeceutical eye creams designed to minimize puffiness and bags under the eyes. Witch hazel allergy should be suspected in patients with periorbital swelling who have begun using a new eye area cosmeceutical.

The Compositae family comprises a group of plants that have sensitizing capabilities. *Arnica montana* is an important medicinal plant that has been reported to cause allergic contact dermatitis (Fig. 21.3). Screening patients with sesquiterpene lactone mix, found on the traditional dermatologic patch test tray, may miss some of these reactions and therefore testing to the plant or other

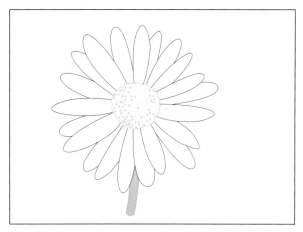

Fig. 21.4 Bisabolol is a chamomile extract found in products designed for sensitive skin and may be a rare cause of allergic contact dermatitis

chemical constituents of the plant is recommended. Chamomile, another member of the Compositae family, is also a cause of allergic contact dermatitis (Fig. 21.4). This is interesting given the fact that a chamomile extract, known as bisabolol, is used as an anti-inflammatory in cosmeceutical moisturizers. However, echinacea and marigold are two members of this family that have not been reported to cause allergic contact dermatitis. This indicates that there must be subtle differences in each of these plant extracts accounting for the presence or absence of the dermatitis-causing allergen.

Sunscreens

Our attention now turns to another common category of cosmeceuticals that can cause contact dermatitis known as sunscreens. Sunscreens are added to cosmetic and cosmeceutical products and are the cause of irritant contact dermatitis, allergic contact dermatitis, and photoallergic contact dermatitis. There are several classes of sunscreens including para-aminobenzoic acid (PABA) and its esters, cinnamates, salicylates, benzephenones, anthranilates, and dibenzoylmethanes to which contact dermatitis have been reported. Irritant contact dermatitis is the most common adverse reaction to sunscreens, but reports of allergic and photoallergic contact dermatitis are present in the literature. PABA is the most common cause of photoallergic reactions, but pure PABA is no longer used in currently marketed sunscreens. Patch testing and photo patch testing are necessary to confirm the diagnosis in suspected cases of allergic contact

dermatitis to sunscreen ingredients. Sunscreens can be closed patch tested 'as is'. However, most sunscreens contain a 'cocktail' of active ingredients to provide broad spectrum sun protection. It is best to contact the sunscreen manufacturer through the Cosmetic Industry On Call brochure, as discussed previously, to obtain individual raw material sunscreen actives for patch testing.

Fragrances

Many cosmeceutical products are fragranced and an allergic or irritant reaction may be due to the fragrance component. Fragrances are the most common cause of allergic contact dermatitis to cosmetics. Patch testing to fragrance is typically done via a fragrance mix that contains the individual fragrance ingredients listed in Box 21.1.

Several authors have suggested the addition of other essential oils to the current fragrance mix, such as sandalwood, narcissus, jasmine, and ylang ylang to enhance the detection of fragrance allergy. If testing to the fragrance mix and these other chemicals is negative and a fragrance allergy is still suspected, patch testing to other fragrances on extended series should be considered.

Unfortunately, product labeling can be misleading as no specific information regarding fragrance components is usually listed on cosmeceutical products manufactured for sale in the USA. Product labels simply list 'fragrance' in the ingredient disclosure. Even if patch testing allows identification of specific fragrance allergen, labels do not typically list individual fragrance components. This makes management of the fragrance allergic patient difficult.

To further complicate matters, there are several fragrance chemicals such as benzyl alcohol, benzaldehyde, and ethylene brassylate that can have

---

Constituents of the fragrance mix

- Cinnamic alcohol
- Cinnamic aldehyde
- Hydroxycitronellal
- Isoeugenol
- Eugenol
- Oakmoss absolute
- Amylcinnamic alcohol
- Geraniol

Note: Each of these fragrance ingredients is present at a concentration of 1% in petrolatum

Box 21.1 Constituents of the fragrance mix

other functions in addition to being a fragrance component. These chemicals can still be used in a product labeled 'fragrance free' if they provide other functions in addition to fragrance in the cosmeceutical. This is often the case with botanical extracts that are frequently not listed as fragrance ingredients because they are used for their medicinal properties and not for the ability to impart fragrance. Patients who are allergic to fragrance should also be instructed to avoid botanical preparations. Initial avoidance of all fragrances is recommended for at least 4–6 weeks, and then if necessary, or desired, introduction of one fragranced product at a time can be initiated. Each product should be used for approximately 2 weeks prior to introducing another fragrance or fragranced product. Physicians must educate patients to the fact that unscented does not mean no fragrance exists, just that it cannot be smelled. Many times unscented products contain masking fragrances designed to mask the chemical odor of the formulation.

Preservatives

Preservatives used to prevent bacterial growth and oxidation in cosmeceutical products are the second most common cause of allergic contact dermatitis. Preservatives are found in all cosmeceutical products. Formaldehyde, formaldehyde releasers such as quaternium-15, DMDM hydantoin, diazolidinyl urea, and imidazolidinyl urea are common allergens. Quaternium-15 is the most frequently found preservative causing allergic contact dermatitis in cosmeceuticals.

The parabens are widely used cosmeceutical preservatives and are felt to be very safe. The most common parabens used are ethyl, butyl, methyl, propyl and isobutyl paraben. Although these are generally a well tolerated class of preservatives, there are isolated reports of allergic contact dermatitis to parabens. However, given the widespread use of these preservatives, the rate of sensitivity is low. Thus, patients with suspected preservative allergies should be advised to select cosmeceuticals that use parabens for preservation.

Methylchloroisothiazolinone (MCI/MI, Kathon CG, Euxyl K 100) is another preservative used in cosmetic preparations that can cause allergic contact dermatitis. The rate of sensitivity as determined by the North American Contact Dermatitis Group is 2.9%. Allergic contact dermatitis to this chemical was initially reported in Europe where the chemical

was first introduced. However, with increased usage in the USA, reports of allergy to this chemical have been made. At present, methylchloroisothiazolinone is used mainly in rinse-off products such as hair shampoos and conditioners where the short contact time minimizes the chances of an allergic reaction. However, there are a variety of sensitive skin moisturizers that contain this ingredient, which may be problematic.

Patch Testing

The gold standard for diagnosing an allergic contact dermatitis to any product including cosmeceuticals is patch testing. This is a simple easy office procedure that can be extremely helpful in determining the cause of a patient's dermatitis (Fig. 21.5). Obviously, other causes of the patient's reaction including irritant contact dermatitis, contact urticaria,

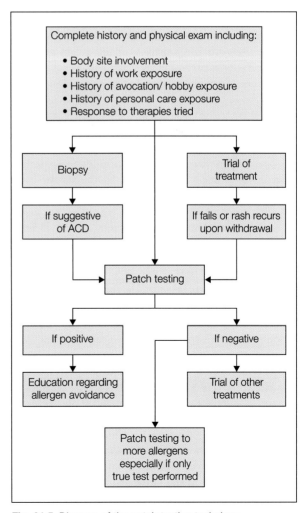

Fig. 21.5 Diagram of the patch testing technique

acneiform eruptions, rosacea, seborrheic dermatitis, atopic dermatitis, perioral dermatitis, and other skin disorders must be considered. However, in the patient who does not respond to traditional methods of treatment, or who has a persistent or localized dermatitis, or a dermatitis that flares after discontinuation of a treatment regimen, the diagnosis of allergic contact dermatitis should be considered and patch testing should be performed. It is important to note that most patients, and even experienced specialists within the field of allergic contact dermatitis, are unable to reliably and consistently identify the causative allergen prior to patch testing based on history and physical examination alone.

The procedure of patch testing requires an interest and level of suspicion on the part of the clinician as well as a set of allergens in the office. First the physician must take a thorough history detailing the products the patient uses, including make-up, moisturizers, natural products the patient might be using as well as the method of application, and removal of these products. Natural products that a patient uses are frequently omitted when giving a history. Patients often falsely assume that something natural could not be the cause of their problem. They should be reminded that poison ivy is natural and causes many people significant skin problems.

Once the allergens to be tested have been chosen, a nurse within the office, who has been trained on the application of patch testing, applies the patches. This involves applying allergens to the upper back and taping them in place. The allergens applied can be obtained from several different companies including Allerderm (manufacturers of TRUE Test, Petaluma, CA, USA), Chemotechnique Diagnostics (Malmo, Sweden) and Trolab/Pharmascience (Canada). The TRUE Test is a reasonable starting place for patch testing but studies have shown that expanded sets of allergens are more successful in identifying a causative allergen in the patient who suffers from allergic contact dermatitis. Therefore, if considering the diagnosis of allergic contact dermatitis, expanded testing is often helpful, particularly if the TRUE test is unrevealing. If expanded allergen series are not available, referral to a center specializing in patch testing may be necessary if the suspicion of allergic contact dermatitis remains. It is usually possible to obtain the specialized allergens required by contacting the company as listed in the Cosmetic Industry On Call brochure. Most companies can also provide informa-

tion on how to formulate and apply the patches, as well as providing the Material Safety Data Sheet (MSDS) for specific chemical information about the substance.

The initial patches should be kept in place and kept dry for 48 hours. The patches are then removed and a map of the allergens is drawn on the back. The patient should return for a second reading from 96 hours to 1 week later to assess for delayed reactions which are well documented in the literature. If a second reading is not performed, several allergic reactions may be missed (Box 21.2).

As many of the cosmeceuticals are relatively new and standardized allergens are not available, testing to the products themselves can be helpful. If the product is intended to be a leave-on product, it can be tested as is. However, if the product is a rinse-off product intended to be diluted with water, the product must be diluted prior to application so as to avoid irritant reactions. There are guides available to help determine the appropriate dilutions of such products. Controls must be done when using patient products for testing. The standard negative control used is generally petrolatum. It may also be worthwhile to include a positive irritant, such as sodium lauryl sulfate, if an irritant reaction is suspected for comparison.

If an allergic reaction is identified, the patient should be instructed on allergen avoidance, and label reading. The dermatitis can take 6–8 weeks to resolve despite avoidance and patients should be reassured during this time period. A database called the Contact Allergen Replacement Database is available to members of the American Contact Dermatitis Society through the society web page (www.contactderm.org) and can be very helpful in identifying products free of a patient's known allergens. The physician types in the chemicals the patient tested positive to and

Responses in patch test reading	
1/– +	macular erythema only
+	= weak (nonvesicular) reaction ; erythema, infiltration, possibly papules
++	= strong (edematous or vesicular) reaction
+++	= extreme (spreading, bullous or ulcerative) reaction
IRR	= irritant morphologic appearance
–	= negative reaction
NT	= non tested

Box 21.2 Responses in patch test reading

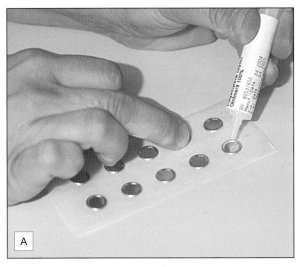

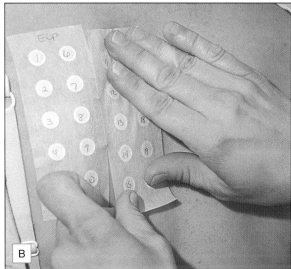

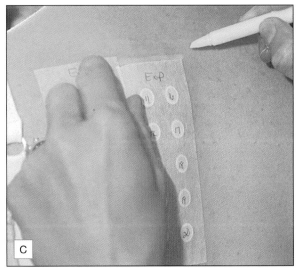

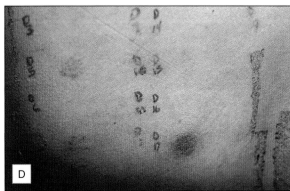

Fig. 21.6 Patch testing. (**A**) Allergen is placed in metal Finn chambers. (**B**) Numbered allergens are placed on upper back. (**C**) Orientation marks are placed for allergen identification upon removal. (**D**) Positive patch test is present at site D17

the database provides a listing of products free of these chemical ingredients. The database is extensive but is limited by the products entered into the database. It is updated once yearly. It can prove helpful in identifying products a patient can use and is a helpful resource for patients.

Cosmeceuticals are an increasingly popular arena in the skin care market. Even these products, many containing natural ingredients and intended to enhance beauty, can cause an allergic or irritant contact dermatitis. Contact dermatitis to these products has been reported though not with high frequency. As more people use cosmeceuticals, an increase in adverse reactions might be expected. Fortunately, the cosmetic industry is early to recognize problems

and reformulate to minimize consumer difficulties. Nevertheless, the possibility of allergic contact dermatitis should be considered. Patch testing is an important tool to identify and confirm the possible cause of an adverse reaction to a cosmeceutical (Fig. 21.6).

Further Reading

Bazzano C, De Angeles S, Kleist G, Maedo N 1996 Allergic contact dermatitis from topical vitamins A and E. Contact Dermatitis 35:261–262

De Groot AC 1994 Patch testing, 2nd edn. Elsevier, New York

De Groot AC 1998 Fatal attractiveness: the shady side of cosmetics. Clinics in Dermatology 16:167–179

Frosch PJ, Johansen JD, Menne T, Pirker C, Rastogi SC, Andersen KE 2002 Further important sensitizers in patients sensitive to fragrances. Contact Dermatitis 47:279–287

Kiken D, Cohen D 2002 Contact dermatitis to botanical extracts. American Journal of Contact Dermatitis 13:148–152

Kim B, Lee Y, Kang K 2003 The mechanism of retinal-induced irritation and its application to anti-irritant development. Toxicology Letters 146:65–73

Mowad C 2001 Patch testing for cosmetic allergens. Atlas of Office Procedures 4:551–563

Paulsen E 2002 Contact sensitization from Compositae-containing herbal remedies and cosmetics. Contact Dermatitis 47:189–198

Scheinman P 2001 Exposing covert fragrance chemicals. American Journal of Contact Dermatitis 12:225–228

Scheman A 2000 Adverse reactions to cosmetic ingredients. Dermatologic Clinics 18:685–698

Thomson K, Wilkinson S 2000 Allergic contact dermatitis to plant extracts in patients with cosmetic dermatitis. British Journal of Dermatology 142:84–88

Wolf R, Wolf D, Tuzun B, Tuzun Y 2001 Contact dermatitis to cosmetics. Clinics in Dermatology 19:502–515

Part 3

The Application of Cosmeceuticals to Dermatologic Practice

This section of the volume is intended to integrate the cosmeceutical concepts discussed in earlier chapters into ancillary treatments that may be used by the dermatologist in recommending possible useful ingredients to patients. Frequently patients will inquire about the over-the-counter technologies that may supplement prescription treatments, or they may simply wish to select the moisturizer that would provide an optimal benefit. There are many concoctions available for purchase, which may be bewildering to the patient and dermatologist alike.

There are a number of dermatologic conditions that may respond to the cosmeceuticals presented in this text: wrinkles and fine lines, facial redness, dyspigmented skin, oily skin, dry skin, and acne. Cosmeceutical actives may be of benefit when used in cleansers, toners, and moisturizers. In most cases, they do not replace prescription therapy, but may be useful in the maintenance phase of disease treatment for conditions such as dyspigmentation and acne. Other conditions, such as oily skin, have no safe efficacious long term prescription therapy for the average patient making cosmeceuticals the only treatment option. Facial redness, beyond that induced by diseases such as rosacea, remains a therapeutic enigma. Here cosmeceuticals represent an important adjuvant for reducing inflammation induced by the use of common hygiene products. Cosmeceutical actives may also provide barrier enhancement in patients with dry skin where compensating for environmental factors and adjusting the skin biofilm may be necessary to maintain an optimal appearance.

Wrinkles and Fine Lines

22

Zoe Diana Draelos

This chapter deals with those ingredients that are marketed for the purpose of improving the appearance of fine lines and wrinkles. The ingredients have been divided into several categories based on function: botanical antioxidants, vitamin antioxidants, and cellular regulators (Tables 22.1, 22.2, 22.3). These ingredients represent the most popular cosmeceuticals placed in moisturizers designed to minimize fine lines and wrinkles. It is important to remember that the effects of the moisturizing ingredients cannot be separated from those of the cosmeceutical active in most cases. Nevertheless, moisturizers are the most common cosmeceutical wrinkle treatment currently available.

There are two major types of wrinkles that characterize the aging face: wrinkles at rest and wrinkles in motion. Moisturizers are effective only for wrinkles at rest. Even though there have been some moisturizer additives that claim to modulate neuromuscular junction activity, such as dimethyl-aminoethanol (DMAE) and hexapeptides, for all practical purposes moisturizers function to minimize the appearance of fine facial lines due to dehydration. These are the tissue paper appearing

Botanical antioxidants		
Cosmeceutical	**Effects on skin physiology**	**Patient selection comments**
Soy	Flavonoid antioxidant with estrogenic effect, genistein and daidzein	Improves skin thickness
Curcumin	Polyphenol antioxidant with tetrahydrocurcumin, used as a natural preservative	Slight burning sensation possible on application
Green tea	Polyphenol antioxidant with epigallocatechin	Must be used freshly brewed or stabilized with BHT as oxidizes to brown color rapidly, useful as a photoprotectant
Silymarin	Flavoinoid antioxidant with silybin, silydianin, and silychristine	May be useful topically in photosensitive individuals
Pyncogenol	Phenol and phenolic acid antioxidant	Useful in supplementing antioxidant effects of vitamins C and E
Lutein and lycopene	Carotenoid antioxidant	Best consumed orally in fresh picked ripe tomatoes
Rosmarinic acid	Polyphenol antioxidant	Found in high concentration in fresh rosemary leaves
Hypericin (St John's wort)	Polyphenol antioxidant	Must not be consumed orally in large quantities
Ellagic acid (pomegranate fruit)	Polyphenol antioxidant	Marketed as potent antioxidant for topical and oral use

Table 22.1 Botanical antioxidants

Vitamin antioxidants		
Cosmeceutical	**Effects on skin physiology**	**Patient selection comments**
Vitamin E	Alpha tocopherol active primary skin antioxidant form	Primary substance responsible for the prevention of oxidation of cell wall lipids, poor topical penetration
Vitamin C	L-ascorbic acid, secondary skin antioxidant form peroxidation	Regenerates vitamin E to active form to prevent cell membrane lipid, poor topical penetration beyond epidermis
Niacinamide	Decreases protein glycation to function	Nonirritating exfoliant
Alpha lipoic acid	Antioxidant	Synthesized by body in mitochondria, not a true vitamin
Ubiquinone	Antioxidant	Synthesized by body, not a true vitamin, regenerates vitamin E
Idebenone	Antioxidant	Newer form of ubiqiunone with stronger cutaneous antioxidant effects
Retinol	Vitamin A	May be irritating at high concentration above 1%, must be stabilized for activity
Retinyl propionate	Vitamin A ester	Less Irritating than other topical retinoids
Retinyl palmitate	Storage form of vitamin A	Weak biologic activity, sometimes used as product antioxidant preservative

Table 22.2 Vitamin antioxidants

Cellular regulators		
Cosmeceutical	**Effect on skin physiology**	**Patient selection comments**
Fibroblast growth factors	Fibroblast spent culture media containing numerous unknown fibroblast secreted substances, such as epidermal growth factor, transforming growth factor beta, and platelet derived growth factor	Unusual smell imparted to moisturizer product, does not appear to promote growth of other skin lesions
Signal peptides	Pentapeptide Pal-KTTKS, collagen I fragment that downregulates collagenase production	Used in 4–6 ppm in moisturizers, clinical data lacking
Neurotransmitter peptides	Hexapeptide argireline, inhibits neurotransmitter release to decrease muscle movement and wrinkles	Attempts to mimic effect of botulinum toxin on muscles, clinical data lacking

Table 22.3 Cellular regulators

lines commonly present on the upper cheeks. Lines of dehydration can be improved within 24–48 hours accounting for some of the cosmeceutical claims promising wrinkle reduction in a short time frame. Fine facial lines can be accentuated by accumulated corneocytes, which cannot be adequately hydrated. This is why some of the wrinkle reducing cosmeceuticals contain vitamin exfoliants, such as niacinamide, and low level acids, such as lactic acid or lactobionic acid.

The larger question is whether wrinkles and fine lines can be reduced through more permanent mechanisms, since neither moisturization nor exfoliation benefits are long lasting. The best method of wrinkle reduction is restoration of lost collagen and elastic fibers that account for thinning skin. There is some extrapolation that cosmeceutical retinoids, such as retinol, retinyl propionate, and retinyl palmitate may have some of the collagen regeneration benefits of prescription tretinoin. Yet, these benefits cannot be discussed fully in a cosmetic arena. Other methods of wrinkle reduction include restoration of the underlying bone and subcutaneous fat that support the skin. Some of the most concerning folds of the aging face are not from moisturization defects or collagen loss, but rather due to skin that drapes over a shrinking suboptimal framework. Unfortunately, cosmeceuticals can do nothing for this type of facial fold.

Facial Redness

23

Zoe Diana Draelos

Facial redness can be due to a variety of dermatologic causes including rosacea, physiologic flushing, telangiectasias, eczema, seborrheic dermatitis, psoriasis, irritant contact dermatitis, etc. All of these conditions have in common activation of the inflammatory cascade, which results in vasodilation and the recruitment of white blood cells. Facial redness is minimized by cosmeceuticals functioning as anti-inflammatories and barrier enhancers. Table 23.1 lists those cosmeceuticals that are currently used in moisturizers designed to improve facial redness. At present, there are no good cosmeceutical vasoconstrictors to deal with the vasoactive component of facial redness.

Notice that the facial redness cosmeceuticals fall into several categories. There are those, such as aloe vera and prickley pear, that can function as a mucilage to put a protective coating over the skin minimizing the effects of barrier damage. Aloe vera further is rich in choline salicylate, a well known anti-inflammatory present in aspirin. This is the second category of cosmeceuticals for facial redness, the naturally occurring anti-inflammatories. Bisabolol and allantoin also fall into this category as the most commonly used natural anti-inflammatory agents. The third category involves those substances that decrease facial redness by improving the skin barrier. Panthenol, also known as vitamin B_5, is an example

Cosmeceuticals to minimize facial redness		
Cosmeceutical	**Effects on skin physiology**	**Patient selection comments**
Prickley pear	Mucilage rich in mucopolysaccharides forms protective film	Extract used in moisturizers, usually does not provide mucilage properties
Aloe vera	Mucilage containing 99.5% water and a mixture of mucopolysaccharides and choline salicylate	Salicylate component functions as topical anti-inflammatory, since mucilage properties lost in most moisturizer formulations
Bisabolol	Chamomile extract preparing by distillation	Potent anti-inflammatory in moisturizers
Allantoin	Comfrey root or synthetic manufacture from uric acid	Used commonly in sensitive skin formulations
Panthenol	Barrier enhancing humectant	Used to hydrate the skin and prevent barrier damage
Tea tree oil	Polyphenols	May cause allergic contact dermatitis
Evening primrose oil	Polyphenols	Purported to be of benefit in atopic dermatitis
Ginkgo biloba	Polyphenol fraction	Ginkgolides, bilobalides are active anti-inflammatories
Green tea	Polyphenols	Epigallocatechin, epigallocatechin-3-gallate are active anti-inflammatories
Saw palmetto	Polyphenols	High concentration needed for efficacy
St John's wort	Polyphenols	High concentration needed for efficacy

Table 23.1 Cosmeceuticals to minimize facial redness

of a humectant that decreases skin dehydration and improves barrier function. A better functioning barrier will also aid in facial redness reduction. Finally, the last category is the anti-inflammatory polyphenols, which are quite numerous. The best studied of these polyphenols is green tea, which is the most potent. Many cosmeceuticals for facial redness combine a variety of polyphenols to obtain the final formulation.

Designing a facial cosmeceutical treatment regimen for patients with facial redness can be a challenge. The major problem is that products are introduced to and withdrawn from the marketplace with great rapidity. For this reason, rather than discussing specific product names, I have presented a facial skin care maintenance routine demonstrating which product type should contain which cosmeceutical active to be most effective. These recommendations are listed in Box 23.1. Patients can take this list to the cosmetic counter or spa and select those products that contain the ingredients listed.

Skin care ingredient recommendations for facial redness

1. Cleanser selection
Product description:
Synthetic detergent mild liquid cleanser with excellent rinsability. Removal of any soap residue is critical to preventing irritation. Recommend a product labeled as a sensitive skin foaming face wash.
Cosmeceutical ingredient:
None in particular, since the short contact time during cleansing would do little for facial redness.
Rationale:
Mild cleanser to clean skin while minimizing barrier damage.

2. Toner or astringent selection
These are liquid products designed to either remove any unwashed soap residue, increase sebum removal, or provide a mild skin moisturizer. These products evaporate quickly from the skin surface and may provide a sensory stimulus that results in flushing and redness. All sensory stimuli should be avoided in patients with facial redness and toners or astringents are not recommended.

3. Moisturizer selection
Product description:
Cream rather than lotion with minimal water or other vehicle to evaporate from face. Avoid propylene glycol, glycolic acid, salicylic acid, strong fragrances, and products with extensive botanical cocktails. These may evoke facial stinging.
Cosmeceutical ingredients:
Allantoin, bisabolol, and panthenol.
Rationale:
Allantoin and bisabolol form the basis for many of the sensitive skin claims in moisturizers, time tested effective ingredients for reducing inflammation. Panthenol is a nonsticky humectant to enhance stratum corneum hydration and prevent or minimize barrier damage.

4. Sunscreen selection
Product description:
Thicker lotion or cream sunscreen labeled for sensitive skin with SPF 15. Avoid gels, water resistant products, and sticky high SPF products.
Cosmeceutical ingredient:
Zinc oxide or titanium dioxide.
Rationale:
Chemical sunscreens absorb UV radiation and transform it to heat, which may invoke facial flushing and vasodilation. Physical sunscreens mainly reflect UV radiation preventing photoaging without a sensory component.

5. Treatment moisturizer selection
Product description:
Cream moisturizer with petrolatum, dimethicone, low levels of glycerin to prevent transepidermal water loss and increase skin hydration thus enhancing the skin barrier.
Cosmeceutical ingredient:
Green tea.
Rationale:
Of all the polyphenols, green tea is the most potent anti-inflammatory and demonstrates the highest efficacy.

Box 23.1 Skin care ingredient recommendations for facial redness

Dyspigmented Skin

24

Zoe Diana Draelos

Unwanted pigmentation of the skin is a difficult dermatologic condition to treat. Epidermal pigment is accessible to a variety of cosmeceutical actives, but dermal pigmentation does not reliably respond to any topical therapies. The cosmeceuticals available for decreasing pigmentation include vitamins, botanical extracts, penetration enhancers, and hydroquinone. None of these substances can reliably produce decreased pigmentation in persons of all skin types. Usually, a variety of complimentary actives to lighten skin produce the best results.

Table 24.1 lists the cosmeceuticals that are currently in the literature for pigment lightening. This table is useful when planning patient therapy, since it lists the mechanism of action and any pertinent patient selection comments. Hydroquinone has always been the mainstay of pigment lightening treatment, however it is an unstable radical that can produce irritation and has a cytotoxic effect on melanocytes. For this reason, hydroquinone is not allowed in skin lightening products sold in Japan. There is concern that hydroquinone may also be removed from the

Cosmeceuticals for dyspigmentation		
Cosmeceutical	**Effects on skin physiology**	**Patient selection comments**
Niacinamide	Inhibition of melanosome transfer from melanocytes to keratinocytes	No irritation, weak skin lightening agent
Retinol	Inhibits tyrosinase, interferes with pigment transfer	Mild irritation, weak skin lightening agent
Ascorbic acid (vitamin C)	Interacts with copper ions at tyrosinase active site	Magnesium-L-ascorbic acid-2-phosphate is more stable form, weak skin lightening agent
Kojic acid	Tyrosinase inhibitor from fungus	Mildly irritating and a possible allergen
Glabridin	Tyrosinase inhibitor from licorice	No cytotoxicity, no irritation, most common skin lightener in US cosmetics
Arbutin	Glycoside that inhibits tyrosinase from bearberry fruit	Less potent than kojic acid, must be used in combination with other skin lightening agents
Paper mulberry	Tyrosinase inhibitor from mulberry tree roots	Low irritation, same potency as kojic acid, not commercialized in USA
Soy	Fresh milk inhibits PAR-2 pathway and melanosome transfer	Only present in fresh soy milk, difficult to stabilize
Azelaic acid	Dicarboxylic acid derived from *Pityrosporum ovale* that is tyrosinase inhibitor	Slight stinging upon application, effective skin lightening agent

Table 24.1 Cosmeceuticals for dyspigmentation *Continued*

Cosmeceuticals for dyspigmentation—cont'd		
Cosmeceutical	**Effects on skin physiology**	**Patient selection comments**
Aloesin	Aloe vera derivative that is competitive inhibitor of DOPA oxidation, noncompetitive inhibitor of tyrosine	Weak skin lightening agent
Glycolic acid	Sugar derived alpha hydroxy acid that increases exfoliation of pigmented skin, penetration enhancer of other skin lightening actives	Irritating at high concentrations, may induce postinflammatory hyperpigmentation
Hydroquinone	Tyrosinase inhibitor, cytotoxic	Highly reactive radical, very irritating, effective skin lightening agent

Table 24.1, cont'd Cosmeceuticals for dyspigmentation

market at some point in the United States, as well. This has spurred research into a variety of vitamin and botanical pigment lightening agents. Of these, kojic acid, glabridin, and azelaic acid show the most promise by all functioning as tyrosinase inhibitors. Best results are achieved when these agents are used in combination with penetration enhancers, such as glycolic acid, and pigment lightening vitamins, such as niacinamide and retinol. Care must be taken not to induce irritation that may result in postinflammatory hyperpigmentation, especially in persons of darker skin color.

The optimal treatment for facial dyspigmentation is the use of a topical prescription skin lightening agent, such as 4% hydroquinone or mequinol, in combination with a retinoid, such as tretinoin or tazarotene. Since barrier damage can occur with all prescription skin lightening agents, a cosmeceutical moisturizer containing kojic acid, glabridin, and/or azelaic acid can be applied to prevent postinflammatory hyperpigmentation from xerosis while providing additional pigment lightening effects.

25 Oily Skin

Zoe Diana Draelos

Oily skin is a challenge for the dermatologist since there is a fine balance between removing enough sebum to get rid of facial shine while not inducing temporary skin dehydration. Many patients with oily skin are tempted to use strong detergent cleansers to remove sebum, however the intercellular lipids are also damaged yielding the appearance of dry skin. It is not possible for a cleanser to separate between sebum and intercellular lipids, thus a cleanser should be selected that minimizes barrier damage. Barrier damage is a problem created by many acne medications that contain skin irritants such as benzoyl peroxide or retinoids. Table 25.1 lists some of the cosmeceutical ingredients that might be helpful in products designed for oily skin.

These cosmeceuticals should be used in a stepwise fashion to obtain the best oil control results for a given patient, since each works on a different mechanism. Box 25.1 is a flowchart detailing how to use these substances in products combined to yield optimal results. This basic flowchart can be used to customize cosmeceutical treatment for patients depending on their degree of sebum production and gender.

Cosmeceutical actives for oily skin		
Cosmeceutical	**Effects on skin physiology**	**Patient selection comments**
Niacinamide	Reduces amount of sebum collected on skin surface	Used topically in oil reducing moisturizers
Polymer absorbing beads	Bead uses Van der Waals' forces to absorb and hold oil in polymer sphere	Used in moisturizer to hold and absorb oil that reaches the skin surface
Salicylic acid	Oil soluble exfoliant that can enter sebum rich pore mileu	Used as an astringent to remove oily residue from skin surface and follicular ostia
Witch hazel	Astringent containing tannins from leaves obtained by steam distillation	Used to remove excess sebum from face in a tonic as an astringent
Papaya	Papain proteolytic enzyme removed from fruit and applied to skin surface	Enzyme removes oil and desquamating corneocytes from skin surface
Soy	Fresh soy milk fraction contains phytoestrogen genistein	Thought to be an antiandrogen hormonally reducing oil production
Retinol	Naturally occurring form of vitamin A functioning as a retinoid	Thought to produce a drying effect on skin similar to prescription retinoids on a lesser level

Table 25.1 Cosmeceutical actives for oily skin

Flowchart for oil control

Step 1: Cleansing
Salicylic acid-containing foaming face wash.

Rationale:
Mild synthetic detergent cleansing with oil soluble chemical exfoliant functioning in and around the follicular ostia.

Step 2: Toner application
Witch hazel astringent over oily T-zone (entire forehead, between eyebrows, and nose).

Rationale:
Additional sebum removal from oily facial areas missed by mild cleanser without damaging the barrier of drier facial sites.

Step 3: Cosmeceutical moisturizer application
Niacinamide and/or retinoid (retinol, retinyl proprionate) moisturizer.

Rationale:
Decreased surface presence of sebum.

Step 4: Oil absorption
Polymer bead oil absorbing cream.

Rationale:
Polymer beads to hold sebum as secreted to minimize facial shine.

Step 5: Oil control cosmetics
Oil absorbing facial powder.

Rationale:
Talcum powder applied to absorb remaining sebum.

Box 25.1 Flowchart for oil control

Dry Skin

26

Zoe Diana Draelos

Dry skin is an area where cosmeceuticals play an important role both in enhancing the efficacy of prescription medications and in preventing disease relapse. In a world where the medical and social benefits of cleansing are well recognized, dry skin can result both from endogenous and exogenous causes. No matter what the cause, the appearance, functioning, and feel of dry skin can be effectively improved through the use of cosmeceuticals. Table 26.1 organizes the cosmeceutical actives such that the dermatologist can select which ingredients might be most beneficial in a moisturizer for a given patient. The table has been broken into the subgroups of occlusives, humectants, stratum corneum modifiers, and emollients.

A quality moisturizer should contain ingredients from each of the subgroups to improve the skin barrier through many different complementary mechanisms. The goals of moisturization are to increase skin water content, improve skin smoothness, and decrease symptoms of itching, stinging, and burning. The water content of the skin can be improved by retarding transepidermal water loss while increasing the flux of water from the dermis to the epidermis. The best agent at decreasing transepidermal water loss is petrolatum, however it must be combined with silicone and mineral oil to decrease its stickiness. Water flux from the dermis to the epidermis is accomplished through the use of humectants; usually glycerin is used as the primary humectant in combination with a secondary agent. Finally, the skin must be made to appear smooth through the use of emollients that fill in the gaps between the desquamating corneocytes.

Cosmeceutical actives for dry skin		
Cosmeceutical	**Effects on skin physiology**	**Patient selection comments**
A: Occlusive moisturizing		
Petrolatum	Rapidly reduces transepidermal water loss (TEWL) by 99%	Most effective for extremely dry skin, greasy, decreases scaling appearance
Mineral oil	Reduces TEWL by approximately 40%	Less greasy than petrolatum, does not cause acne
Lanolin	Mimics human sebum	Common cause of allergic contact dermatitis, not used in hypoallergenic formulations
Lanolin alcohol	Similar to lanolin, but branched molecule provides smooth skin feel	Excellent at smoothing skin surface, common cause of allergic contact dermatitis
Liquid paraffin	Provides protective film, reduces TEWL	Excellent hand and foot moisturizer for hand dermatitis and dyshidrosis
Carnauba wax	Provides protective film somewhat thinner than liquid paraffin	Same as liquid paraffin, naturally derived ingredient
Dimethicone	Reduces TEWL without greasy feel	Excellent for acne and sensitive skin patients, hypoallergenic, noncomedogenic, nonacnegenic
Cyclomethicone	Thicker silicone than dimethicone	Same as dimethicone

Table 26.1 Cosmeceutical actives for dry skin

Continued

Cosmeceutical actives for dry skin—cont'd		
Cosmeceutical	**Effects on skin physiology**	**Patient selection comments**
B: Humectant		
Propylene glycol	Attracts water from viable epidermis and dermis to stratum corneum	Not good on abraded or sensitive skin as can cause stinging
Glycerin	Most effective humectant available to increase stratum corneum hydration	If used in too high concentration will create sticky feeling on skin, especially under high humidity conditions
Hyaluronic acid	Used as a secondary humectant	May be used to supplement glycerin to decrease stickiness
Panthenol	Vitamin B$_5$ is the most effective vitamin humectant	May be used to supplement other humectants
Sodium PCA	Considered part of natural moisturizing factor for skin	May be used to supplement glycerin to decrease stickiness
C: Stratum corneum modifying		
Ceramides	Naturally present as part of intercellular lipids	Improves skin barrier in atopic dermatitis
Cholesterol	Naturally present as part of intracellular lipids	Should be balanced with free fatty acids and ceramides
Urea	Increases water binding sites on dehydrated keratinocytes	Hydrates callouses and keratin debris
Lactic acid	Decreases corneocyte adhesion	Enhances desquamation of corneocytes in icthyosis
D: Emollient		
Cetyl stearate	Smoothes desquamating corneocytes	Most common emollient, nongreasy skin smoothing effect
Dicaprylyl maleate	Used to dissolve UV sunscreens in moisturizing formulations	Provides excellent smooth skin feel
C12–15 alkyl benzoate	Fills in spaces between desquamating corneocytes	Less waxy feel on skin than paraffin

Table 26.1, cont'd Cosmeceutical actives for dry skin

While each of the previously discussed ingredients are considered cosmeceuticals, the recent ability to artificially synthesize ceramide 3 has decreased the cost of this raw material such that it can now be used in facial moisturizers to speed barrier repair. Urea and lactic acid are also useful cosmeceuticals. Urea is unique in that it can open up the water binding sites on keratin thereby hydrating dry, callused skin. This hydration of the hardened keratin allows for softening and easier removal of callus material and improved appearance of xerotic skin characterized by retained dehydrated keratinocytes. Lactic acid is also helpful in the treatment of xerosis and photoaged skin, since it dissolves the intercellular keratinocyte bridges encouraging desquamation.

Moisturizers are true cosmeceuticals. They have the ability to profoundly alter the structure and function of the skin. Their true main role is to enhance or maintain the water content of the skin, but they are also the most efficient vehicle for delivering sun protection and other actives. The majority of the unique actives discussed in this book are applied to the skin in some type of moisturizer. This is due to the fact that moisturizers are applied on a daily basis to the entire face, providing an ideal vehicle to transport the active to the face. Furthermore, moisturizers contain both water soluble and oil soluble ingredients into which either hydrophilic or lipophilic actives can be dissolved. For this reason, an understanding of moisturizers is key to understanding cosmeceuticals.

Acne

27

Zoe Diana Draelos

Acne can be treated both with topical and oral medications that may fall into either the prescription or over-the-counter (OTC) categories. Cosmeceuticals, of course, are OTC products that can alter some of the mechanics of acne formation. It is also possible that some cosmeceutical ingredients may even cause comedogenic acne. Substances that appear on the lists of comedogenic ingredients include cocoa butter, isopropyl myristate, industrial quality mineral oil, industrial quality petrolatum, and vegetable oils. No current cosmetic manufacturer would consider using anything but cosmetic grade mineral oil and petrolatum. Industrial grades are cheaper, but may also contain tar contaminants. These tar contaminants are comedogenic, possibly accounting for some of the older reports regarding the comedogenicity of

mineral oil and petrolatum. However, this data is quite outdated and no longer pertinent to modern formulations. For all practical purposes, the concept of acne cosmetica is no longer germane.

Pomade acne, on the other hand, is a viable concept. Pomade acne afflicts the skin along the hairline in individuals who use these styling products to add shine, moisturization, and manageability to chemically straightened hair. Both olive oil and cocoa butter are still used in some of the older pomade formulations on the market. Pomade acne can be prevented through the avoidance of these substances and the use of high quality, pure cosmetic grade raw materials.

The cosmeceuticals that are useful adjuvants in the treatment of acne are listed in Table 27.1.

Cosmeceuticals for acne therapy		
Cosmeceutical	**Effects on skin physiology**	**Patient selection comments**
Salicylic acid	Exfoliation induced on the skin surface and in the follicular ostia, anti-inflammatory	Potent comedolytic suitable for sensitive skin
Glycolic acid	Exfoliation on the skin surface	Comedolytic best for photoaged skin
Lactobionic acid	Exfoliation on the skin surface with humectant and antioxidant effects, lower irritation profile	Moisturizing and comedolytic properties
Retinyl propionate	Possibly converted to biologically active retinoic acid in the skin, low irritation profile, stable	Mild retinoid effect suitable for sensitive skin
Retinol	Possibly converted to biologically active retinoic acid in the skin, more irritation possible, less stable	Mild retinoid effect suitable for photoaged skin
Niacinamide	Enhanced exfoliation without low pH due to NADPH pathway	Oil reduction and exfoliation effects combined, appropriate for sensitive skin
Zinc	Anti-inflammatory	May be used both orally and topically as antiacne treatment

Table 27.1 Cosmeceuticals for acne therapy

Salicylic acid, sometimes referred to as a beta hydroxy acid, is the mainstay of OTC acne treatments. It is an oil soluble active able to penetrate into the sebum rich milieu of the pore. Within the pore, it is able to loosen the comedonal plug and may exert some low level anti-inflammatory effects. It is a valuable ingredient for the treatment of acne and can be incorporated into cleansers, moisturizers, and facial foundations. Its ability to induce exfoliation has also allowed salicylic to function as an antiaging/acne ingredient for women with both needs. Glycolic acid, an alpha hydroxy acid, is used similarly, however it is a water soluble active that is not quite as potent a comedolytic. The last hydroxy acid acne cosmeceutical is lactobionic acid, a polyhydroxy acid that is used in the treatment of acne for patients with sensitive skin. It is not a potent comedolytic, but can function as a humectant preventing barrier damage from acne medications.

The OTC retinoids are gaining popularity for the treatment of acne, in addition to photoaging. Small amounts of both retinyl propionate and retinol may be converted to tretinoin in the dermis. Tretinoin is an established prescription active for the treatment of acne through the elimination and prevention of microcomedones. The enzymatic machinery that transforms the OTC retinoids into prescription retinoids is the rate limiting factor. Nevertheless, the daytime wear of stable retinoids in the form of moisturizers may be helpful in acne patients.

The last two actives discussed in this text that may be helpful in acne are niacinamide and zinc. Topical niacinamide is a molecule with many diverse cutaneous effects. This may be due to the fact that it is a key substance in the NADPH pathway responsible for the energy producing machinery of every cell. Niacinamide is useful to enhance cutaneous exfoliation, decrease sebum production, and treat acne. It is used both orally and topically in cosmeceuticals designed to minimize acne inflammation. The role of zinc is similar, in that it too is used orally and topically for acne inflammation.

Several ingredients have been touted for acne that are not listed in Table 27.1. One ingredient is triclosan, an antibacterial found in surgical hand scrubs, antibacterial soaps, deodorant soaps, and rinseless hand antiseptics. While triclosan is found in several cosmeceutical acne treatment lines, it is not very effective at reducing the *Propionibacterium acnes* counts and is not listed for this reason. There are a variety of botanicals that have been touted for their acne effect, which is primarily anti-inflammatory in nature. These ingredients are better at reducing facial redness and are discussed in Chapter 23 for this reason.

Part 4

Cosmeceutical Myths

There are many myths that surround cosmeceuticals. Some of these myths are perpetuated by patients who are unable to rationalize cause and effect without the assistance of a dermatologist. Other myths are conceived by marketing departments more concerned with cosmeceutical product appeal than medical accuracy. Nevertheless, it is the role of the dermatologist to dispel these myths and help patients use good medical science to direct their skin care. This section provides succinct information to aid the dermatologist toward this end.

Acne Cosmeceutical Myths

28

Zoe Diana Draelos

The purpose of this chapter is to dispel some of the commonly held myths regarding acne cosmeceuticals. These myths may be held by dermatologists and patients alike. They are perpetuated by the popular press and exuberant marketing efforts that present ideas or concepts that seem to make common sense but cannot be verified by the scientific method. This chapter presents the material by first stating the acne cosmeceutical myth and subsequently exploring where the truth may lie. The acne myths discussed were collected from the authors and editors of this text by canvassing dermatologists in their respective practices and dermatology training programs. It is hoped that this material serves to further cosmeceutical science by providing concise analyses to frequent acne misconceptions.

Cosmeceuticals Do Not Produce Acne If Labeled Noncomedogenic and Nonacnegenic

Similar to hypoallergenic, noncomedogenic and non-acnegenic are marketing claims carrying no implied regulation (Fig. 28.1). They were also developed to create a new consumer image for cosmetic lines designed to minimize acne. In order to make the claim noncomedogenic, rabbit ear or human come-dogenicity testing should be undertaken. Both the animal and the human model are based on the presence of new comedone formation after the exposure of skin to the finished cosmetic. Human testing is considered to be more accurate, but the results are highly dependent on the skill of the contract testing laboratory. Acnegenic claims are based on human use testing and the evaluation of volunteer subjects following product use for an increase in the presence of acne. Many manufacturers, however, make noncomedogenic and nonacnegenic claims based on the safety profiles of the individual ingredients in

the formulation. This is inaccurate. Noncomedogenic and nonacnegenic claims should be made based on clinical testing of the finished formulation. The dermatologist should still consider all products labeled noncomedogenic or nonacnegenic as problematic.

Mineral Oil is Comedogenic

Mineral oil is one of the most common ingredients in skin care products and colored cosmetics (Fig. 28.2). It is a light weight inexpensive oil that is odorless and tasteless. One of the common concerns regarding the use of mineral oil is its presence on several lists of comedogenic substances. These comedogenic lists were developed many years ago, yet remain frequently quoted in the dermatologic literature. There are several important points to consider. First, there are different grades of mineral oil. There is industrial grade mineral oil, which is used as a machine lubricant, that is not of the purity required for skin application. Cosmetic grade mineral

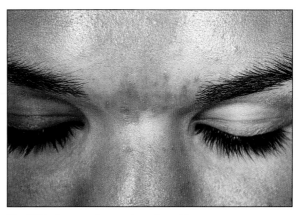

Fig. 28.1 Acne and comedone formation can occur even with products bearing the noncomedogenic and nonacnegenic label

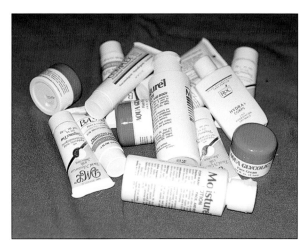

Fig. 28.2 Numerous dermatologist-recommended facial moisturizers contain mineral oil

oil is the purist form without contaminants. Industrial grade mineral oil may be comedogenic, but cosmetic grade mineral oil is not. Quality manufacturers only purchase quality products from quality suppliers who guarantee the quality of the materials they provide. I believe that cosmetic grade mineral oil is noncomedogenic and I have never found it to be comedogenic in any of the testing I have performed for the skin care industry.

Sunscreens Produce Acne

Many patients note the occurrence of 'breakouts' following the use of sunscreens. These patients typically present with perifollicular papules and pustules in a random distribution over the face. This eruption appears within 24 to 48 hours after wearing a facial sunscreen. I have not performed biopsies on patients who develop this problem, but I would like to put forth a hypothesis based on my knowledge of how sunscreens function.

Most of the sunscreens on the market today are based primarily on UVB absorbing ingredients, such as octylmethoxycinnamate, oxybenzone, homosalate, etc. Many also have UVA absorbing ingredients, such as avobenzone, titanium dioxide, or zinc oxide, as secondary sunscreens. All of the UVB sunscreens and avobenzone function by transforming ultraviolet radiation to heat energy through a process known as resonance delocalization. This heat energy is appreciated by many patients who will state that they do not like wearing sunscreens, since the gels or lotions make them feel hot. In some patients, I

believe that the increased sweating induced by the sunscreens accompanied by the warm sunny weather cause increased activity by the eccrine glands. This may cause miliaria rubra that may be magnified by the occlusive nature of the water resistant, rubproof product. Thus, I believe that much of the problem with sunscreen induced breakout is the formation of papules or pustules around the eccrine duct ostia without the sebaceous gland involvement that characterizes true acne.

Vitamin E Capsules Improve the Appearance of Scars

A common practice among lay persons is to break open a vitamin E capsule and massage the oil over scars to improve their cosmetic appearance. I do not believe that this is a medically sound practice. The vitamin E present in vitamin capsules is intended for oral administration with subsequent absorption across the digestive mucosa. The vitamin E is dissolved in vegetable oil, which may be comedogenic. Furthermore, vitamin E administered in this fashion cannot be absorbed through the skin. The main benefit is the massaging action, which may be beneficial to the scar. I would recommend a moisturizer designed for skin application as a massage product rather than oral vitamin E capsules.

Glycolic Acid Application Can Reduce Pore Size

Glycolic acid is a water soluble chemical exfoliant. It cannot enter the oily milieu of the pore and thus does not exfoliate within the pore. Glycolic acid may improve the smoothness of the skin surface creating the illusion of reduced pore size, but it cannot measurably reduce pore size. As a matter of fact, there is no cosmeceutical ingredient that can measurably reduce pore size. Salicylic acid is an oil soluble chemical exfoliant that can remove debris from the pore creating the appearance of skin smoothness, but it too cannot measurably reduce pore size. It is important to distinguish between real pore size reduction and an improved cosmetic appearance. Figure 28.3 demonstrates the appearance of pores containing keratotic debris. Removal of this debris with a salicylic acid peel can improve the appearance of the pores and can shrink the size of dilated pores due to debris presence, but the physical size of the pore cannot be altered.

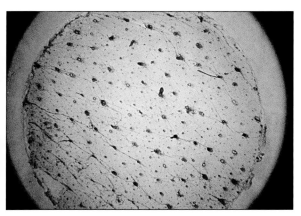

Fig. 28.3 The appearance of pores containing keratotic debris. Removal of this debris with a salicylic acid peel can improve the appearance of the pores and can shrink the size of dilated pores due to debris presence, but the physical size of the pore cannot be altered

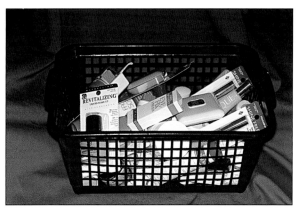

Fig. 28.4 There is no scientifically proven dermatologic benefit to the use of complex regimens for skin care

Tretinoin Topically Aids in the Treatment of Acne Scarring

Whether tretinoin aids in the treatment of acne scarring is rather controversial, even among dermatologists. Tretinoin normalizes follicular keratinization, which improves comedonal, pustular, and superifical papular acne. This effect may smooth out the skin around acne scars simply by treating the acne. Tretinoin also increases collagen production after extended use, which may improve acne scarring. The degree to which tretinoin improves pitted acne scarring has never been quantified and more research is needed in this area. However, it is unlikely that this research will be forthcoming from the pharmaceutical industry, since tretinoin is now generic and there is currently no indication for acne scarring, only acne treatment.

A Complex Skin Care Regimen of Multiple Cleansers, Moisturizers, and Ancillary Skin Care Products is Necessary for Clear Skin

There are many different approaches to skin care. There is the no nonsense bar of soap and water twice daily approach and the 20 step skin care routine approach. Which is better? I am not sure I know the answer. In Japan, skin care is a complex ritual of multiple cleansers, toners, and moisturizers. The Japanese also feel that they have the most sensitive skin of all races and the incidence of atopic dermatitis is dramatically rising in their country. Is this due to the use of extensive skin care products? I also do not know the answer to this question. But, there is no doubt that the more the skin is manipulated, the more opportunity there is for problems to arise. Perhaps the old adage of everything in moderation is the best advice, even when it comes to skin care (Fig. 28.4).

Breakouts After the Age of 30 in Women are Rare and Will Benefit from Special Skin Care

Acne after age 30 is actually becoming more and more common in women. The cause of this trend is not totally known, but appears to be related to fluctuating hormones and the onset of the premenopause and the perimenopause. This supposition is based on the observation that the acne is not characterized by open and closed comedones, but rather inflammatory papules and pustules. Since these lesions are deep seated within the lower epidermis and dermis, it is not possible for special skin care routines to have a dramatic effect. Thus, the use of oral antibiotics and hormonal therapies, such as birth control pills or estrogen replacement therapy, are the best options for acne control. Cosmetics and skin care products have little effect.

Cosmeceutical Antiaging Myths

29 *Zoe Diana Draelos*

The most numerous dermatologic myths relate to cosmeceuticals and their ability to improve the appearance of facial aging. Notice that the word 'appearance' is always used when referring to the effects of cosmeceuticals on wrinkling. This is due to the fact that improving appearance insures that claims made regarding the cosmeceutical active are perceived as cosmetic in nature and not pharmaceutical. Claims regarding improving appearance deal with how an active alters looks and not function. Yet, there are some claims and myths that seem to continue due to their consumer and marketing appeal. These cosmeceutical antiaging myths represent the most common patient questions encountered by the practicing dermatologist.

Expensive Moisturizers are More Effective

For many consumers, price equates with quality. This may be true for some commercial purchases, but is not necessarily true for moisturizers. The most expensive part of any facial moisturizer is the fragrance, the bottle, and the packaging. None of these contribute to the efficacy of the moisturizer, only the aesthetic appeal. A quality moisturizer should cost less than $30 a bottle and products priced above this amount are selling more than skin efficacy. A quality moisturizer should contain an occlusive agent, a humectant, and some form of silicone. Ideally, it should also contain a sunscreen to provide the added benefit of sun protection. No moisturizer in any price range will improve the wrinkling on the lower face demonstrated in Figure 29.1.

Moisturizers Remove Wrinkles

Moisturizers do not remove wrinkles, they simply minimize their appearance. The role of moisturizers in reducing wrinkles is primarily through increased skin hydration. The moisturizer contains an occlusive agent, such as petrolatum, mineral oil, or dimethicone, which prevents transepidermal water loss from the skin surface and increases the water content of the skin. This increased water content decreases or even eliminates wrinkles that are due to stratum corneum barrier defects. Barrier repair will prevent the wrinkles from recurring and the moisturizer creates an environment to initiate barrier repair. Thus, moisturizers do not remove wrinkles (Fig. 29.2), they simply can provide an environment to reverse dehydration due to stratum corneum barrier defects.

Cosmeceuticals Can Produce Beneficial Effects on Facial Muscles to Improve Skin Tone

The first cosmeceutical introduced to produce an effect on facial muscles was DMAE, which is dimethylaminoethanol. It is a releaser of acetylcholine, a neurotransmitter required for muscle movement.

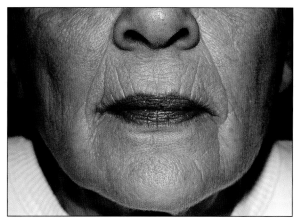

Fig. 29.1 No moisturizer can improve perioral wrinkling that is due to muscles of facial expression, loss of facial subcutaneous fat, and facial osteoporosis

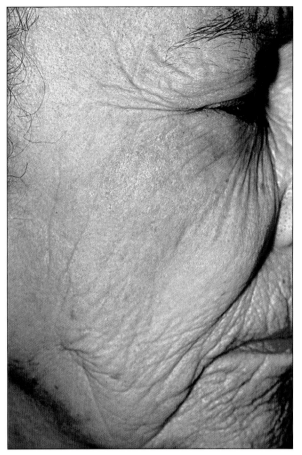

Fig. 29.2 Coarse wrinkles on the lateral face do not improve with moisturization, since they are not due to cutaneous dehydration

Another group of cosmeceuticals, composed of engineered peptides, claims to interrupt the neuro-muscular junction and relax facial muscles, functioning in a manner opposite to DMAE. The peptide is intended to mimic the effect of botulinum toxin. In conclusion, much research and many clinical studies remain to be done on these cosmeceuticals designed to increase or relax facial muscle tone.

Bleaching Creams Can Improve Brown Spots Quickly

Unfortunately, no botanical, hydroquinone or mequinol-based bleaching cream can quickly improve the appearance of brown spots. Most products take at least 6 weeks and possibly even 3 months to work. This is because none of the bleaching cream actives is effective at removing melanin pigment from the skin. They all work by interrupting one step in the pathway of melanin synthesis or melanosome transfer. This means that the bleaching creams are shutting down new pigment production while the old pigment is being dispersed by traditional physiologic mechanisms.

Bleaching creams are most effective when used on the face due to enhanced penetration through thin skin. Neck, chest, and forearm hyperpigmentation respond even more slowly to treatment due to the decreased penetration of the active (Fig. 29.3).

Glycolic Acid Peels Must Hurt to be Effective

There is a misnomer that the 'no pain, no gain' philosophy applies to both muscles and the skin. While muscles must be exercised to the point of exhaustion to promote increased muscle mass, this is not the case with the skin. Any procedure that induces pain is injuring the skin. Sometimes dermatologists injure the skin for what are considered to be medically beneficial reasons, but injury is still occurring. For example, glycolic acid peels are intended to exfoliate the outer layer of skin removing unwanted melanin pigment and producing smoother skin with better color (Fig. 29.4). However pain may indicate that the skin has been injured and the resulting inflammation may actually worsen skin color through postinflammatory hyperpigmentation. Peels that are intended simply to remove the stratum corneum should not hurt. Thus, glycolic acid peels do not have to hurt to be effective.

DMAE was originally introduced as a homeopathic nutritional supplement for individuals with Alzheimer's disease and children with attention deficit disorder (ADD). The highest natural food source of DMAE is salmon, which explains the recent interest in diets incorporating several servings of the fish weekly.

The idea of using DMAE to improve the appearance of the facial skin is based on the concept that the facial skin must cover a bed of facial muscles. If the underlying muscle layer is contracted and firm, the skin has a better framework over which to lay. This may create an improved facial appearance, which is sometimes characterized by the cosmetic phrase 'better skin tone'. The first several times that DMAE is applied a skin tingling sensation is present, however this disappears with continued use. It is unclear whether accommodation occurs to topical cosmeceuticals intended to alter muscle function with time.

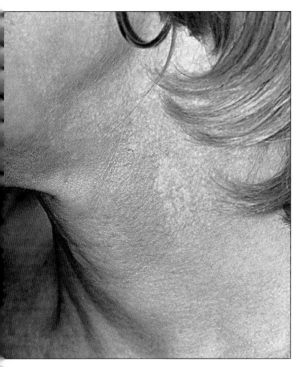

Fig. 29.3 Neck hyperpigmentation is extremely difficult to treat with bleaching creams

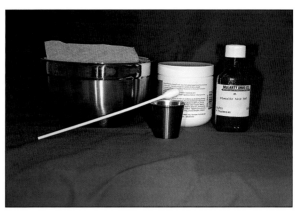

Fig. 29.4 The typical equipment used to administer a mild facial peel

Cosmeceuticals Need to Penetrate the Skin Barrier to Work

Cosmeceuticals can function in many different skin compartments. Petrolatum, mineral oil, and dimethicone function on the skin surface and must not penetrate the skin. Retinoids do not function on the skin surface and must penetrate into the dermis to reach the retinoid receptors to have an effect. As this book demonstrates, cosmeceuticals are a diverse category of actives and each must be considered separately. Not all cosmeceuticals must penetrate the skin barrier to work.

Topical Formulations of Vitamins and Supplements are Similar to Pills in Effectiveness for Skin Improvement

The comparison between the efficacy of oral vitamins and supplements and topical vitamins and supplements is an ongoing area of controversy in the aesthetic and cosmetic world. However, I believe there is little room for dispute in medical circles that oral consumption of vitamins and supplements is far superior in efficacy to topical application. Yet, there are some effects of topical

vitamins that cannot be achieved with oral ingestion. For example, topical vitamin E is an effective emollient allowing a rough skin surface with stratum corneum disruption to feel smooth and soft to the touch. Oral consumption of vitamin E cannot enhance skin texture, since vitamin E internally can only function as an antioxidant. Thus, there are unique topical and internal benefits to various vitamins.

Vitamin Containing Products Can Reverse Photoaging

There are many cosmeceutical skin care preparations containing the antioxidant vitamins A, C, and E. It is interesting to note that no vitamin claims are made for most of these products. No cosmeceutical claims to reverse photoaging with these vitamins because that constitutes a drug claim and the FDA would send a warning letter to the company asking them to either stop making the claim or remove their product from the market. Most cosmeceuticals simply claim that they contain the vitamin and the consumer is left to decide the topical vitamin benefits. Thus, vitamins containing products can 'help reduce the appearance of photoaging', but cannot 'reverse photoaging'.

Retinol in Over-The-Counter Preparations Works Like Prescription Tretinoin

Retinoids are a complex family of cosmeceuticals covered in Chapter 6. Retinol is the retinoid vitamin form that is necessary for vision. If the retinol is properly stabilized, it is possible that the skin can enzymatically convert small amounts of retinol to tretinoin. While this is theoretically possible, it has never been quanititated.

A Sunscreen with an SPF Above 15 Does Not Provide Additional Photoprotection

Sunscreens above SPF 15 do actually provide additional photoprotection, but the increase in the amount of photoprotection provided is small. The percent UVB photoprotection provided by a given SPF rating is summarized in Table 29.1.

Notice that an SPF 4 sunscreen blocks 75% of the UVB radiation, but an SPF 15 sunscreen blocks 93%. This is a substantial improvement in photoprotection, however the percent increase in UVB protection decreases as the SPF increases such that an SPF 30 product only has 4% more photoprotection than an SPF 15 product. Thus, dermatologists typically recommend SPF 15 sunscreens to combine product function with aesthetic characteristics, since higher SPF products tend to be sticky due to increased concentration of the sunscreen actives. Higher SPF products may provide value in patients with unique medical UVB photosensitive disorders.

It is important to remember that the single most common reason sunscreens fail is due to incomplete film formation over the skin surface. This may be due to uneven application or migration of the sunscreen over the skin surface. Figure 29.5 is a 400× video microscope of the appearance of a sunscreen containing facial foundation on the skin surface. Notice how the film has begun to separate 2 hours after application. This means that the sunscreen will not deliver the SPF labeled amount of sun protection after 2 hours. Frequent reapplication of sunscreen products is essential to achieving adequate sun protection.

Self-Tanning Cosmeceuticals Provide Sun Protection

Self-tanning cosmeceuticals are based on dihydroxyacetone (DHA) as the active. DHA is a 3-carbon sugar that is manufactured as a white, crystalline hygroscopic powder. It interacts with amino acids, peptides, and proteins to form chromophobes known as melanoidins. Melanoidins structurally have some similarities to skin melanin. The browning reaction that occurs when DHA is exposed to keratin protein is known as the Maillard reaction. DHA is technically categorized as a colorant or colorless dye. It is added in concentrations of 3–5% to self-tanning preparations. Lower concentrations of DHA produce mild tanning while higher concentrations produce greater darkening. This allows self-tanning products to be formulated in light, medium, and dark shades.

The depth of color produced by self-tanning products is enhanced by increasing the protein content of the stratum corneum. As might be expected, skin areas with more protein stain a darker color. For example, keratotic growths such as seborrheic keratoses or actinic keratoses will hyperpigment. Protein rich areas of the skin, such as the elbows, knees, palms, and soles, also stain more deeply. DHA does not stain the mucous membranes, but will stain the hair and nails. The chemical reaction is usually visible within 1 hour after DHA application, but maximal darkening may take 8–24 hours.

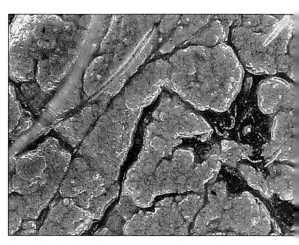

Fig. 29.5 A 400× video microscope image of facial foundation on the skin surface

UVB photoprotection provided by a given SPF rating	
SPF rating	**% UVB radiation blocked**
4	75
8	88
15	93
30	97
45	98

Table 29.1 UVB photoprotection provided by a given SPF rating

DHA is a nontoxic ingredient both for ingestion and topical application. It has a proven safety record with only a few reported cases of allergic contact dermatitis. Unfortunately, the browning reaction does not produce adequate photoprotection. At most, self-tanning preparations may impart an SPF of 3–4 to the skin for up to 1 hour after application. The photoprotection does not last as long as the artificial tan. The brown color imparts limited photoprotection at the low end of the visible spectrum with overlap into the UVA portion of the spectrum. DHA used to be approved as a sun protective agent in combination with lawsone, however the new sunscreen monograph has removed this ingredient largely due to its lack of popularity. However, DHA remains popular as a safe alternative to a sun induced tan, but for all practical purposes should be considered by the dermatologist as providing no sun protection.

Botanical Cosmeceutical Myths

30

Zoe Diana Draelos

There are numerous botanical cosmeceutical myths. This may be due in part to the aura that plants are natural, preservative-free, healthy, holistic, relaxing, restoring, healing, etc. Certainly, the plant kingdom is a rich source of active ingredients. Plants have adapted to thrive in an environment rich in UV radiation. It is for this reason that humans look to plants for solutions to oxidative insults. Plant extracts provide a rich source of antioxidants and anti-inflammatories. However, a major dermatologic question is whether the plant materials are more effectively consumed or topically applied. Most of the botanicals used in cosmeceuticals have been highly processed to allow their efficient addition to moisturizers and other topically applied products. Cosmeceuticals typically take the form of creams, lotions, serums, and solutions. Botanicals must be liquids or powders to easily blend into an esthetic formulation of this type. This chapter examines some of the more common cosmeceutical myths, providing insight into their fallacies.

Hypoallergenic Botanical Cosmeceuticals Do Not Produce Allergic Reactions

The term hypoallergenic is a marketing term meaning 'reduced allergy' not 'nonallergenic'. This term was first popularized by Clinique cosmetics, a division of Estee Lauder, for advertising purposes to create a unique image for this new makeup line. There are no governmental guidelines that apply to the hypoallergenic concept. Dermatologists should consider hypoallergenic cosmetics as a source of allergic contact dermatitis for all patients (Fig. 30.1). It is hoped that companies making the hypoallergenic claim have conducted repeat insult patch testing as part of their product safety assessment, but this cannot always be assumed.

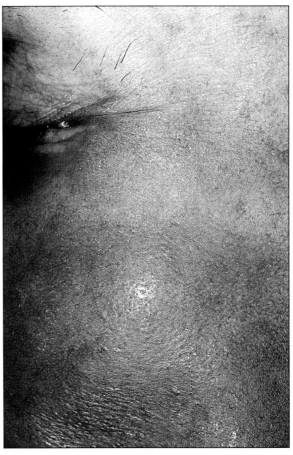

Fig. 30.1 Allergic contact dermatitis to a hypoallergenic product

Preservative-Free Botanical Cosmeceuticals Produce Less Skin Reactions

Many products are now claiming to be better for the skin because they are 'preservative-free'. This is a somewhat meaningless term, since all products must contain preservatives (Fig. 30.2). Preservatives

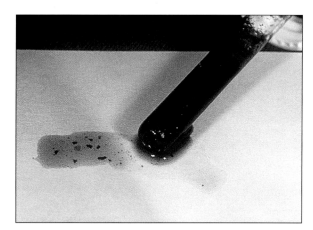

Fig. 30.2 All topical vitamin C preparations must contain a preservative to prevent oxidation of the ascorbic acid and darkening of the product

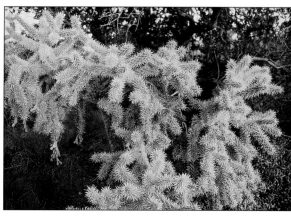

Fig. 30.3 Cactus extract is usually a high processed material, since cactus spines would not be acceptable for topical application

fall into several categories. There are preservatives that are classified as antioxidants. These are substances designed to prevent the rancidity of the oils in the formulation and prevent the breakdown of coloring agents. Common antioxidant preservatives that perform this function are tocopheryl acetate and retinyl palmitate and ascorbic acid. These are of the same family as the topical vitamin E, A, and C additives that many companies are claiming prevent skin oxidation. Oxidation is a universal event leading to aging of any living or biologically derived material. However, tocopheryl acetate, retinyl palmitate, and ascorbic acid in the concentrations used for product preservation do not have much biologic activity for the prevention of skin oxidation.

Another category of preservatives comprises those aimed at preventing microbe contamination, whether the source is a bacteria, yeast, or fungi. These are substances such as phenoxyethanol, Kathon-CG, Bronopol, parabens, etc. All formulations that contain water must contain some type of preservative to maintain purity on the shelf, whether it is called a preservative or not. Some clove extracts, such as eugenol, have preservative characteristics and 'natural' formulations may use ingredients for this purpose. Some traditional preservatives, such as phenoxyethanol, have a rose fragrance and may have their stated purpose as a fragrance, even though they are functioning as a preservative. Most companies use a preservative in anhydrous formulations, even though it may not be necessary.

In summary, there is no such thing as a 'preservative-free' formulation, unless it is pure petrolatum. Preservatives may have other functions or may be natural ingredients with preservative properties, but all products must be protected against contamination and oxidation.

Botanical Cosmeceuticals are Natural

There is a misconception that all botanical cosmeceuticals are natural because they are derived from plant sources. Most botanical actives were first discovered and isolated from plant sources, but are no longer obtained from plants. This is far too expensive in most cases. Many botanical extracts are modified and chemically synthesized to obtain a form that can be easily incorporated into a skin moisturizer. Ground-up leaves or cactus spines (Fig. 30.3) typically do not create an aesthetic feel when sprinkled in a moisturizer and undergo extensive processing to create a liquid or fine powder suitable for cosmeceutical use. An excellent example is allantoin, botanically obtained from the root of the comfrey plant. However, most allantoin used as an anti-inflammatory agent in sensitive skin cosmeceuticals is obtained from uric acid. It is bioidentical to the plant derived allantoin, but synthesized in a chemical plant not grown by 'mother nature'. Thus, the claim that botanicals are natural is meaningless. All chemicals are in some sense natural, since they are derived from materials present on the earth.

Botanically Derived Fragrances Do Not Cause Allergic Contact Dermatitis

Many of the newer botanically derived fragrances entering the market claim to be 'hypoallergenic'.

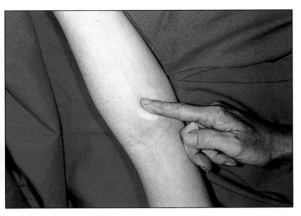

Fig. 30.4 Use testing in the antecubital fossa is an excellent method for evaluating possible ingredient allergy in sensitive skin patients

Remember that the term hypoallergenic means reduced allergic potential and not zero allergic potential. Also remember that hypoallergenic refers to a reduced incidence of allergic contact dermatitis and not a reduced incidence of vasomotor rhinitis or other untoward nasal or respiratory effects from the perfume. Botanically derived fragrances can most certainly cause allergic contact dermatitis in the sensitized patient. I usually have my patients apply the new hypoallergenic perfume in one antecubital fossa for five nights in a row prior to more liberal application to avoid widespread allergic contact dermatitis (Fig. 30.4).

Botanical Cosmeceuticals Can Reduce Sebum Production

Many skin care products on the market today contain botanical ingredients that claim to decrease facial sebum. Sometimes it is unclear from the label whether the appearance of sebum is reduced or whether the production of sebum is decreased. One mechanism for reducing the appearance of facial oil is to adsorb the sebum into 1–30 µm diameter polymer spheres composed of three monomers: isobornyl methacrylate (IBMA), lauryl methacrylate (LMA), and divinylbenzene (DVB). The DVB serves to crosslink the IBMA and LMA to form a three dimensional copolymer network capable of absorbing liquid oil soluble substances. This technology was originally developed to control industrial organic solvent spills.

The sebum is absorbed by the polymer through imbibition, since the oil can be absorbed, but not released. This is due to the sebum being held inside the polymer with Van der Waals forces, creating a strong attraction without chemical bonding. Thus, the oil can be imbibed, but not released when the polymer is saturated or squeezed. The polymer can expand up to six times its volume during the sebum absorbing process. This is one of the few proven technologies that can decrease the appearance of facial sebum but it is not botanically based; however botanicals can be added to the formulation to make a claim. There is some preliminary evidence that niacinamide can reduce sebum production, but further study is warranted. Bascially, there is no true botanical that can reliably reduce sebum.

Antiperspirants Contain Chemicals that are Not Naturally Derived and are Therefore Damaging to the Sweat Glands

Metal salts of aluminum and/or zirconium form the active agent in all commercially marketed antiperspirants, which are considered over-the-counter drugs by the United States Food and Drug Administration (FDA). Essentially, the metal salt forms a reversible physical obstruction in the duct of apocrine and eccrine sweat glands reducing perspiration by 40–60%. These aluminum salts have an acidic pH of 3.0–4.2. Thus, formulation is critically important to create an antiperspirant that minimizes skin irritation.

Botanicals and Mineral Cosmetics are Safe and Do Not Cause Acne

Botanicals are plant derived materials and mineral cosmetics contain pigments derived from rock sources. Botanicals and mineral cosmetics are no more or less likely to produce acne than any other raw materials. They must undergo the same comedogenicity testing and clinical testing as any other ingredient. Their safety must be demonstrated in a cosmetic chemistry laboratory and cannot be assumed (Fig. 30.5).

Face Masks with Botanicals Improve Skin Tone

Face masks are creams or pastes that are applied to the face for a limited period of time ranging from 5 to 30 minutes followed by removal. They largely impart aesthetic benefits to the skin. Face masks can be based on quick drying polymers, clay, or botanicals. Polymer face masks occlude the skin and

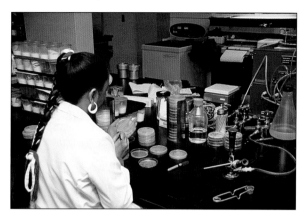

Fig. 30.5 Laboratory testing is critical to determine the cutaneous safety

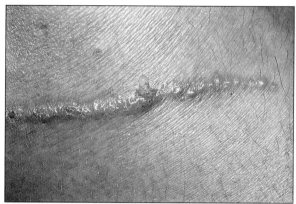

Fig. 30.6 Poison ivy is a natural ingredient not considered safe for skin application

have a temporarily moisturizing effect. They are peeled from the face as one sheet. Clay face masks are typically used to absorb oil and are rinsed down the drain. Botanical face masks are dried plant ingredients packaged in a pouch to which water is added to create a paste for facial application. They too are rinsed from the face using water.

The main question here is the issue of skin tone. This term is a marketing term that has little dermatologic meaning. Well toned muscles are strong, quick, and hard to fatigue. These terms do not apply to the skin. I believe that skin tone is a concept combining tactile smoothness, even color, and even texture. I do not believe that the short term application of botanical face masks can produce this benefit, yet they may provide a pleasant period of aromatic relaxation desirable to some consumers.

All Natural Ingredients are Safer in Skin Care Products

It is hard to know exactly what 'all natural ingredients' constitutes. All natural has come to mean actives derived from the plants and minerals of the earth. But isn't everything we see in our world derived from the plants and minerals of the earth? Something that is chemically altered still has its basis in the plants and minerals of the earth. Thus, this term is basically marketing jargon with little medical credibility. All natural ingredients are not necessarily safer in skin care products. Even poison ivy which causes an intense allergic contact dermatitis is 'natural' (Fig. 30.6).

Numerous Botanicals in Cosmeceuticals are Better

There is an unspoken rule in cosmeceutical formulation that if one active ingredient is good, 20 active ingredients are great. This had led to the botanical cocktails present in many facial moisturizing products. A quick read through the label reveals at least 10 different plant extracts. Why are they all there? Many times the botanical cocktail is purchased from a supplier with the intent to create a pleasant fragrance from the botanical mixture. Other times the cosmetic formulator selects the concoction to meet some marketing or media needs at the time. Botanical cocktails are extremely problematic for the dermatologist who is trying to figure out which ingredient is the cause of a patient's allergic contact dermatitis (Fig. 30.7). For this reason, I typically recommend that my patients avoid facial moisturizers that contain numerous botanical extracts.

Cleansers with Ground Botanical Materials are Good for Deep Cleaning Pores

A number of botanical facial cleansers contain ground fruit pits, leaves, or other abrasive substances for the purpose of cleaning the pores (Fig. 30.8). In fact it is impossible to clean the sebaceous gland and the duct. Only the follicular ostia of the pilosebaceous unit can be accessed from the skin surface. This means that these facial scrubs can basically only mechanically exfoliate the skin surface and the follicular ostia. Comedonal plugs sticking above the skin surface might be removed, as well as any

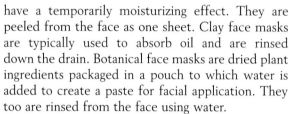

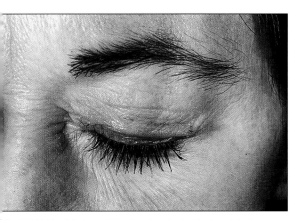

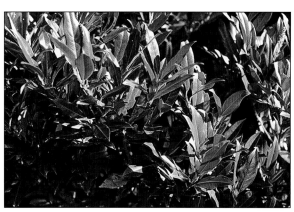

Fig. 30.7 Eyelid dermatitis due to a botanical moisturizer where the exact cause would be difficult to ascertain

Fig. 30.8 Leaves are used in botanical facial scrubs to abrade the skin surface and induce mechanical exfoliation

desquamating corneocytes. It is possible to scrub too hard with fruit pits and induce sensitive skin or milia. For patients who wish to mechanically exfoliate, I recommend one of the scrubs with the dissolving sodium tetrahydrate decaborate granules that wear away with continued scrubbing. This prevents the obsessive-compulsive patient from inducing skin damage.

Part 5

New Research in Cosmeceuticals

The realm of cosmeceuticals is in its infancy. Many of the cosmeceuticals of the future are only concepts today based on actives that are being synthesized with the aid of sophisticated biologic techniques. Novel actives that are identified through gene array technology will use biologic effects to drive identification and purification of substances that enhance skin functioning. Many new actives have already been identified in the categories of antioxidants and hydroxy acids. Novel delivery systems will also aid in targeting cosmeceuticals to specific locations on and within the skin. This section of the text offers a glimpse of the future.

31

Gene Array Technology and the Search for Cosmeceutical Actives

Bryan B. Fuller, Brian K. Pilcher, Dustin R. Smith

Introduction

The number of cosmeceutical products on the market which claim a variety of beneficial effects on skin structure and function is growing rapidly with new product introductions occurring almost daily. Products which claim effectiveness in stimulating collagen and elastin production, blocking activity of matrix metalloproteinases, and slowing down the aging process are widely available and most advertise that 'scientific research' is behind their development. The development of truly efficacious cosmeceuticals involves:

1. The use of a rigorous cell and molecular biology-based screening program to identify active compounds with the desired biological activity (e.g. collagen I, III, or VII gene stimulation).
2. The application of this screening program to determine that the identified 'active' ingredient does NOT also produce undesirable biologic effects on skin cells (e.g. stimulate the MMP-1 gene activity).
3. The development of topical formulations which can be shown by skin percutaneous absorption analysis to deliver sufficient amounts of the 'active' ingredient across the stratum corneum and down to the target cells to achieve the required biological effect.
4. The use of double blind, placebo controlled clinical studies with a sufficient number of patients to generate statistically significant data on product efficacy.

Since the first step in developing an effective cosmeceutical product is to demonstrate that the putative 'active' ingredient not only produces the desired biological action but also does not have any deleterious effect on skin structure or function, it would be advantageous to have access to a single biologic screening tool that could accomplish both needs simultaneously. Such a screening method would allow one to predict a compound's efficacy prior to undertaking any laborious formulation development and before conducting expensive clinical studies. The use of gene array technology fulfills these requirements

Basic Principles of Gene Array Analysis

All cells in the body continuously produce a specific set of proteins that defines the structure and function of that particular cell type. For example, liver cells produce unique hormone receptors for glucagon and insulin, while kidney cells produce proteins for the vasopressin receptor, and for those involved in ion transport. These proteins are coded for by genes that produce unique mRNAs and, thus, each cell type expresses a unique 'footprint' of these mRNAs. Under certain conditions such as ultraviolet radiation (UVR), hormone influence, and aging, this profile of mRNA expression changes as do the proteins coded for by these 'messengers'. Thus, for example, in young skin, dermal fibroblasts express mRNA for the proteins collagen I, III, and VII, whereas in aged skin the fibroblasts produce less mRNA for the collagens but more mRNA for the enzyme MMP-1 (matrix metalloproteinase 1; collagenase 1), which destroys collagen. With the advent of modern molecular biology gene arrays, it is now possible to isolate a 'pool' of mRNA from cells expressing different phenotypes (e.g. young and old human fibroblasts) and from an analysis of these mRNAs, determine which genes are being expressed or repressed in different cell types or in cells exposed to different conditions. Gene arrays are filters or glass slides to which are bound small pieces of known and unknown (EST–expressed sequence tags) human genes. Typical nylon gene array filters may contain over

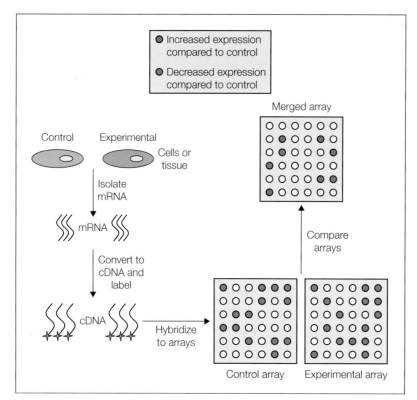

Fig. 31.1 Sequence of steps in gene array analysis. Yellow stars on the cDNAs represent radioactive or fluorescent label. Colored circles on the control and experimental arrays represent mRNAs that are expressed, while white circles represent mRNAs that are not expressed

5000 different gene sequences on a single filter and some arrays have been designed with specific tissues or diseases in mind. For example, a gene filter has been designed to which over 4000 'skin specific' genes have been bound, allowing one to assess the effects of biologic modifiers such as hormones, cytokines, and ultraviolet radiation on the expression of genes important in skin.

The sequence of steps involved in a gene array analysis is shown in Figure 31.1. The first step involves isolating mRNA from cells that represent the 'control' group, and from cells exposed to some experimental condition, such as ultraviolet irradiation ('experimental' group). The mRNA preparation from each group is then reverse transcribed into 'complementary DNA' (cDNA), which is more stable and hybridizes better to DNA than mRNA. This cDNA is then labeled with either a radioisotope or a fluorescent tag so that each unique cDNA can be detected and identified at the conclusion of the experiment. Once the cDNAs have been tagged, they are incubated with the gene array filter (e.g. the 'skin specific' array) so that hybridization between a given cDNA and its complementary DNA on the

array can occur. Once hybridization is complete, any unbound cDNA is washed away and the hybridized cDNA is detected and quantified. Since the location and identity of each gene on the filter is known, by comparing the quantified spots on the array produced from the 'control' group to those spots that are produced in 'experimental' array, one can determine if a particular gene in the experimental group is upregulated or downregulated relative to the control group. Given the complexity of gene arrays, a computer software program is used to aid in the quantification and analysis of the large amount of data that is obtained. The software produces an 'overlay' image of both gene array filters, calculates the difference in expression level for each gene between the control and experimental groups, and then converts this relative expression data into a color image. Typically, a gene that is upregulated in the experimental group relative to the control group is shown as a green spot on the computer generated image while genes that are downregulated are shown in red. An example of the use of this technology in the identification of a novel antiaging and anti-inflammatory active is discussed below.

Application of Gene Arrays to the Identification and Characterization of AntiAging and Anti-inflammatory Bioactive Molecules

As results from microarray technology have become more reliable and reproducible over the last few years, it has become possible to determine the effects of candidate 'bioactive' molecules on skin cells with increased confidence. Furthermore, the use of microarrays has expanded from basic research studies for candidate compound identification to screening tissue samples in a clinical setting to determine an individual's susceptibility to certain diseases such as cancer. Due to the vast amount of data obtained from one particular experiment (e.g. 5500 genes of interest on one DNA filter), it is advantageous to only select a highly restricted set of 'critical' genes of interest for investigation. For example, if anti-inflammatory activity is desired one might investigate the regulation of genes such as COX-2 (PGE-2 producing gene), IL-1α, IL-6, IL-8, and TNF-α. Alternatively, if an antiaging bioactive was desired one would focus on the expression of extracellular matrix genes such as collagens, elastin, and proteoglycans combined with the inhibition of matrix degrading proteases such as collagenase and the gelatinases. Microarray technology also offers the opportunity to identify new beneficial effects that would have not been discovered otherwise using typical single gene experiments.

We have used gene array technology to identify unique compounds that have antiaging and/or anti-inflammatory effects in multiple skin cell types. In one study we assessed the ability of a novel nitrone spin-trap compound to modulate the expression of aging-related genes in older human dermal fibroblasts. The fibroblasts were grown in the presence (Experimental) or absence (Control) of the compound, CX-412, for 48 hours at which time the mRNA from each cell culture group was isolated, converted to a complementary DNA (cDNA), labeled with radioactive nucleotides, and hybridized to IntegriDerm DermArray gene filters. These microarray filters contain over 4400 unique cDNAs specifically chosen due to their expression in skin cells and relevance to dermatologic research. Genes that are commonly expressed in skin are spotted in duplicate at different sites on the gene filters to provide an estimate of reproducibility of the hybridization reac-

CX-412 induced changes in expression of inflammation and age-related genes

Upregulated by CX-412
- Tissue inhibitor of metalloproteinases 1 (TIMP-1)
- Tissue inhibitor of metalloproteinases 2 (TIMP-2)
  Type I collagen
  Type II collagen
  Type III collagen

Downregulated by CX-412
- Collagenase 1 (MMP-1)
- 72 kDa gelatinase (MMP-2)
- Urokinase-type plasminogen activator (uPA)
- Tissue-type plasminogen activator (tPA)
- Plasminogen activator inhibitor I (PAI-1)
- Plasminogen activator inhibitor II (PAI-2)
- Chemokine receptor I
- Activated leukocyte cell adhesion molecule
- Interleukin 1b
- Interleukin 6
- Interleukin 13 receptor
- Fibroblast growth factor-2 (bFGF)

Box 31.1 CX-412 induced changes in expression of inflammation and age-related genes: IntegriDerm DermArray: dermal fibroblast gene expression

tion. The hybridization images are imported into a computer program that normalizes the data set and provides a color coded picture of which expressed genes in the CX-412 treated fibroblasts were upregulated (coded in green) or downregulated (coded in red) relative to the untreated fibroblast cultures (Figure 31.2C). Figures 31.2A and B show the actual filter images of the hybridized radioactive cDNAs which were upregulated or downregulated by the spin-trap, CX-412.

After quantifying the level of all expressed genes in control and CX-412 treated cells, we found that aged fibroblasts treated with CX-412 shifted their expression patterns from matrix destruction to matrix production (Box 31.1). For example, inhibition of the matrix metalloproteinases collagenase 1 and 92 kDa gelatinase was noted while the naturally occurring inhibitors of MMPs, TIMP-1, and TIMP-2 were upregulated. Furthermore, the expression of collagen types I, II, and III were enhanced in fibroblasts. In addition to age related genes we also found that certain inflammation associated genes, including uPA, tPA, PAI-1, IL-1α, and IL-6 were markedly inhibited by the spin-trap compound tested.

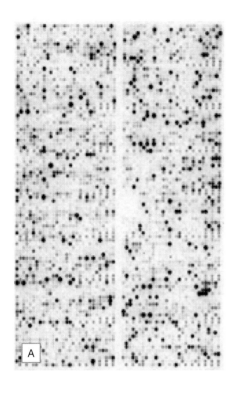

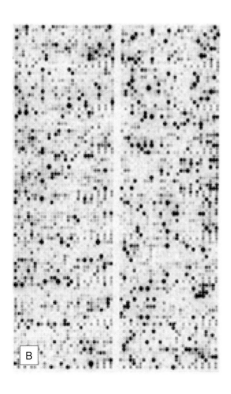

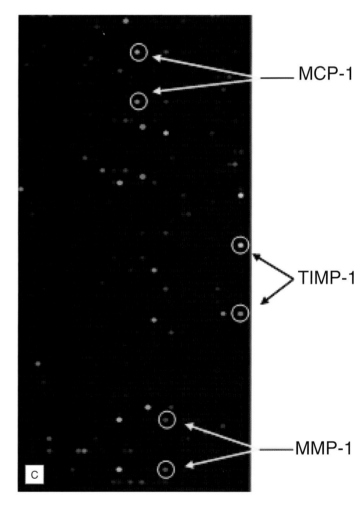

Fig. 31.2 IntegriDerm gene array results in fibroblasts treated with Cutanix Compound, CX-412. cDNA from cells treated with control (**A**) or CX-412 (**B**) was hybridized to gene array nylon membranes. Following hybridization, the blots were developed using a Packard Cyclone phosphorimager. (**C**) The computer generated comparison image showed that CX-412 reduced the expression of monocyte chemotactic protein (MCP-1) and collagenase-1 (MMP-1) as evidenced by the red hybridization spots, but induced the expression of tissue inhibitor of metalloproteinase-1 (TIMP-1) as evidenced by the green hybridization spots

Summary

The use of gene array technology allows one to obtain, from a small number of experiments, a wealth of information on specific genes that are both stimulated and repressed by any compound being considered for cosmeceutical development. The technique can be used to identify new drug candidates for treating such dermatologic diseases as psoriasis, atopic dermatitis, seborrheic dermatitis, and even actinic keratoses, and as shown above is useful for identifying compounds that can reduce, delay, or even reverse the skin aging process. Finally, gene arrays provide an opportunity to quickly analyze cosmeceutical 'actives' and botanical extracts currently in skin care products to determine what positive and negative effects these 'actives' may actually have on skin function.

Further Reading

Baldi P, Hatfield GW, Hatfield WG 2002 DNA microarrays and gene expression: from experiments to data analysis and modeling. Cambridge University Press, Cambridge

Curto EV, Lambert GW, Davis RL, Wilborn TW, Dooley TP 2002 Biomarkers of human skin cells identified using DermArray® DNA arrays and new bioinformatics methods. Biochemical and Biophysical Research Communications 291:1052–1064

Fisher GJ, Kang S, Varani J, et al 2002 Mechanisms of photoaging and chronological skin aging. Archives of Dermatology 138:1462–1470

Floyd RA, Hensley K, Forster MJ, Kelleher-Andersson JA 2002 Nitrones, their value as therapeutics and probes to understand aging. Mechanisms of Ageing and Development 123:1021–1031

Gerhold D, Caskey C T 1996 It's the genes! EST access to human genome content. Bioessays 18: 973–981

Herlaar E, Brown Z 1999 p38 MAPK signaling cascades in inflammatory disease. Molecular Medicine Today 5:439–447

Johnston M 1998 Gene chips: array of hope for understanding gene regulation. Current Biology 8:R171–174

Okubo K, Matsubara K 1997 Complementary DNA sequence (EST) collections and the expression information of the human genome. FEBS Letters 403:225–229

32

Future Cosmeceuticals of Dermatologic Importance

Neil S. Sadick

Introduction

Utilization by patients of new and innovative cosmeceutical agents is ever expanding. Correlations and trends between in vitro and in vivo results have produced better objective scientific evaluation of the true efficacy of these newer agents. Thus, new and innovative molecules have been developed. Two new cosmeceuticals are genomically derived DNA skin care and a new generation of superpotent antioxidants (AO), for example genestein and idebenone.

Antioxidants

The skin is dependent upon AOs to protect it from oxidant stress generated by sunlight and pollution. The mechanism of action of antioxidants includes the ability to scavenge reactive oxygen species in response to ultraviolet exposure. The new generation antioxidant botanicals quench singlet oxygen and reactive oxygen species, such as superoxide anions, hydroxy radicals, fatty peroxy radicals, and hydroperoxides.

Recently two new metalloproteinase kinase genes, ERK and JNK, have been found to play an important role in oxidative free radical ultraviolet induced damage. The genes can regulate the decreased activation of metalloprotein kinases (MAPs). This can subsequently lead to the decreased production of collagenase, gelatinase, stromelysin, and other metalloproteinases (Fig. 32.1).

Botanical antioxidants are playing an increasing role in this regard. They can be classified into one of three categories: flavonoids, carotenoids, and polyphenols. Flavonoids possess a polyphenolic

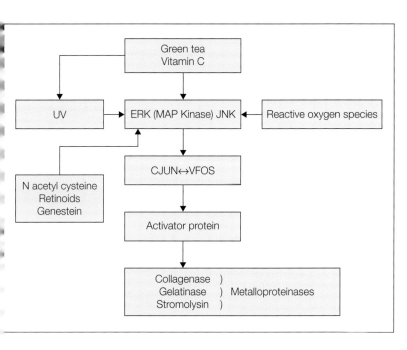

Fig. 32.1 Free radical theory of aging

structure that accounts for their antioxidant, UV protection, and metal chelation abilities. Genestein is another such example. Carotenoids are chemically related to vitamin A, which encompasses all of the naturally occurring retinol derivatives. The third group, polyphenols, comprises the largest group of botanical antioxidants.

Antioxidants are unstable compounds, which allows them to function in redox reactions. However, this instability makes them difficult to formulate into acceptable stable skincare products. AOs also are often colored and in addition may require accelerated delivery systems which allow them to penetrate to maximal skin levels in appropriate concentrations. Finally, AOs must have strong photoprotective effects, including reduction of erythema, reduction of sunburn cell formation, and reduction of DNA changes.

Genestein

Background

Genestein is a soybean isoflavone with diverse biologic activities. It was first isolated from soy beans in 1931. It is a potent antioxidant, a specific inhibitior of protein tyrosine, kinase, and phytoestrogens. In recent years, increasing evidence has emerged from many investigators that this natural ingredient exhibits preventative and therapeutic effects on breast and prostate cancers, postmenopausal syndrome, osteoporosis, and cardiovascular diseases in animals and humans. Multiple studies over the past decade have shown that genestein has significant antiphotocarcinogenic and antiphotoaging effects. Genestein has significant effects in terms of inhibition of chemical carcinogenesis and ultraviolet induced skin carcinogenesis and photoaging in mice as well as photodamage in humans. The mechanism of action involves protection of oxidative and photodynamically damaged DNA, downregulation of UVB activated signal transduction cascades, and antioxidant activities.

Biologic activities (Box 32.1)

Genestein is known to have estrogenic effects; however, the estrogenic potency is much weaker than physiologic steroids, being only about 1/10 000 to 1/50 000 that of estriol or estradiol.

Genestein exhibits antioxidant properties preventing the hemolysis of red blood cells by dialuric acid

Biologic effects of genestein

- Potent antioxidant
- Inhibitor of tyrosine kinase
- Phytoestrogen
- Inhibits oncogene activation post UVB radiation
- Protection of oxidative and photodynamically damaged DNA
- Downregulation of UVB activated signal transduction cascades

Box 32.1 Biologic effects of genestein

or H_2O_2 and inhibiting microsomal lipid peroxidation induced by Fe^{2+}-ADP complex and NADPH. Genestein and related isoflavones also inhibit the NADH oxidase and respiratory chain in rat liver mitochondria. Finally, genestein has been found to be the most potent inhibitor of p450 mediated activation of benzo[a]pyrene among all isoflavones.

In addition, genestein has been shown to have multiple beneficial effects on systemic health. It has been used as an alternative to treat menopausal syndrome in women, based upon a study in Asian females. These individuals consume more soy in their diets and have fewer symptoms of menopausal syndrome. Genestein has also been proposed as a treatment for osteoporosis in postmenopausal women and elderly men.

A number of studies have also shown that such consumption of soy isoflavone is associated with a decreased incidence of cardiovascular disease, reduction in low density lipoproteins, and increase in high density lipoproteins. This has also been found in women on soy protein diets containing high concentrations of isoflavones.

Genestein has been found to have chemopreventative and anticancer activities. It has been shown to inhibit the activity of tyrosine protein kinase (TPK), topoisomerase II (Topo II), and ribosomal S6 kinase (RS6K) in cell culture. It has also been shown to inhibit the growth of the *ras* oncogene and decrease PD6F induced c-*fos* and c-*jun* expression in fibroblasts.

Effect of genestein on photocarcinogenesis and photoaging (Box 32.2)

Although numerous in vitro studies have shown that genestein has potential anticancer properties as stated above, evidence is lacking on the effect on skin carcinogenesis, although there is strong scientific support for its potential. Genestein has been shown to inhibit UVR induced oxidative DNA damage in purified DNA and cultured cells and blocks UVB induced c-*fous* and c-*jun* protooncogene expression in mouth skin. It has also been shown to inhibit EGF-R phosphorylation and metalloproteinase in human skin independent of its sunscreen effect.

Genestein has been shown to inhibit UVB induced skin carcinogenesis in mice (Fig. 32.2). In a complete photocarcinogenesis study mice were clinically exposed to 0.3 KJ/m^2 of UVB twice weekly following topical application. Genestein dose dependent inhibition of skin carcinogenesis by more than 90% occurred, substantiating topical genestein's capability for inhibiting UVB induced skin carcinogenesis.

Genestein has also been shown to inhibit UVB induced acute and chronic photodamage in mouse skin. In an acute sunburn study, mice were irradiated with daily UVB (1.8 KJ/m^2) for 10 days. Topical application of 5 μmol of genestein 60 minutes before each UVB irradiation completely blocked UVB induced acute sunburns. In a chronic UVB exposure study mice were irradiated with UVB twice weekly (0.3 KJ/m^2) for 4 weeks. Chronic exposure to low dose UVB increased roughness and wrinkling in mice. Application of genestein prior to and post UVB exposure alleviated photodamage, with pre-UVB application showing stronger effects. Histologic evaluation showed that genestein inhibited epidermal hyperplasia, acanthosis, and nuclear atypia induced by UVB (Fig. 32.3). Protective effects were histologically confirmed by quantifying the epidermal thickness and elastic fiber density. The above experiments substantiate that genestein substantially blocks the subacute and chronic UVB induced cutaneous damage and histologic alterations related to photoaging.

Genestein has been shown to protect human skin against UVB induced photodamage. Genestein was applied to the dorsal skin of six human male subjects skin types II–IV, 60 minutes before and 5 minutes after UVB irradiation. The skin was photographed and quantified for erythema index by optical chromometry. Application of 5 μmol genestein per cm^2 substantially blocked erythema induced by different doses of UVB radiation, whereas post-UVB application showed very little protection of cutaneous erythema. The results of this study showed that pre-UVB application of genestein significantly inhibited both cutaneous erythema and discomfort, whereas post-UVB application improved discomfort with minimal effect on erythema (Fig. 32.4).

In addition, genestein has been shown to protect against PUVA induced photodamage in the mouse skin model. Morphologic and histologic damage were minimized with pretreatment topical application. The effects were mediated by inhibition of PUVA induced apoptotic pathways.

Finally, genestein appears to block UVB induced skin burns in humans as well as PUVA induced photodamage. The antipromotional activities are primarily associated with the anti-inflammatory pathway, downregulation of PTK activities, and expression of cell proliferation associated protooncogenes

Idebenone

Idebenone is another newly developed antioxidant. The future promise of idebenone is based on sunburn cell assays, photochemiluminescence, primary and secondary oxidative product assays, and evaluation of damage to UVB irradiated keratinocytes. Idebenone was found to be a powerful antioxidant compared to tocopherol, ubiquinone, ascorbic acid, and alpha lipoic acid (Table 32.1).

Ongoing clinical studies are underway to evaluate its efficacy in vivo. These studies are comparing the protective capacity of commonly used antioxidant ingredients. Correlation and trends between the study results allow for the establishment of a standardization testing protocol to quantify the oxidative stress protection capacity of the substances studied.

In Table 32.1, each study represents a total possible score of 20 points. There were five independent studies; thus a total possible score of 100 points (20 × 5). The points assigned to an antioxidant in each study was dependent on their relative efficacy to protect against oxidative stress in that study. the overall points was then the total of each independent study score for each antioxidant, thereby representing the overall efficacy of the antioxidant

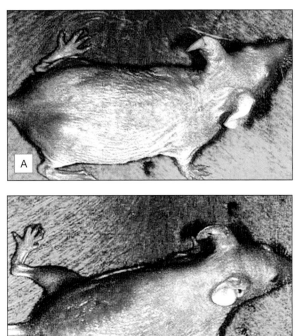

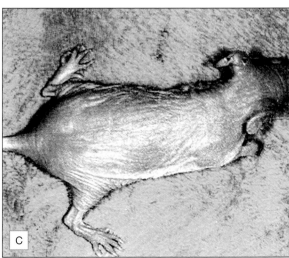

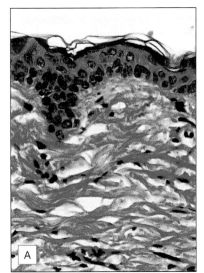

Fig. 32.2 (**A–C**) Effect of genestein on UVB induced acute skin burns in mice

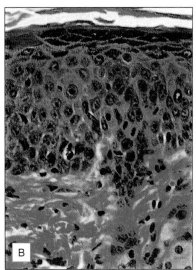

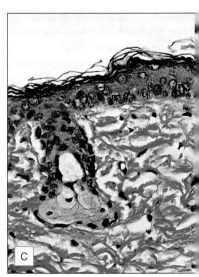

Fig. 32.3 (**A–C**) Effect of genestein on histological alterations in mice exposed to UVB

Mechanism of aging based upon the free radical treatment of oxidative stress						
Test	**Idebenone**	**Tocopheraol**	**Kinetin**	**Ubiquinone**	**Ascorbic acid**	**Lipoic acid**
Sunburn cell assay	20	16	11	6	0	5
Photochemiluminescence	20	20	10	15	20	5
Primary oxidative products	16	10	20	5	3	4
Secondary oxidative products	19	17	10	12	12	20
UVB-irradiated keratinocytes	20	17	17	17	17	7
Total points	**95**	**80**	**68**	**55**	**52**	**41**

Table 32.1 Mechanism of aging based upon the free radical treatment of oxidative stress

to protect against environmental oxidative stress, or sometimes as it is referred,the 'EPF' or 'Environmental Protector Factor' of the antioxidant. The results of the various studies show that idebenone performed as an efficient antioxidant most consistently.

Analysis Based DNA Skin Care

Now that the human genome has been sequenced, genetic variations among individuals can be analyzed to determine interindividual variations. This new field of study is called pharmacogenomics and analyzes genetic variations in individual responses to drugs. Advances in pharmacogenomics enable the identification of drugs effective for an individual and the most effective dosage. This area of study also has implications in skin care.

Recently, genetic research has identified specific genes and other information provided by an individual's DNA that are relevant to the health and aging of skin. For example, those genes and other genetic markers indicate propensity for collagen and elastin breakdown, irritation potential, tolerance for environmental irritants, and ability to counteract damaging free radicals. Thus, an individual's DNA profile can provide information about skin behavior and skin deficiencies. Furthermore, genetic variations among individuals greatly affect how a person responds to particular active ingredients in skincare formulations. To maximize efficacy, skincare formulations can now be formulated based upon an individual's unique genetic makeup.

To obtain genetic material, Skin DNA Test is administered. It is performed using a DNA Test Kit that contains four sterile cotton swabs. DNA samples are obtained by swabbing the inner cheek. Once the swabs are dry, they are placed inside a

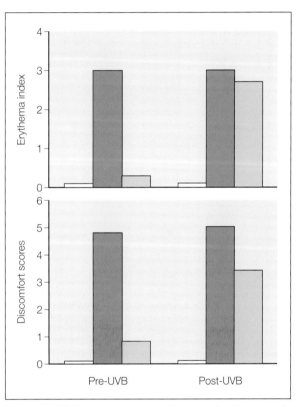

Fig. 32.4 Effect of genestein on UVB induced erythema and discomfort in human skin

DNA swab collection envelope and sealed. The DNA sample, containing thousands of epithelial cells, is analyzed. The DNA profile is determined via polymerase chain reaction, whereby a small amount of DNA is amplified approximately one million times. The amplification allows scientists to identify and test various genetic markers through microarrays. The results are put into a proprietary, computerized formulating system.

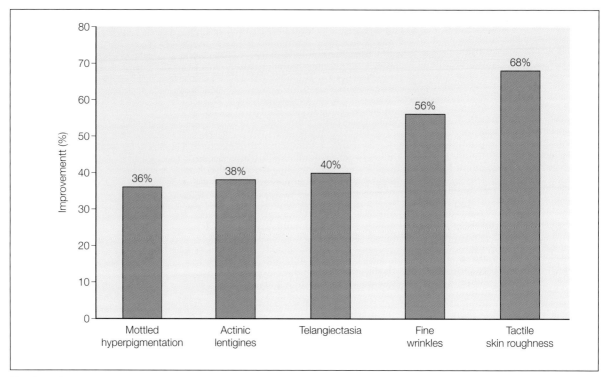

Fig. 32.5 Clinical signs of aging in facial skin: percentage improvement over baseline with 24 weeks' usage

Among the genetic markers analyzed are information from both nuclear DNA and mitochondrial DNA Special focus is placed on linking data from the hypervariable regions 1 and 2 of the D-loop region of the mitochondrial genome to matrix metalloproteinase (MMP) activity. This activity is known to degrade collagen, elastin, and other proteins in the skin. A 24 week clinical study showed improvement in fine wrinkles (56%), actinic lentigines (38%), mottled (blotchy) hyperpigmentation (36%), telangiectasia (40%), and tactile skin roughness (68%). The treatment was well tolerated by the subjects with no adverse effects (Fig. 32.5).

Conclusion

The next generation of cosmeceuticals may focus on high efficacy antioxidants, such as genestein and idebenone, which appear to protect against ultraviolet induced cell damage, decrease the incidence of skin cancer, and may help reverse the photoaging process. Genome based DNA technologies represent a new approach to skin care. Both new technologies may have a role in the photoaging armamentarium of the practicing dermatologist when further scientific studies substantiate their efficacy.

Further Reading

Akiyama T, Ishida J, Nakagawa S, et al 1987 Genestein, a specific inhibitor of tyrosine-specific protein kinases. Journal of Biological Chemistry 262:5592–5595

Albertazzi P, Pansini F, Bonaccorsi G, et al 1998 The effect of dietary soy supplementation on hot flashes. Obstetrics and Gynecology 1998;91:6–11

Arora A, Nair MG, Strasburg GM 1998 Antioxidant activities of isoflavones and their biological activities in liposomal system. Archives of Biochemistry and Biophysics 356:133–141

Brezeinski A, et al 1997 Short-term effects of phytoestrogens-rich diet on postmenopausal women. Menopause 42:89–94

Cai Q, Wei H 1996 Effects of dietary genestein on antioxidant enzyme activities in Sencar mice. Nutrition and Cancer 25:1–7

Correa P 1981 Epidemiological correlations between diet and cancer frequency. Cancer Research 41:3685–3690

Draelos Z 2003 Botanical antioxidants. Cosmetics and Dermatology 16:46–48

Fotsis T, Pepper M, Adlercerutz H, et al 1993 Genestein, a dietary-derived inhibitor of in vitro angiogenesis. Proceedings of the National Academy of Sciences USA 90:2690–2694

Gyorgy P, Murata K, Ikehata H 1964 Antioxidants isolated from fermented soybeans (tempeh). Nature 203:870–872

Kang S. Chung JH, Lee JH, et al 2003 Topical N-acetyl cysteine and genistein prevent ultraviolet-light-induced signaling that leads to photoaging in human skin in vivo. Journal of Investigative Dermatology 120:835–841

Kapiotis S, Hermann M, Held I, et al 1997 Genestein, the dietary-derived angiogenesis inhibitor, prevents LDL oxidation and protects endothelial cells from damage by atherogenic LDL. Arteriosclerosis, Thrombosis and Vascular Biology 17:2868–2874

Kiguchi K, Constantinou A, Huberman E 1990 Genestein induced cell differentiation and protein-linked DNA strand breakage in human melanoma cells. Cancer Communications 2:271–278

Lee EH, Cho SY, Kim SJ, et al 2003 Ginsenoside Fl protects human HaCat keratinocytes from ultrarole +B induced apoptosis by maintaining constant levels of Bcl-2. Journal of Investigative Dermatology 121:607–613

Li D, Yee JA, McGuire MH, Yan F 1999 Soybean isoflavones reduces experimental metastasis in mice. Journal of Nutrition 29:1075–1078

Messina M, Barnes S 1991 The role of soy products in reducing risk of cancer. Journal of the National Cancer Institute 83:541–546

Monon LG, Kuttan R, Nail MG 1998 Effect of isoflavone genestein and daidzein in the inhibition of lung metastasis in mice induced by B16F-10 melanoma cells. Nutrition and Cancer 30:74–77

Okura A, Arakawa H, Oka H, Yoshinari T, Monden Y 1988 Effect of genestein on topoisomerase activity and on the growth of [VAL 12] Ha-ras-transformed NIH 3T3 cells. Biochemical and Biophysical Research Communications 157:183–189

Pinnell SR 2003 Cutaneous photodamage, oxidative stress and topical antioxidant protection. Journal of the American Academy of Dermatology 48:1–19

Pratt DE, Di Pietro C, Porter WL, Giffee JW 1981 Phenolic antioxidants of soy protein hydrolyzates. Journal of Food Science 47:24–25

Tham DM 1998 Potential health benefits of dietary phytoestrogens: a review of the clinical, epidemiological and mechanistic evidence. Journal of Clinical Endocrinology and Metabolism 83:2223–2235

Wang Y, Yaping E, Zhang X, et al 1998 Inhibition of ultraviolet B induced c-fos and c-jun expression by genestein through a protein tyrosine kinase-dependent pathway. Carcinogenesis 19:649–654

Wei H, Bowen R, Zhang X, Lebwohl M 1998 Isoflavone genestein inhibits the initiation and promotion of two-stage skin carcinogenesis. Carcinogenesis 19:1509–1514

Wei H, Cai Q, Rhan R 1996 Inhibition of Fenton reaction and UV light-induced oxidative DNA damage by soybean isoflavone genestein. Carcinogenesis 17:73–77

Yamaguchi M, Goa YH 1998 Genestein inhibits bone loss. Biochemical Pharmacology 55:71–76

Zwiller J, Sassone-Corsi P, Kakazu K, Boyton AL 1991 Inhibition of PDGF-induced c-jun and c-fos expression by a tyrosine protein kinase inhibitor. Oncogene 6:219–221

33

The Next Generation Hydroxy Acids

M. Elizabeth Briden, Barbara Green

Introduction

The polyhydroxy acids (PHAs) represent the next generation of alpha-hydroxyacids (AHAs) for use in cosmetic and dermatologic skin care. Structurally similar to traditional AHAs, the polyhydroxy acids provide antiaging and skin smoothing effects comparable to AHAs, while offering several therapeutic advantages. PHAs are less irritating to skin compared to AHAs, and cause less stinging and burning. PHA compatibility with clinically sensitive skin types has previously been demonstrated in patients diagnosed with atopic dermatitis and rosacea. PHAs also enhance the skin barrier; an important fact for patients with compromised skin conditions. In addition, these molecules function as humectants and moisturizers, as well as provide antioxidant chelation effects due to their polyhydroxy structure. PHAs, however, do not increase sun sensitivity but they do provide free radical scavenging effects. Multiple skin benefits are provided by PHAs, making them important cosmeceuticals.

The polyhydroxy acid structure

Polyhydroxy acids are organic carboxylic acids, which possess two or more hydroxyl groups on an aliphatic or alicyclic molecular structure. When one of the hydroxyl groups occurs in the alpha position, the PHA is a polyhydroxy AHA (Fig. 33.1). Because they share the common AHA structure, PHA compounds have the ability to provide skin effects similar to traditional AHAs, such as glycolic acid.

Gluconolactone: a Representative PHA

Gluconolactone (gluconic acid delta lactone) is a nontoxic, naturally occurring component of the skin. The molecule's somewhat larger size (molecular

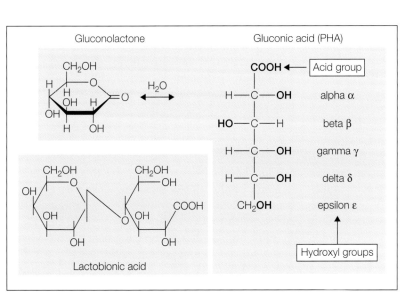

Fig. 33.1 PHAs: gluconolactone and lactobionic acid

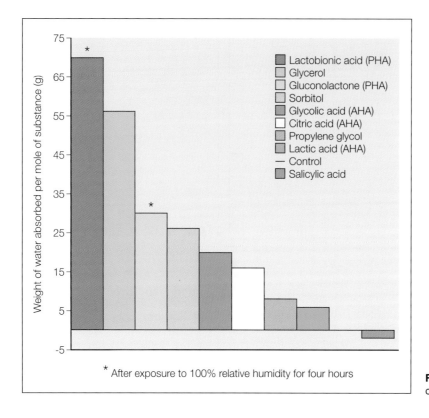

Fig. 33.2 Water-binding properties of PHAs

Legend:
- Lactobionic acid (PHA)
- Glycerol
- Gluconolactone (PHA)
- Sorbitol
- Glycolic acid (AHA)
- Citric acid (AHA)
- Propylene glycol
- Lactic acid (AHA)
- — Control
- Salicylic acid

y-axis: Weight of water absorbed per mole of substance (g)

*After exposure to 100% relative humidity for four hours

weight 178 vs. 76 for glycolic acid) facilitates a gradual penetration into skin, thus minimizing irritation. The smaller molecule of glycolic acid penetrates the skin more rapidly, often causing stinging and burning. Gluconolactone's potential for increased hydration is attributed to humectant properties of the multiple hydroxyl groups, which can attract and hydrogen bond water (Fig. 33.2).

Antioxidant and free radical scavenging effects of gluconolactone

The antioxidant properties of gluconolactone are evident in food and drug substances, in which gluconolactone has been shown to inhibit oxidation and help maintain product integrity (Fig. 33.3).

Bernstein et al demonstrated that gluconolactone provides free radical scavenging effects comparable to other well known compounds such as ascorbic acid and alpha-tocopherol using an in vitro model of cutaneous photoaging. In this model, compounds are measured for their ability to prevent ultraviolet induced activation of an elastin promoter in skin via free radical scavenging activity. An increase in

the expression of elastin promoter causes an abnormal deposition of poorly structured elastic material in skin—the condition known as solar elastosis. Maximum protection by free radical scavengers occurs at a rate of approximately 50%; the other 50% is caused by direct UV damage to cells and cellular DNA. Results of the study indicated that gluconolactone provided up to 50% protection against UV radiation. This effect could not be explained by UV screening alone, and therefore was attributed to gluconolactone's ability to chelate oxidation promoting metals possibly via the direct free radical scavenging effects of gluconolactone.

Clinical effects of gluconolactone

Studies have demonstrated many different clinical benefits of the PHAs including antiaging and skin firming effects that are comparable to commonly used AHAs, with reduced irritation potential (Fig. 33.4). In addition, significant antiaging benefits have been observed in various ethnic skin types including African-American, Asian, and Hispanic. Separately, in a vehicle controlled, double blind evaluation, 14%

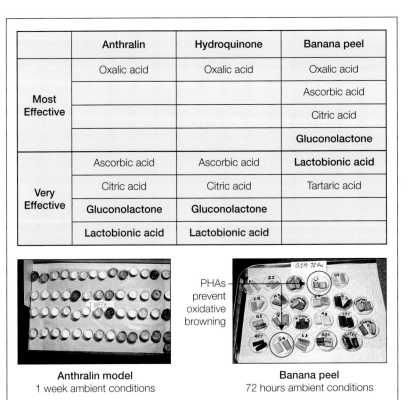

	Anthralin	Hydroquinone	Banana peel
Most Effective	Oxalic acid	Oxalic acid	Oxalic acid
			Ascorbic acid
			Citric acid
			Gluconolactone
Very Effective	Ascorbic acid	Ascorbic acid	**Lactobionic acid**
	Citric acid	Citric acid	Tartaric acid
	Gluconolactone	**Gluconolactone**	
	Lactobionic acid	**Lactobionic acid**	

PHAs prevent oxidative browning

Anthralin model
1 week ambient conditions

Banana peel
72 hours ambient conditions

Fig. 33.3 Antioxidant effects of PHAs

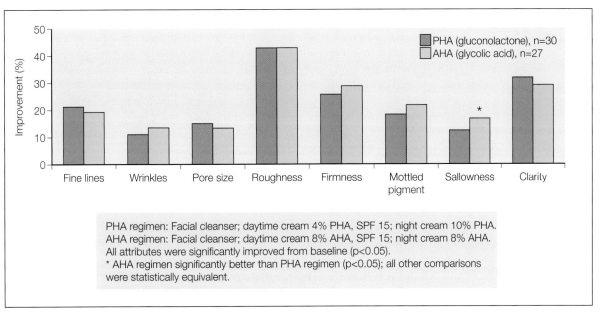

PHA regimen: Facial cleanser; daytime cream 4% PHA, SPF 15; night cream 10% PHA.
AHA regimen: Facial cleanser; daytime cream 8% AHA, SPF 15; night cream 8% AHA.
All attributes were significantly improved from baseline ($p < 0.05$).
* AHA regimen significantly better than PHA regimen ($p < 0.05$); all other comparisons were statistically equivalent.

Fig. 33.4 Antiaging effects of AHAs and PHAs. Clinical grading, week 12: mean relative percentage improvement compared to baseline

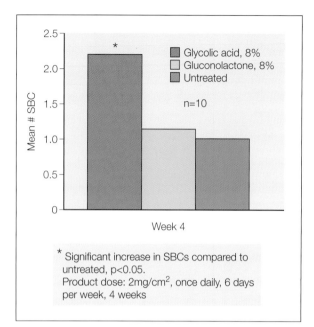

*Significant increase in SBCs compared to untreated, p<0.05.
Product dose: 2mg/cm^2, once daily, 6 days per week, 4 weeks

Fig. 33.5 Sun sensitivity model: mean sunburn cell count (sunburn cell count per high power field)

gluconolactone solution was shown to provide anti-acne effects with less irritation than 5% benzoyl peroxide lotion on individuals with mild to moderate acne. These findings are most likely related to the epidermal cell turnover enhancement effects of PHAs and possibly the antioxidant effects. PHAs are compatible with traditional acne medications including tretinoin. This is illustrated in a clinical study utilizing a 15% (pH 3.3) gluconolactone containing cream in combination with the daily use of tretinoin gel 0.1%.

Effects of hydroxyacids on skin barrier integrity were evaluated in a vehicle controlled, double blind clinical study. Unlike AHAs (glycolic acid and lactic acid), antioxidant PHAs were shown to strengthen stratum corneum barrier function as measured by transepidermal water loss and colorimetry. Clinically, this finding may help to explain data that revealed a lack of increased sun sensitivity with PHA use. The PHAs gluconolactone and glucoheptonolactone did not cause an increase in the formation of sunburn cells following exposure to UVB in the testing model employed by the Cosmetics, Toiletries and Fragrances Association (CTFA) and the Food and Drug Administration (FDA) (Fig. 33.5).

Lactobionic Acid: a Complex PHA

Lactobionic acid is a complex PHA formed by the oxidation of lactose (milk sugar). It is composed of one molecule of the sugar D-galactose and one molecule of D-gluconic acid (i.e. gluconolactone, a PHA). Lactobionic acid is termed a 'complex' PHA due to the attachment of an additional sugar unit to the traditional PHA structure (Fig. 33.1).

One component of the lactobionic acid molecule is gluconic acid, a PHA with multiple beneficial effects on skin as described above. Galactose, the second component of lactobionic acid, is a naturally occurring sugar that is utilized by human skin during dermal proteoglycan and procollagen synthesis. In addition, in vitro wound healing studies indicate that galactose may play a role in wound healing.

Antioxidant and other uses of lactobionic acid

Lactobionic acid is currently used in the pharmaceutical industry as a counter ion (e.g. erythromycin lactobionate, calcium lactobionate) to minimize irritation. In addition, lactobionic acid is a key antioxidant chelator in organ transplant preservation solutions that are used to suppress tissue damage caused by hydroxyl radicals during organ storage and reperfusion. Lactobionic acid reportedly inhibits hydroxyl radical production by forming a complex with Fe(II).

The antioxidant properties of lactobionic acid have also been studied in food and drug substances, demonstrating the capacity to inhibit the oxidation of readily oxidizable drugs including anthralin and hydroquinone, as well as banana peels (Fig. 33.3). Since oxidation and UV induced free radicals are a cause of skin aging, the potent antioxidant benefits of lactobionic acid may play an important role in its antiaging effects.

Lactobionic acid: skin protector

Investigative work in the field of organ preservation has revealed that lactobionate is a cryptic inhibitor of matrix metalloproteinase (MMP) enzymes obtained from human liver effluents during transplantation. Protective benefits in skin are both feasible and enticing because MMPs are responsible for the degradation of the skin's extracellular matrix and structural integrity. MMPs also cause or contribute

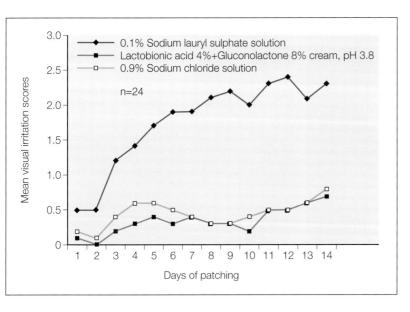

Fig. 33.6 Irritation assessment of PHA formulation. Cumulative irritation study: 14 day occlusive patch test

to wrinkle formation, skin laxity, and visible telangiectasia. Naturally occurring tissue inhibitors of MMPs protect the skin from degradation by these enzymes. Nonetheless, MMP activity in skin increases with UV exposure and advancing age leading to the visual and morphologic signs of photodamage. The use of lactobionic acid to inhibit MMPs may provide a benefit to photoaged skin.

Topical uses of lactobionic acid

Lactobionic acid provides antiaging benefits to skin beyond traditional AHAs due to its unique chemical structure and molecular composition. As a result of the multiple hydroxyl groups, lactobionic acid is a strong humectant, with the ability to attract and retain water better than common humectants including glycerin and sorbitol (Fig. 33.2). It also forms a unique gel matrix during the drydown process as a result of its strong water retention properties.

PHA formulations of lactobionic acid in combination with gluconolactone are nonirritating (Fig. 33.6). These combinations have also exhibited strong antiaging effects including marked improvements in skin clarity (260%, $P < 0.05$) and notable skin plumping effects (9.7%, $P < 0.05$). A second, independent clinical study revealed significant improvements in

skin roughness (33%, $P < 0.05$) and pore size (60%, $P < 0.05$), while demonstrating excellent skin tolerance. No subjects reported burning or stinging throughout the study and there was a significant (50%, $P < 0.001$) reduction in erythema (Fig. 33.7).

Use of PHAs in the Dermatologist's Office

PHAs are an important cosmeceutical. They are efficacious, nonirritating, antioxidant humectants with antiaging properties. PHAs can be used solely in skin care regimens or adjunctively with topical drug therapies for the treatment of inflammatory skin conditions including psoriasis, rosacea, acne, keratosis pilaris, and seborrheic dermatitis. They are especially useful to help control skin discomfort when using topical medications that are drying or irritating. PHAs can be combined with skin lightening ingredients to effectively diminish hyperpigmentation (Fig. 33.8).

PHAs are well suited for use in combination with cosmetic procedures. They can be used to help smooth and condition the skin before and after laser resurfacing, microdermabrasion, intense pulsed light treatments, and chemical peel procedures. In this capacity, PHAs provide antioxidant and moisturization benefits while contributing to the antiaging and therapeutic effects of these procedures.

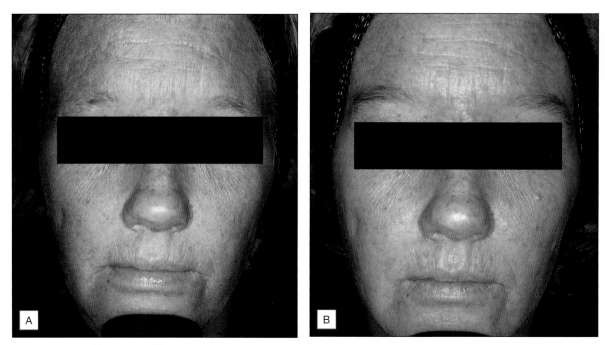

Fig. 33.7 Before (**A**) and after (**B**) a 12 week clinical study to assess the effects of a lactobionic acid + gluconolactone gel (total 8%) when used twice daily. Skin shows marked improvement in skin clarity, texture, and pore size after 12 weeks

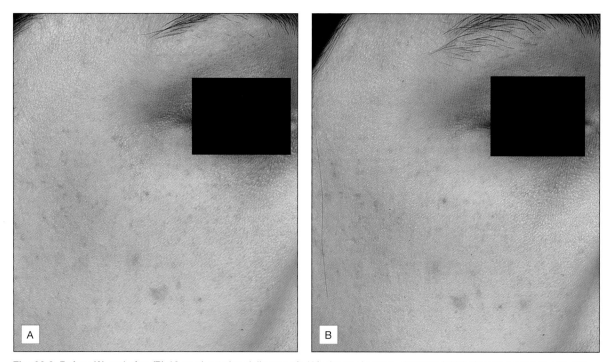

Fig. 33.8 Before (**A**) and after (**B**) 12 weeks, twice daily use of: 4% gluconolactone cleanser (pH 3.4); skin lightener with 5% lactobionic acid, 5% gluconolactone, 2% hydroquinone, 3% kojic acid (pH 3.9); 4% gluconolactone day lotion SPF 15 (pH 3.9); 15% gluconolactone night cream (pH 3.3). Skin shows reduced pigmentation, with increased clarity and smoothness

Summary

There are many applications for PHAs in cosmetic and therapeutic skin care. PHAs represent the hydroxy acids of the future with their nonirritating, humectant, and antioxidant effects. PHAs are a cosmeceutical that can be used alone or with various topical medications and cosmetic procedures to smoothe, condition, and improve photoaged skin.

Further Reading

Berardesca E, Distante F, Vignoli GP, Oresajo C, Green B 1997 Alpha hydroxy acids modulate stratum corneum barrier function. British Journal of Dermatology 137:934–938

Bernstein EF, Brown DB, Schwartz MD, Kaidbey K, Ksenzenko SM 2004 The polyhydroxy acid gluconolactone protects against ultraviolet radiation in an in vitro model of cutaneous photoaging. Dermatologic Surgery 30:1–8

Charloux C, Paul M, Loisance D, Astier A 1995 Inhibition of hydroxyl radical production by lactobionate, adenine, and tempol. Free Radicals in Biology and Medicine 19:699–704

Edison BL, Green BA, Wildnauer RH, Sigler ML 2004 A polyhydroxy acid skin care regimen provides antiaging effects comparable to an alpha-hydroxyacid regimen. Cutis 73(suppl 2):14–17

Green BA, Edison BL, Wildnauer RH, Sigler ML 2001 Lactobionic acid and gluconolactone: PHAs for photoaged skin. Cosmetic Dermatology Sep:24–28

Grimes PE, Green BA, Wildnauer RH, Edison BL 2004 The use of polyhydroxy acids (PHAs) in photoaged skin. Cutis 73(suppl 2): 3–13

Hunt MJ, Barnetson R StC 1992 A comparative study of gluconolactone versus benzoyl peroxide in the treatment of acne. Australasian Journal of Dermatology 33:131–134

Kossi J, Peltonen J, Ekfors T, Niinikoski J, Laato M 1999 Effects of hexose sugars: glucose, fructose, galactose and mannose on wound healing in the rat. European Surgical Research 31:74–82

NuSkin International, Inc 2004 Data on file

Thibodeau A 2000 Metalloproteinase inhibitors. Cosmetics and Toiletries 115:75–76

Upadhya GA, Strasberg SM 2000 Glutathione, lactobionate, and histidine: cryptic inhibitors of matrix metalloproteinases contained in University of Wisconsin and histidine/tryptophan/ketoglutarate liver preservation solutions. Hepatology 31:1115–1122

Van Scott EJ, Yu RJ 2002 Hydroxy acids: past, present, future. In: Moy R, Luftman D, Kakita L (eds) Glycolic acid peels. Marcel Dekker, New York, pp 1–14

Wilhelmi BJ, Blackwell SJ, Mancoll JS, Phillips LG 1998 Creep vs. stretch: a review of the viscoelastic properties of skin. Annals of Plastic Surgery 41:215–219

34 Novel Transdermal Cosmeceutical Delivery Systems

Carla G. Nugent

Introduction

This chapter discusses the newly developed methods of delivering cosmeceutical actives to the skin transdermally. While there is no officially recognized category of product as 'cosmeceutical', common usage suggests that a cosmeceutical ingredient is a substance used for cosmetic purposes which performs its function by interacting with the skin rather than merely sitting on the surface of the skin. Thus it is important to understand the factors affecting both interaction of substances with the skin and the delivery of substances to various sites within the skin. Historically delivery systems have been developed for the delivery of drugs either to the skin (topical delivery) or through the skin to the underlying tissues and the general circulation (transdermal delivery) and the cosmetic industry can learn from these developments and apply the technology to improve the activity of cosmeceutical products. During the development of topical and transdermal drug products much has been learned about the nature of substances that will penetrate the skin and the effects that the vehicle in which they are delivered will have on penetration.

Transdermal delivery systems (TDSs) are designed to enable the passage of drug molecules across intact skin in a controlled manner. There are two major factors that determine transdermal delivery success: the biologic properties of the skin and the physiochemical properties of the cosmeceutical and delivery system.

Advantages of drug delivery via the skin and the use of TDSs are: (i) better efficacy with less risk of side effects due to more constant delivery of active; (ii) avoidance of first-pass metabolism by the liver; (iii) ease of use; (iv) ability to target a particular area; and (v) enhanced compliance. The disadvantages of drug delivery via the skin and the use of TDSs are: (i) localized skin irritation; (ii) limitation to molecules small enough to pass through the skin; and (iii) a complex manufacturing process that is inefficient and costly.

TDSs can be divided into two categories: passive and active transport systems. The passive systems have been well studied and are currently internationally widely marketed both in the cosmetic and the pharmaceutical arena. Active systems are relatively newer and have had limited marketing.

Passive vs. Active Transdermal Delivery Systems

Passive transdermal systems used in the pharmaceutical realm rely on medications diffusing through the skin based on a concentration gradient as the driving force. Penetrating substances may either concentrate in the stratum corneum or penetrate into the epidermis, from where they will diffuse into the dermis. Once in the dermis the penetrating substance can then either diffuse deeper into local tissues or can enter the capillaries and be taken into the bloodstream for a systemic effect. While in many cases systemic delivery is desirable for drugs, the objective with cosmeceuticals is to deliver them into the stratum corneum or superficial epidermis. Passive transdermal delivery can be enhanced by occluding the skin with patch devices, or with occlusive ointments and creams, or by chemical penetration enhancers. Patch devices create a drug reservoir on the surface of the skin, whereas nonocclusive systems rely on the partitioning of a matrix of drug and/or vehicle establishing the drug reservoir within the skin.

Active transdermal systems require a physical force to disrupt the normal skin barrier and thus allow passage of molecules that otherwise would not permeate the skin or would permeate only very slowly. Some such techniques involve the use of electrical current or electrical potential and this can be used to deliver ionized compounds along a charge gradient. Other techniques for disrupting the barrier include ultrasound radiofrequency waves and microneedles. These active TDSs are currently under development and may someday be capable of delivering large molecules, such as proteins and growth modulators, through the skin. Active transdermal delivery currently is divided into four categories as presented in Box 34.1.

The technology that has been used for cosmeceutical preparations are passive transdermal delivery systems, e.g. patches, creams, and lotions which were adapted from the pharmaceutical industry. Since the introduction of the transdermal patches into the cosmeceutical market, there has been a technology plateau and relatively little breakthrough in innovations regarding new penetration enhancers or delivery systems. With the recent emphasis of getting active cosmeceutical to penetrate the outer layer of the skin, application of new TDS

technology is very attractive since it provides the opportunity to transport molecules into the skin that might otherwise not permeate sufficiently to provide their beneficial effects.

Novel Transdermal Cosmeceutical Delivery Systems

Recent research has led to the identification of novel transdermal delivery systems by use of Generally Recognised As Safe (GRAS) chemical penetration enhancers which are currently used as topical sunscreening agents. Examples of chemical penetration enhancers in this group are padimate O, octyl salicylate (Fig. 34.1), and octyl methoxycinnamate. These substances are approved as sunscreens with maximal topical concentrations of 8.0, 5.0, and 7.5%, respectively in the USA, Europe, Japan, and Australia. Over their many years of use as topical sunscreens these agents have shown a very low incidence of local skin reactions.

Other researchers have observed that a commercial sunscreen lotion significantly increased ($P < 0.01$) the in vitro diffusion of benzene across human epidermis when the lotion was used to pretreat the skin. The researchers were unsure as to what component(s) of the chemical sunscreen (Coppertone 25 sunblock lotion) were responsible for the penetration enhancement. An ingredient search revealed that the sunscreen formulation in question contained octyl methoxycinnamate and octisalate, and it may have been these components which functioned as the penetration enhancer.

These new sunscreen chemical penetration enhancers warrant further attention because they are safe and effective given the findings in a recent study. It is also fortuitous that their general use as

---

Active transdermal cosmeceutical delivery systems

1. Iontophoresis (low-voltage electric transport of lower molecular weight cosmeceutical actives into the skin)
2. Electroporation (high voltage pulses administered for short periods to transport large cosmeceutical molecules into the skin)
3. Phonophoresis (topically applied ultrasound to enhance skin penetration of cosmeceutical actives)
4. Microneedles (an array of microscopic needles impregnated with a cosmeceutical active at their tips are pressed into the skin)

Box 34.1 Active transdermal cosmeceutical delivery systems

Properties of octyl salicylate

Structure[a]	M.Wt[a]	logP[a]	Physical form[a]	Solubility[a]
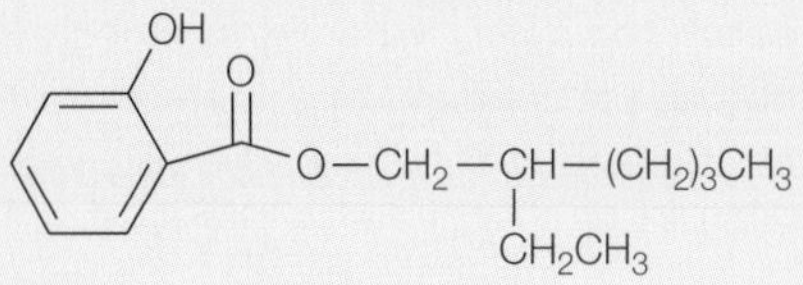	250.3	5.97	Non-volatile, colorless to pale yellow liquid, characteristiically bland odour	Insoluble in water; freely soluble in absolute ethanol

Fig. 34.1 The chemical structure of octyl salicylate

sunscreen agents allows ready entry into the current market. However, the ability of these sunscreen actives to enhance chemical penetration may warrant their restriction in certain work environments where toxins might accidentally be spilled or aerosolized on the skin. Further finite dose exposure studies are needed to verify the significance of any potential risk from these penetration enhancers.

The incorporation of octisalate and octyl methoxycinnamate into cosmeceutical delivery systems provides 'patch performance without a patch' and offers the advantage of low skin irritation with greater ease of use avoiding unsightly patches. It also simplifies the manufacturing method.

While these 'sunscreen' enhancers can be incorporated into conventional delivery systems such as patches, ointments, lotions, creams and gels, they also lend themselves to a novel form of delivery—a spray. For this novel spray delivery system to work, the drug and chemical penetration enhancer would need to rapidly partition into the skin while the volatile vehicle component of the spray evaporated into the atmosphere. Figure 34.2 depicts this concept of 'forced partitioning' into the stratum corneum from a topical spray, and the subsequent formation of a drug/penetration enhancer reservoir within the stratum corneum.

A major determinant of the rate and extent of cosmeceutical and penetration enhancer uptake into the skin will be their underlying affinity for the stratum corneum. The main factors affecting this uptake process are the log P of the compound

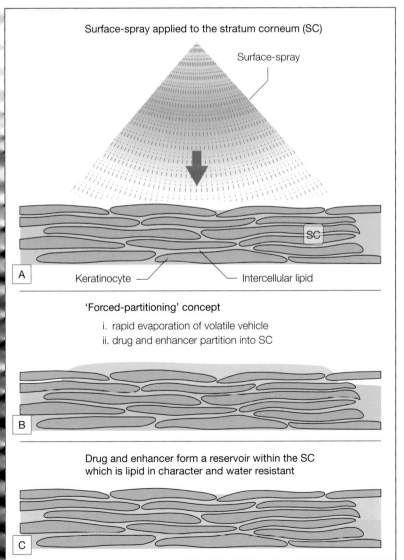

Surface-spray applied to the stratum corneum (SC)

Surface-spray

SC

A   Keratinocyte — / — Intercellular lipid

'Forced-partitioning' concept
   i. rapid evaporation of volatile vehicle
   ii. drug and enhancer partition into SC

B

Drug and enhancer form a reservoir within the SC which is lipid in character and water resistant

C

Fig. 34.2 Transdermal partitioning effect

(P = the partition coefficient), its stratum corneum lipid solubility, and protein binding. The degree of skin substantivity is primarily dependent upon the cosmeceutical actives' aqueous water solubilities and affinity for the skin. Provided the cosmeceutical actives have both low water solubility and high affinity for the skin, they are unlikely to be removed from the skin under normal bathing conditions.

Summary

Novel TDSs are important for antiaging cosmeceutical applications. This technology shows promise in allowing active ingredients, including those not able to be delivered previously, to not only be delivered within the epidermis, but also specifically into a targeted location.

It will be possible using this new TDS technology to deliver key cosmeceutical actives to target locations, allowing for simultaneous multiaction effects, while also creating a prolonged and sustained reservoir.

Further Reading

Bangha E, Elsner P, Kistler GS 1996 Suppression of UV-induced erythema by topical treatment with melatonin (N-acetyl-5-methoxytryptamine). A dose response study. Archives of Dermatological Research 288:522–526

Bernstein EF, Underhill CB, Lakkakorpi J, et al 1997 Citric acid increases viable epidermal thickness and glycosaminoglycan content of sun-damaged skin. Dermatologic Surgery 23:689–694

Corish J, Corrigan OI, Foley D 1990 The iontophoretic transdermal delivery of morphine hydrochloride and other salts across excised human stratum corneum. In: Proceedings of the Conference on Prediction of Percutaneous Penetration, London

Davis AF, Hadgraft J 1993 Supersaturated solutions as topical drug delivery systems. In: Walters KA, Hadgraft J (eds) Pharmaceutical skin penetration enhancement. Marcel Dekker, New York, pp 243–267

Davis DP, Daston GP, Odio MR, York RG, Kraus AL 1996 Maternal reproductive effects of oral salicylic acid in Sprague–Dawley rats. Toxicology Letters 84:135–141

Draelos ZD 1995 Cosmetics in dermatology. Churchill Livingston, New York, pp 83–85

Dreher F, Denig N, Gabard B, Schwindt DA, Maibach HI 1999 Effect of topical antioxidants on UV-induced erythema formation when administered after exposure. Dermatology 198:52–55

Eichler O, Sies H, Stahl W 2002 Divergent optimum levels of lycopene, beta-carotene and lutein protecting against UVB irradiation in human fibroblasts. Photochemistry and Photobiology 75:503–506

Francoeur ML, Golden GM, Potts PO 1990 Oleic acid: its effects on stratum corneum in relation to (trans)dermal drug delivery. Pharmaceutical Research 7:621–627

Funk JO, Dromgoole SH, Maibach HI 1995 Sunscreen intolerance. Dermatologic Clinics 13:473–481

George DJ, Sharp AM 2000 Exposure assessment. In: Weiner ML, Kotkoskie LA (eds) Excipient toxicity and safety. Marcel Dekker, New York, p 291

Giacomoni PU, Rein G 2001 Factors of skin ageing share common mechanisms. Biogerontology 2:219–220

Harrison's principles of internal medicine, 13th edn, 1994 McGraw-Hill

Hayden CJ, Benson HAE, Roberts MS 1998 Sunscreens: toxicological aspects. In: Roberts MS, Walters KA (eds) Dermal absorption and toxicity assessment. Marcel Dekker, New York, pp 561–588

Higuchi WI, Yu C 1987 Prodrugs in transdermal delivery. In: Kydonieus AF, Berner B (eds) Transdermal delivery of drugs, vol 3. CRC Press, Boca Raton, FL, p 65

Hoppe U, Bergemann J, Diembeck W, et al 1999 Coenzyme Q10, a cutaneous antioxidant and energizer. Biofactors 9(2–4):371–378

Itoh T, Xia J, Magavi R, Nishihata T, Rytting JH 1990 Use of shed snake skin as a model membrane for in vitro percutaneous penetration studies: comparison with human skin. Pharmaceutical Research 7:1042–1047

Kuiper GGJM, Lemmen JG, Carlsson B, et al 1998 Interaction of estrogenic chemicals and phytoestrogens with estrogen receptor β. Endocrinology 139:4252–4263

Labrie F, Luu-The V, Labrie C, Pelletier G, El-Alfy M 2000 Intracrinology and the skin. Hormone Research 54:218–229

Langer R 2004 Transdermal drug delivery: past progress, current status and future prospects. Advanced Drug Delivery Reviews 56:557–558

Leopold CS, Lippold BC 1995 An attempt to clarify the mechanism of the penetration enhancing effects of lipophilic vehicles with differential scanning calorimetry (DSC). Journal of Pharmacy and Pharmacology 47:276–281

Morgan TM, Finnin BC 1999 Transdermal penetration enhancers: applications, limitations, and potential. Journal of Pharmaceutical Sciences 88:955–958

Morgan TM, Parr RA, Reed BL, Finnin BC 1998 Enhanced transdermal delivery of sex hormones in swine with a novel topical aerosol. Journal of Pharmaceutical Sciences 87:1219–1225

Morgan TM, Reed BL, Finnin BC 1998 Enhanced skin permeation of sex hormones with novel topical spray vehicles. Journal of Pharmaceutical Sciences 87:1213–1218

Morgan TM, Reed BL, Finnin BC 1998 Percutaneous absorption in humans predicted by SAR. In: Proceedings of the 25th International Symposium on Controlled Release of Bioactive Materials, p 6901

Motwani MR, Rhein LD, Zatz JL 2001 Differential scanning calorimetry studies of sebum models. Journal of Cosmetic Science 52:211–224

Murphy EG, Janousek A, Groves GA, Fukuda M, Naganuma M 1997 Regulatory aspects. In: Lowe NJ, Shaath NA, Pathak MA (eds) Sunscreens. Development, evaluation, and regulatory aspects. 2nd edn. Marcel Dekker, New York, pp 201–260

Niezgoda JA, Cianci P, Folden BW, et al 1997 The effect of hyperbaric oxygen on a burn wound model in human volunteers. Plastic and Reconstructive Surgery 99:1620–1625

Reed BL, Morgan TM, Finnin BC 2001 US Patent 6,299,900, Dermal penetration enhancers and drug delivery systems involving same. 9 October

Shah MG, Maibach HI 2001 Estrogen and skin. An overview. American Journal of Clinical Dermatology 2:143–150

Soula A, Richard V, Labrie F, Labrie C 2000 Exclusive androgenic effect of dehydroepiandrosterone in sebaceous glands of rat skin. Journal of Endocrinology 166:455–462

Treffel P, Gabard B 1996 Skin penetration and sun protection factor of ultra-violet filters from two vehicles. Pharmaceutical Research 13:770–774

Ueng SW, Lee SS, Lin SS, et al 1998 Bone healing of tibial lengthening is enhanced by hyperbaric oxygen therapy. Journal of Trauma 44:676–678

Walters KA, Brain KR, Howes D, et al 1997 Percutaneous penetration of octyl salicylate from representative sunscreen formulations through human skin in vitro. Food and Chemical Toxicology 35:1219–1225

White EL, Reed BL, Finnin BC 1997 Effect of padimate O, octyl salicylate and laurocapram on the thermal profile of a model stratum corneum lipid mixture. In: Proceedings of the Australian Pharmaceutical Science Association Conference, Sydney, Australia, p 45

Summary

What is the future of cosmeceuticals?

Zoe Diana Draelos

This volume has covered the wide variety of cosmeceuticals currently present in the marketplace from the standpoint of the dermatologist. The topic is introduced by Albert Kligman, the father of cosmeceuticals, commenting on how he conceived of this unique concept. The text then turns its attention to the issues that define the realm of cosmeceuticals before embarking on an in depth discussion of the major ingredients currently part of this category. These ingredients are then presented in flowchart format to guide the physician through the use of these ingredients for medical and aesthetic purposes while discussing some of the more common cosmeceutical myths. Finally, the text takes a brief look at some of the new cosmeceutical technologies emerging at this time. The last issue is now to take a look at the future. What is the future of cosmeceuticals?

No one knows for sure where the cosmeceutical category will go in the next 10, 20, 30 years and beyond, yet some educated conjecture is in order. The regulation under which we are currently operating to define drugs, over-the-counter drugs, and cosmetics was developed in the 1930s. Much progress, both in terms of novel raw materials and skin physiology insights, has occurred during the last 75 years, which has blurred the boundaries between drugs and cosmetics. The Cosmetics and Toiletries Act is badly in need of updating, yet this is not an issue that Congress appears likely to address any time soon. It would be necessary first to update the act prior to the initiation of any development of a new category to define cosmeceuticals. Japan has already taken this step forward, and as a result is far ahead of the USA in terms of cosmeceutical development. Since there is no positive political or economic advantage to creating a recognized cosmeceutical category, I do not foresee any changes in the next 10 years.

The Cosmetics and Toiletries Act was passed when physicians recognized the inclusion of unsafe substances in these products, such as lead and arsenic. At the time the act was passed, the most popular safe cosmeceutical was a topical estrogen-containing moisturizer cream. The cream was very effective, since the estrogenic effect on the skin increased collagen production improving fine wrinkling and enhancing skin smoothness. Today, we are unable to sell creams containing estrogen as cosmeceuticals, but the incorporation of soy as a phytoestrogen into facial moisturizers and cellulite creams continues. Even though we have come very far in our ability to synthesize new raw materials, we still are trying to achieve the same end in the same manner.

Perhaps the most disturbing part of the whole cosmeceutical category issue is the definition of a dermatologic drug as something that alters the structure and function of the skin. This was the language used in the original Cosmetics and Toiletries Act. The act was written at a time when the skin was thought to be nothing more than a covering on the outside of the body with little biologic activity. We now know that the skin is enzymatically and immunologically active, participating in important metabolic functions required to sustain life. We know that the skin is profoundly impacted by many externally applied substances—even water alters the structure and function of the skin. This then leads us to wonder how cosmeceuticals are currently defined.

Cosmeceuticals are currently defined by the claims that are made regarding their intended use. A product that 'eliminates wrinkles' is a drug while a product that 'minimizes the appearance of wrinkles' is a cosmetic, even though they may both contain the same ingredients. It seems rather unscientific to define product functioning based on package labeling and advertising, yet this is our current level of sophistication. Where will we go in the future?

I believe that several things will need to happen before a cosmeceutical category will be developed and the Cosmetics and Toiletries Act updated. At present, I think the skin care industry is satisfied with the current absence of regulation of cosmetic products. The industry basically is self regulated and has done a wonderful job of policing the safety of cosmetic products marketed to consumers. The incidence of irritant and allergic contact dermatitis is extremely low and no major safety issues have arisen as of late. Increased regulation means increased cost and paperwork for the industry, which is not a welcome change. The only advantage of a new cosmeceutical category would be the ability to advertise with greater conviction and conduct more in depth clinical testing. The skin care industry probably will not push for a new cosmeceutical category. Where is the driving force for change?

In my opinion, the driving force for change will come from the vitamin and nutritional supplement industry. These are companies that now market products known as nutraceuticals. Many raw materials incorporated into nutraceuticals are the same ingredients topically applied in cosmeceuticals. At present, it is generally felt that substances appropriate for internal ingestion are also appropriate for topical application. Recently, there has been concern about some of the nutritional supplements containing hormone analogs, stimulants, and other low grade toxic materials. There has also been much in the popular press about the purity of vitamin supplements and the inclusion of biologically active vitamin forms. The nutritional supplement industry is completely unregulated at present. Some major problem will need to develop in the nutraceutical industry resulting in legal proceedings that will cause the US government to set standards. It is likely at that point in time that the nutraceutical standards will also be adapted to cosmeceuticals, thus creating a new category of some sort.

For the present time, many new developments will be forthcoming within the currently defined realm of cosmeceuticals. Drug development techniques and gene array technology will be used to find topical actives that specifically upregulate or downregulate skin functioning, most likely through modulation of the inflammatory cascade. Since the inflammatory cascade is the final common pathway of skin injury and aging, breakthroughs in this area will be significant. New delivery systems will also be developed to deliver higher concentrations of already studied actives and to deliver into the skin actives that currently are incapable of biologic functioning due to penetration problems. Protein sequencing technology will be adapted to skin care and result in the development of cellular messengers that can turn on or off specific biosynthetic pathways. Lastly, the ability to identify individual actives within botanical extracts will result in the large scale synthesis of substances currently too expensive to put in mass market cosmeceuticals.

In summary, I believe that cosmeceuticals will become an ever increasing part of the fund of knowledge of dermatology. We are now only at the beginning of the cosmeceutical story. Cosmeceuticals were derived from the cosmetics industry's desire to go beyond simply adorning the skin. The industry wanted to improve the appearance of the skin by tackling important functional issues to meet the demands of consumers. Now, the cosmeceutical arena needs to learn from the medical arena. The principles of the scientific method must be applied to the clinical study of cosmeceuticals. No longer can in vitro data be used to extrapolate visible clinical results. No longer can 15 subject studies be used to determine the value of a specific ingredient. No longer can trends and not statistical significance be used to confirm the skin effect of a given formulation. Dermatology will move the cosmeceutical story forward and dermatologists will drive the future of cosmeceuticals. This text is a step in that direction, attempting to provide a cosmeceutical knowledge base for the dermatologist.

Subject Index